# Handbook of Physical Measurements

## Second Edition

JUDITH G. HALL
*Professor Emeritus of Medical Genetics and Pediatrics*
*University of British Columbia*

JUDITH E. ALLANSON
*Professor of Pediatrics*
*University of Ottawa*

KAREN W. GRIPP
*Chief, Division of Medical Genetics,*
*A. I. duPont Hospital for Children, Wilmington, Delaware,*
*Associate Professor of Pediatrics,*
*Thomas Jefferson University, Philadelphia, Pennsylvania*

ANNE M. SLAVOTINEK
*Assistant Professor,*
*University of California, San Francisco*

OXFORD
UNIVERSITY PRESS

2007

# OXFORD
UNIVERSITY PRESS

Oxford University Press, Inc., publishes works that further
Oxford University's objective of excellence
in research, scholarship, and education.

Oxford   New York
Auckland   Cape Town   Dar es Salaam   Hong Kong   Karachi
Kuala Lumpur   Madrid   Melbourne   Mexico City   Nairobi
New Delhi   Shanghai   Taipei   Toronto

With offices in
Argentina   Austria   Brazil   Chile   Czech Republic   France   Greece
Guatemala   Hungary   Italy   Japan   Poland   Portugal   Singapore
South Korea   Switzerland   Thailand   Turkey   Ukraine   Vietnam

Published by Oxford University Press, Inc.
198 Madison Avenue, New York, New York 10016

www.oup.com

Oxford is a registered trademark of Oxford University Press

Library of Congress Cataloging-in-Publication Data
Handbook of physical measurements/Judith G. Hall ... [et al.].—2nd ed.
p. ; cm
Rev. ed. of: Handbook of normal physical measurements. 1989.
Includes bibliographical references and index.
ISBN 978-0-19-530149-6
1. Anthropometry—Handbooks, manuals, etc. 2. Genetic
disorders—Diagnosis—Handbooks, manuals, etc. 3. Growth
disorders—Diagnosis—Handbooks, manuals, etc. I. Hall, Judith G. II. Hall, Judith G.
Handbook of normal physical measurements.
[DNLM: 1. Body Weights and Measures—methods—Handbooks. 2. Infant. 3. Child.
4. Growth—Handbooks. 5. Growth Disorders—diagnosis—Handbooks. 6. Reference
Values—Handbooks. WS 39 H23645 2006]
QM28.H23 2006
573.6—dc22        2006040008

9 8 7 6 5 4 3 2

Printed in the United States of America
on acid-free paper

# Preface

This book was compiled to assist care providers in obtaining and documenting accurate physical measurements for pediatric patients, both as an aid to diagnosis and for clinical management. We have chosen to include detailed information for dysmorphologists and clinical geneticists, but the book can also be used by primary care providers or any of the other professionals involved in pediatric care. In this second edition, our main changes have been to update the currently available growth curves for the height, weight, and head circumference of North American and North European infants and children. We have also added a substantial number of growth curves for individuals with known diagnoses that we hope will prove useful for those involved in the care of these children.

# Acknowledgments

We are grateful to the many authors of the original studies. Anne S. would like to thank David and all of her colleagues at UCSF, from whom she took the time.

# Contents

Contents

Contents

# Handbook of Physical Measurements

# Introduction

## Introduction

The purpose of this handbook is to provide a practical collection of reference data on a variety of physical measurements for use in the evaluation of children and adults with dysmorphic features and/or structural anomalies. It has been prepared as a small pocket book so that it can easily be carried by the physician to the ward or "the field." This book is intended for use by those health professionals evaluating individuals with unusual physical features. It is an attempt to provide standards both for comparison and for improved definition of normal patterns of human development and growth.

There is a need for a standardized approach to physical measurement in patients with congential anomalies and syndromes. Until recently the study of children with dysmorphic features has primarily involved qualitative descriptions. This descriptive phase has brought us to a new stage where accuracy and quantitation have become desirable. The definition and delineation of new clinical entities require precise and reproduceable methods. Careful documentation by measurement, in well-known conditions, will allow one to distinguish heterogeneity, learn more about natural history, and provide a basis for the future application of techniques and concepts from developmental biology and molecular genetics.

The real value of a single measurement lies in comparison with a standard. The standard can be an age-related norm, or it can be the individual patient at another point in time. Comparison can also be made of growth of different parts of the body; for example, to see whether head circumference, height, and weight are at the same percentile or at different percentiles. While graphs or tables of standard growth parameters—length, weight, and head circumference—are easy to find, it is often difficult to obtain comparable standards for other body structures. For this reason, we have compiled a comprehensive set of normal curves. For the measurement graphs we have chosen to illustrate percentiles, if available, rather than standard deviations in order to be consistent. Standard deviations do allow comparison of the individual patient to an age-related normal population, but percentiles have the additional advantage of allowing serial growth measurements in the same person and comparison of the growth of different body parts in one individual in a more easily interpretable form (unless of course, the measurements are way below the 3rd or way above the 97th percentile).

We recognize that obtaining precise physical measurement is, in fact, a complex and specialized field in itself. However for routine clinical use, the method must be simple enough to "get the job done." Therefore, we have outlined and illustrated practical and simple methods and have chosen those graphs and tables which, in our experience as practicing clinical geneticists, are the most useful.

## Structure of the Book

We have chosen charts and graphs that are in common use and, as often as possible, have combined sources. Body proportions and norms for one ethnic group may not be appropriate for individuals from other ethnic backgrounds; however, very little ethnic data are available. Each chapter concentrates on a specific body area, and includes

1. an introduction with embryology of that area, the landmarks from which the measurements are taken, the instruments necessary, and the ways in which to obtain the measurements;
2. growth charts;
3. references to which the reader should refer for in-depth understanding of statistics, methodology, anthropometrics, and anthropologic approach.

There is a chapter on the approach to the patient with structural anomalies. A glossary at the end of the book defines many of the terms that have been used in this book.

This book is an attempt to provide an "easy to use" collection of data on physical measurements aimed at better defining congenital anomalies and syndromes. The authors are aware that this collection is incomplete and will need revision, additions, and updating; therefore, suggestions to improve the quality and usability of the book are welcomed.

# Measurement

2

## Why Measurements Are Useful

Growth is the essence of the developing organism. Physical growth starts shortly after fertilization and continues throughout pregnancy, childhood, and adolescence. It may even occur in the adult. Growth of different parts of the body follows a predictable schedule during normal development and maturation. This timetable of development is influenced and controlled by many genetic and environmental factors. Any disturbance in the "normal" sequence of development and growth may lead to disproportion of physical features. These imbalances may be transient and can sometimes be compensated for by later catch-up growth. Most syndromes with dysmorphic features, however, display more or less recognizable patterns of disproportionate growth.

The growth of different parts of the body can be observed and measured at one point in time or over specific periods of time. It can be expressed as a number, a comparison, a percentile, or standard deviation from the norm. The comparison may be either with the growing individual, at different ages (so that one can observe the changes over time), or with standardized normal values (obtained from either cross-sectional or longitudinal studies of a specific group of individuals). One can assess and compare differential growth of the various parts of the body.

Longitudinal studies follow a group of individuals or cohort over time, with standardized measurements obtained at precise intervals. Longitudinal studies are difficult because they include a large number of individuals, who must be measured at set intervals, using the same techniques, and, ideally, by the same person(s). The work involved and the time span are enormous. Longitudinal studies provide data on patterns of growth and growth velocity. Velocity curves are valuable in demonstrating the rate of change of a specific dimension with time.

Cross-sectional studies utilize data obtained from a large number of individuals of the same age, usually collected at one time. Cross-sectional studies are technically less difficult to do because they do not rely on the long-term cooperation of many individuals. Cross-sectional studies

5

are used mainly as standards of physical measurement and provide less information about variability, velocity, or patterns of growth over time.

Statistical methods and data collection methods involved in the construction of normal growth curves will not be discussed further. Details are available in the literature references listed here. It is important for the reader to be aware that the various standards provided in this book often come from different populations using different methodologies and so are not really comparable. Nevertheless, they are the only measurements presently available.

Most syndromes with dysmorphic features show disturbances of growth either of the entire body or of certain body parts. In the past, various unusual features have been expressed in qualitative terms such as: short stature, long fingers, or other terms that imply a comparison with other body proportions. An impression of the patient or a "gestalt" is formed in the reader's mind. The more objective way to assess body proportions is by quantitative measurement. This is especially important when the disturbance in growth involves only a specific body area or can be related to a disease process, because it may give insight into the basic mechanisms underlying the growth disturbance and thus the pathogenesis of the disease.

Comparison of the dimensions obtained in a specific individual or patient with a normal standard curve requires three things:

1. standardized landmarks on the body from which and to which measurements can be taken;
2. standardized methods of taking measurements;
3. standard equipment.

The landmarks that we will use are shown in Fig. 2.1 and will be referred to at the beginning of each measurement section. In general they represent surface landmarks of underlying bony structures that can be palpated easily through the skin. To obtain a minimum degree of accuracy in physical measurement, the examiner should be aware of these landmarks. There are individual anatomical variations, especially in patients with congenital anomalies or syndromes with dysmorphic features. Landmarks for measurements of the head and facial structures will be discussed in detail in Chapter 7.

## Summary

By taking accurate physical measurements we can express and communicate observations on growth, proportion, and disturbance of the developmental process in quantitative terms. Single measurements are

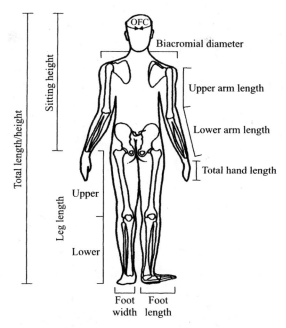

**Figure 2.1**  Body landmarks to and from which measurements can be taken.

meaningless in isolation. They are valuable only in relation to other parameters and in comparison with normal values.

## Anthropometry

Anthropometry is the study of comparative measurement of the human body. A number of precision instruments are available for accurate anthropometric studies. A decision to use these instruments will depend upon the degree of precision that is desired or required.

The pediatrician, physician, medical geneticist, dysmorphologist, or clinician interested in taking precise physical measurements may want to use anthropometric instruments. However, adequate training is necessary to use these devices properly (Fig. 2.2). Most clinics will have an upright measuring device (stadiometer), a supine measuring table, and an infant scale as well as a regular scale. In growth clinics skinfold calipers, orchidometers, and other types of calipers will probably be available. In research centers, such as those dealing with reconstructive surgery of the face, precision instruments for technical measurements are used.

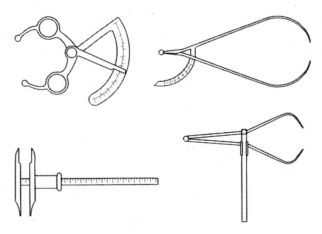

**Figure 2.2** Anthropometric instruments.

In general, the accuracy required to create standard curves in anthropological research under laboratory circumstances will be much greater than the precision that can be expected from the physician who is measuring an unwilling, screaming child in practice. Use of precision instruments usually demands a great deal of cooperation from the patient.

Alternatively, precise physical measurements can be extrapolated from a standardized photograph in a technique called photogrammetric anthropometry. This method is costly, requiring standardized cameras and computarization, and again it is not an everyday, practical approach. Clinical geneticists frequently take photographs to document clinical features. A standard set includes face, front, and side; total body, front, back, and side with palms forward; close-up of hands and feet, and any other unusual features. However, without a reference standard of size in the photograph, they cannot be used for accurate measurements.

For the "field" or ward examination the ordinary tape-measure will be most frequently used. It is important to note that metallic or disposable paper tapes are more reliable for long-term use than cloth tapes. Cloth tapes tend to wear out and become stretched over a period of time. If a cloth tape is used, it should be checked from time to time against a metal or wooden standard.

For a long time there has been a dual measurement system—most European countries used metric units (meters and grams), whereas many physician in the United States used Imperial units (inches and pounds). However, the metric system has become internationally accepted in medicine. In this book, to avoid confusion, most graphs will have both systems

| | |
|---|---|
| millimeter (mm) ÷ 25.4 = inch (in) | inch (in) ÷ 0.039 = millimeter (mm) |
| centimeter (cm) ÷ 2.54 = inch (in) | inch (in) ÷ 0.394 = centimeter (cm) |
| centimeter (cm) ÷ 30.5 = foot (ft) | foot (ft) ÷ 0.033 = centimeter (cm) |
| meter (m) ÷ 0.305 = foot (ft) | foot (ft) ÷ 3.279 = meter (m) |
| meter (m) ÷ 0.915 = yard (yd) | yard (yd) ÷ 1.093 = meter (m) |
| 1 foot (ft) = 12 inches (in); | 1 yard (yd) = 3 feet (ft); 1 yard (yd) = 36 inches (in) |

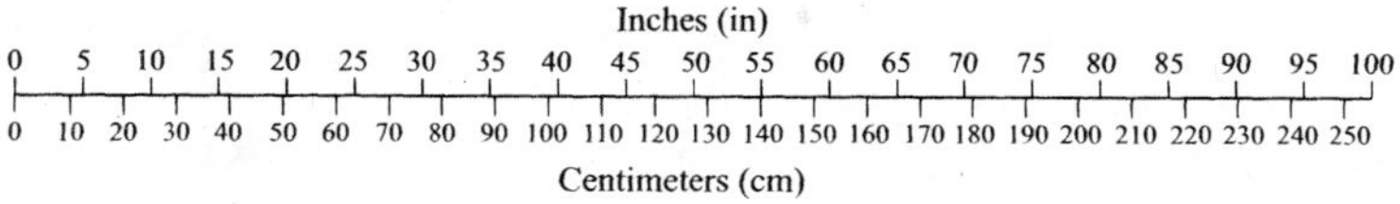

Inches (in)

0  5  10  15  20  25  30  35  40  45  50  55  60  65  70  75  80  85  90  95  100

0  10  20  30  40  50  60  70  80  90  100  110  120  130  140  150  160  170  180  190  200  210  220  230  240  250

Centimeters (cm)

**Figure 2.3**  Linear conversions.

of units. Fig. 2.3 provides the methods to convert centimeters and inches, and Fig. 2.4 gives pounds and kilograms.

Any documentation of measurement(s) should be given together with the age of the individual, the date on which the measurement was obtained, the method used to obtain that measurement, and the name of the person doing the measuring. This makes it easier to compare the values obtained and enables one to anticipate the possible failures of the method employed. In addition, reports or descriptions should include percentiles (or standard deviation) for easy reference and comparison.

**Figure 2.4**  Weight conversions.

| | |
|---|---|
| gram (g) ÷ 28.4 = ounce (oz) | ounce (oz) ÷ 0.035 = gram (g) |
| kilogram (kg) ÷ 0.455 = pound (lb) | pound (lb) ÷ 2.20 = kilogram (kg) |

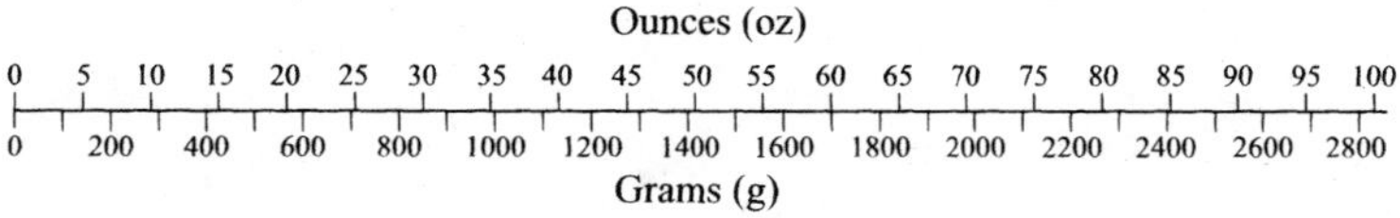

Ounces (oz)

0  5  10  15  20  25  30  35  40  45  50  55  60  65  70  75  80  85  90  95  100

0  200  400  600  800  1000  1200  1400  1600  1800  2000  2200  2400  2600  2800

Grams (g)

## Useful Parameters and Landmarks

Measurements of length, weight, and head circumference are standard measurements of a physical examination. These three measurements are the parameters against which all others are compared. They document growth and body proportions. They should be obtained routinely at every visit to a physician in order to be able to assess longitudinal growth and growth relative to an age- and sex-matched standard. Curves of normal standards of growth, weight, and head circumference are included in every text on pediatrics. They usually start from birth and continue until 18 or 20 years of age. In this book, we have chosen the most commonly used standards and taken the liberty, for practicality, of combining some curves. Although the purist may question this process, we do not think it will markedly affect accuracy in most cases, and we hope the easy utilization of having only one curve will encourage regular and complete measurement. We have included geographic data when available, or markedly different (e.g., North America and North European heights). Unfortunately, ethnic comparisons of most areas of the body are not available.

Ultrasound examination permits monitoring of fetal development (Chapter 15). Routine measurements include biparietal diameter (BPD), crown–rump length, chest circumference, and femur length. These are useful standards with which to observe the well-being of the fetus prior to birth.

Head circumference (OFC) is looked upon as one of the most important measurements in infancy and early childhood, since it reflects intracranial volume and brain growth. The head circumference charts chosen for this book are the ones most widely used. Often centers will have their own OFC charts, related to the population and ethnic groups that they serve (Chapter 6).

When length, weight, or head circumference deviate from the normal growth curve, further investigation is warranted. Many different pathological processes, some of which may be treatable, can lead to growth failure. Discrepancies in growth proportions may provide clues to the pathological process; for instance, chronic infection and renal failure lead to relative loss in weight, while growth hormone deficiency and Cushing syndrome produce relative increase in weight. Usually, by two years of age a child has established a pattern of growth that will predictably follow percentile growth curves. These growth curves, on average, are similar for OFC, height, and weight. During the first year of life a child may change percentile growth curves as he or she establishes an extrauterine growth pattern.

Bone age is an additional parameter of growth that reflects physiological growth. Bone age is determined from radiographs of the hand or other epiphyseal centers (different ones for different ages). If a disturbance of normal growth is suggested, additional X-rays may be necessary (Chapter 13).

Weight and skinfold thickness will be of special value in nutritional problems (Chapter 5).

During adulthood, particular measurements may also reflect an underlying pathological process. Routinely, weight and total body length are measured in the adult, but head size is often excluded because the head usually does not grow in the normal adult. Familial patterns of growth "late-bloomers") and disproportion (large heads or "short waisted") may identify genetically determined influences on growth.

One should always include the measurements of the parents of the child under assessment so that mid-parental parameters can be established for comparison. This is particularly important and appropriate when evaluating deviations from normal of head size and height.

Growth velocity is most rapid immediately after birth and up to three years of age, after which there is a continued deceleration of growth until puberty. The adolescent growth peak in girls is at approximately 12 years, and in boys at approximately 14 years of age. It is useful to compare growth at yearly intervals, although in infancy shorter time intervals will be used because the velocity is greater.

## Measurements in Dysmorphology and Clinical Genetics

The human body is expected to grow predictably and proportionately. The relationship of measurements to each other is expected to be constant at specific ages. These relationships can be expressed as ratios, as an index, or by the use of regression techniques. Those in common use are the relationship between height and weight. They are mainly corrected with the chronological age or the bone age of the patient. These proportions and relationships change dramatically from the fetal period through childhood to adolescence because of various interactions among genetic, hormonal, and environmental factors.

In the study of syndromes with dysmorphic features, we are looking for recognizable signs that help to define and delineate the specific condition. Those recognizable features may be quite different during different life periods. Using Down syndrome as an example, from embryofetal pathology we have learned that manifestation of the Down syndrome phenotype in a fetus depends on the gestational week, and often very few features are present until near birth. Similarly, there is a changing phenotype during childhood and into adulthood, with the typical phenotype of Down syndrome sometimes becoming hard to recognize in the adult.

Because of the change in physical appearance and therefore in the pattern of measurements with time, we can expect that some diseases or disorders will be more obvious and more easily recognized during certain stages of development. The patterns of relative measurements may partly relate to the growth spurts that occur in different organ systems at different times. Theoretically they reflect secondary and tertiary effects of the basic process and underlying pathogenesis.

Measurements of individual body parts can never be separated from general clinical impression or "gestalt." This type of general impression of the patient will usually be obtained by observing the patient for a while before taking specific measurements. The specific measurements and general clinical impression should be integrated with additional factors such as the movement pattern, mode of communication, and type of developmental disability into an overall description and impression.

There is a tendency to neglect the observation and description of the adult patient with malformations, in specific syndromes or even isolated mental retardation. As a consequence, we have limited knowledge of physical changes in syndromes with dysmorphic features as related to the aging process. Study of the natural history of these relationships may lead to a better understanding of the underlying pathophysiology and natural history of the disorders.

# Proportional Growth and Normal Variants

3

## Body Proportions

Body proportions change considerably during fetal and postnatal life. For example, during fetal life the head appears disproportionately large compared with the body. Beginning about eight months *in utero* subcutaneous fat begins to accumulate, and from then until birth the major changes in proportions are due to the accumulation of fat (Fig. 3.1).

The alteration of body configuration is the result of selective regional growth. In infancy the head grows most rapidly, so that during the first year of life, OFC is greater than chest circumference. After the first year, head growth slows down. At birth the limbs are shorter than the trunk; they grow more rapidly and proportions are reversed. Leg growth ceases somewhat earlier than growth of the arms.

The changing proportions are mainly reflected in two ratios. First, the upper/lower segment ratio is the ratio of the distance from the top of

**Figure 3.1**   Body proportions during human development.

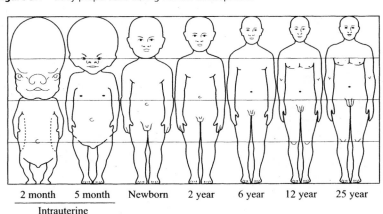

| 2 month | 5 month | Newborn | 2 year | 6 year | 12 year | 25 year |

Intrauterine

the head to the symphysis pubis and the distance from the symphysis pubis to the sole of the foot. At birth, this ratio is about 1.7; at 10 years of age, it is about 1.0; after 10 years of age, the ratio is normally less than 1.0. The second ratio is the comparison of span with height. At birth, the span is over an inch less than height. Normally in boys, the span exceeds standing height by about 10 years of age; in girls normally, span exceeds height at about 12 years of age.

# Height and Length

4

## Introduction

There are two different ways of evaluating height and length. Total body length is the distance between the top of the head and the sole of the foot when the individual is in a recumbent position (lying down) with the foot dorsiflexed (Fig. 4.1). Total standing height is the distance from the highest point of the head to the sole of the foot in the midsagittal plane with the individual standing in an upright position (Fig. 4.5). The head should be held erect with the eyes looking straight forward, so that the lower margin of the bony orbit and upper margin of the external auditory canal opening are in the same horizontal plane (Frankfort plane).

The charts for standard measurement of length or height are ordered in three age groups:

1. length by gestational age at birth (Figs. 4.2–4.4) including twins;
2. birth–4 years (infants are measured in a recumbent position) (Figs. 4.7, 4.9, 4.11, 4.13);
3. 2–18 years (children are measured standing upright) (Figs. 4.8, 4.10, 4.12, 4.14).

## Total Body Length

**Definition**   Length of the supine body.

**Landmarks**   Measure from the top of the head to the sole of the foot with the patient lying on the back with hips and knees extended (Fig. 4.1a, b).

**Instruments**   Ideally, measuring table with engraved measurements, a firm headblock, and a moveable footblock (Fig. 4.1a).

**Position**   For this measurement, ideally, two persons work together. One holds the head of the child, while the other straightens the legs of the child with one hand and moves the footblock toward the heel of the child with

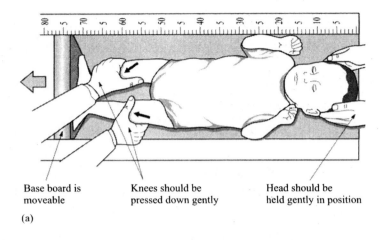

Base board is
moveable

Knees should be
pressed down gently

Head should be
held gently in position

(a)

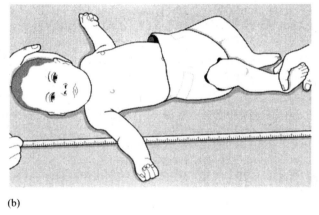

(b)

**Figure 4.1**   Measuring a child less than two years old with a measuring table (a) or tape-measure (b).

the other hand. The top of the head of the patient should be placed against the headboard, eyes looking upward. The ideal head position is with the Frankfort horizontal position held in a vertical plane (i.e., the lower edge of the bony orbit and the upper margin of the external opening of the auditory canal of the ear are in the same vertical plane). The legs, or at least one leg, should be straightened, the ankle at a right angle to the leg with the toes pointing upward. The moveable footboard should be brought in direct contact with the sole of the foot and the measurement read.

**Alternatives**    A less accurate way, when a measuring table is not available, is to mark the sheet or the paper on which the child is lying above the child's head and at the foot, after stretching the patient out. Remove the patient, and measure the distance on the paper or sheet between the markings.

Alternatively, a tape-measure can be placed under the child who is positioned supine on top of or beside the tape (Fig. 4.1b).

**Remarks**    Ideally each measurement should be taken at least twice. The patient should be repositioned between measurements. The experience in clinics dealing with growth problems has shown this to be necessary to obtain accurate measurements of height and length. Measurements in the age group birth to two years are difficult to obtain because the children are sometimes not very cooperative. Thus the measurements may be less accurate in general.

*Small for gestational age* is the term used for newborns who are below the tenth percentile according to their gestational age. Thus, infants less than the tenth percentile in length, even if normal in weight, must be considered small for gestational age.

To determine if babies born prematurely are small for their age, adjustment of their stated age has to be made (the number of weeks they were born prematurely is subtracted from their postnatal age, and the measurement is compared to the corrected age). Premature babies, by definition, are those born before 37 weeks of gestation. Such individuals catch up to normal at about two years of age.

The most widely distributed standard gestational curves are those of Lubchenco et al. (Fig. 4.2). However, compared with North European measurements, they differ considerably after the 37th gestational week. Thus we have also provided the standard curves of Voigt et al. (Fig. 4.4), which are comparable to the gestational age curves of most European centers.

**Pitfalls**    When the head is tipped forward or up, the measurement may be increased. Lack of full extension of the legs or mild contractures of knees or hips, particularly in newborns, will give artificially shortened measurements.

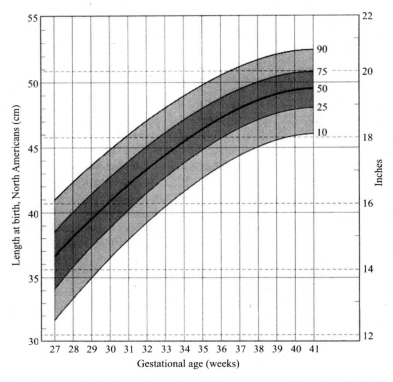

**Figure 4.2**  Length at birth, North Americans, both sexes. From Lubchenco et al. (1963), by permission.

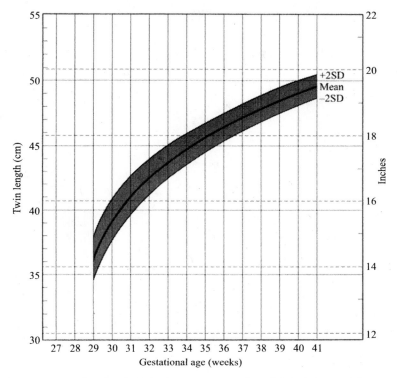

**Figure 4.3**   Twin-length at birth, both sexes. From Waelli et al. (1980), by permission.

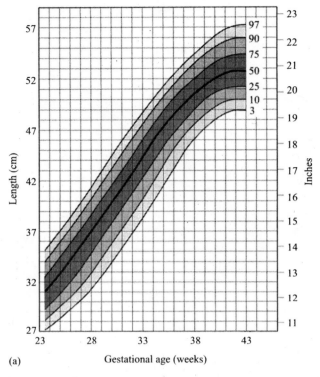

(a)                Gestational age (weeks)

**Figure 4.4(a)** Length at birth, German males born in 1992. Adapted from Voigt et al. (1996).

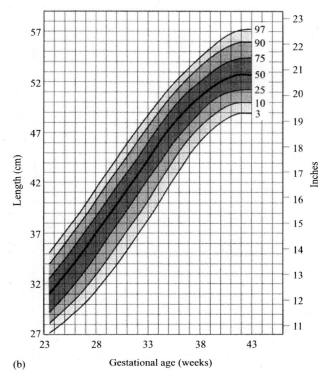

(b)                    Gestational age (weeks)

**Figure 4.4(b)**    Length at birth, German females born in 1992. Adapted from Voigt et al. (1996).

## Standing Height

**Definition**   Total height in the standing position.

**Landmarks**   Top of the head to the soles of the feet. (Fig. 4.5a, b).

**Instruments**   Ideally, a stadiometer (stable, accurate measuring device) with a moveable headboard is used. Alternatively, a type-measure may be fixed to the wall from the floor upward to at least six feet and a right-angle board used to mark the point of greatest height (Fig. 4.5b).

**Position**   The patient should stand upright, with the back against the wall and the head erect (Frankfort horizontal plane), facing forward, and looking straight ahead. The patient should be gently straightened upright; the heels placed together; buttocks and shoulders should be in contact with the wall or measuring device. The moveable headboard is lowered gently until it touches the top of the head. Appropriate clothing should be worn: no socks or shoes (Fig. 4.5).

**Alternative**   A door jamb or the wall and a tape-measure can be used if a stadiometer is not available (Fig. 4.5b). The patient stands straight in the position described above, with heels together against the door jamb. Heels, buttocks, and shoulders should be in contact with the vertical door jamb.

**Figure 4.5**   Measuring standard height with a stadiometer (a) or a tape-measure (b).

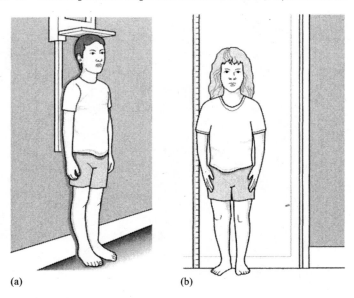

(a)                                    (b)

A book or a ruler can be used to replace the headboard, and the point of greatest height is marked on the door jamb. The total standing height is measured from the floor to the marking on the door jamb or wall.

**Remarks** Repeat the measurement. The patient has to step off after the first measurement and take the position again in between measurements.

The total standing height (upright position) in the 2- to 18-year-old is 1–2 cm less than the total body length (recumbent position). The growth of a normal child usually follows one particular percentile.

Any rapid movements above or below this percentile should be a reason for close follow-up and, if necessary, for further diagnostic procedures.

There are significant differences between the growth charts used in North America and those used for some European countries. The data widely used in North Europe show, for example, that the 50th percentile at one year of age equals the 75th percentile in the North American growth charts. Thus we provided two sets of growth charts, one with North American standards (Figs. 4.7, 4.8, 4.11, 4.12) and one for European standards (Figs. 4.9, 4.10, 4.13, 4.14). It is important to use one or the other standard consistently when making comparisons over time.

**Pitfalls** If the patient is unable to stand, the recumbent length should be measured, recognizing that it will be slightly greater than total standing height.

In individuals with contractures of the legs, the tape is worked along the middle of the patient's leg along the angle of the contracture as in the illustration (Fig. 4.6) to estimate total length.

**Figure 4.6** Measuring an individual with contractures by "walking the tape."

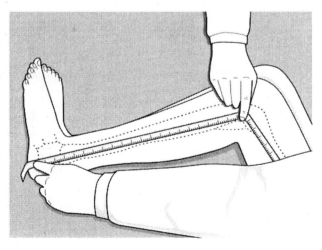

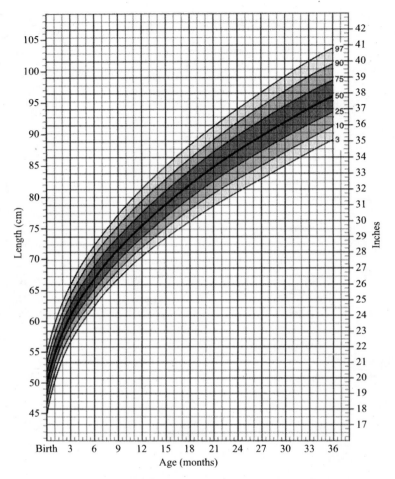

**Figure 4.7**   Length, North American males, birth to three years. Adapted from CDC: http://www.cdc.gov/growthcharts.

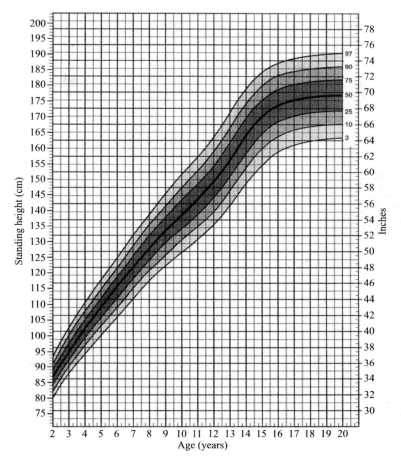

**Figure 4.8** Standing height, North American males, 2 to 20 years. Adapted from CDC: http://www.cdc.gov/growthcharts.

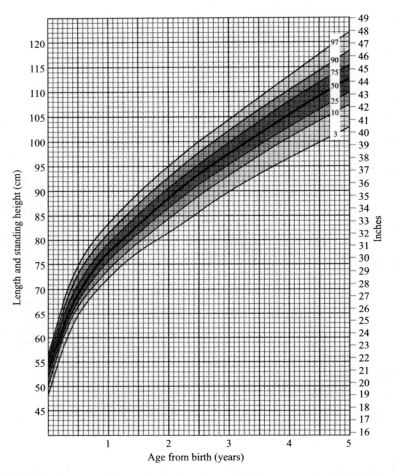

**Figure 4.9** Recumbent length and standing height, North European males, birth to five years. Adapted from Brandt, 1986 (http://www.wachstum-ipep.de/WTK/WTK.html).

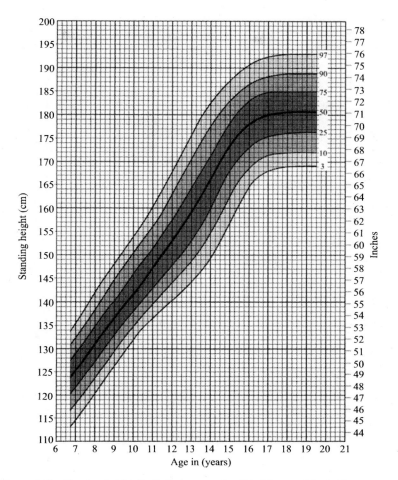

**Figure 4.10** Standing height, North European males, 6 to 19 years. Adapted from Georgi et al.,1996 (http://www.wachstum-ipep.de/WTK/WTK.html).

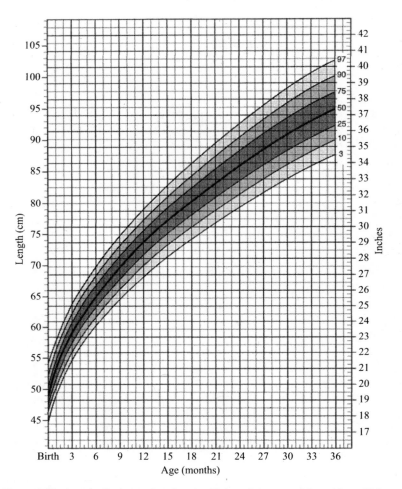

**Figure 4.11**   Length, North American females, birth to three years. Adapted from CDC: http://www.cdc.gov/growthcharts.

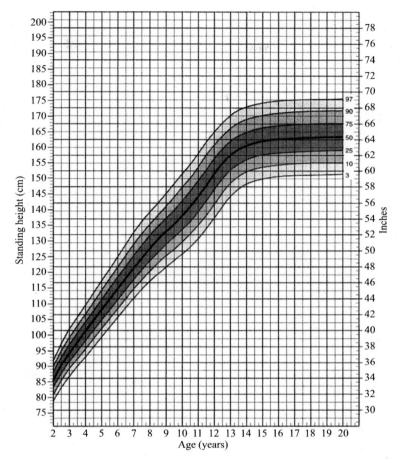

**Figure 4.12** Standing height, North American females, two to twenty years. Adapted from CDC: http://www.gov/growthcharts.

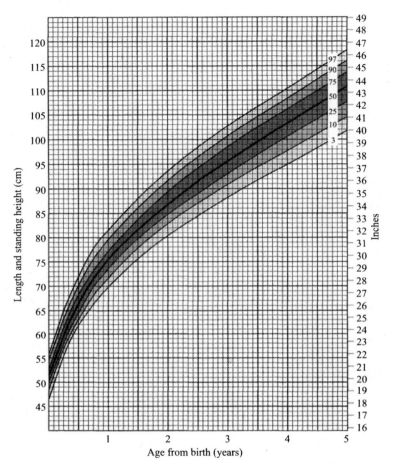

**Figure 4.13**  Recumbent length and standing height, North European females, birth to five years. Adapted from Brandt, 1986 (http:www.watchstum-ipep.de/WTK/WTK.html).

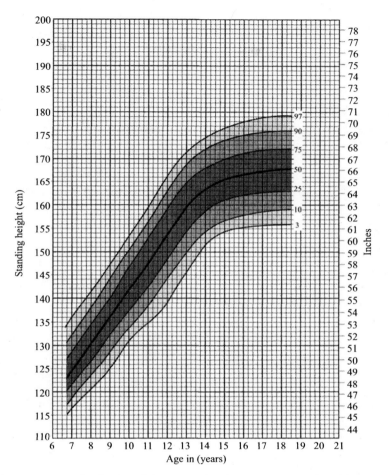

**Figure 4.14** Standing height, North European females, 6 to 19 years. Adapted from Georgi et al., 1996 (http://www.wachstum-ipep.de/WTK/WTK.html).

## Crown–Rump Length

**Definition**    Crown–rump length is the distance from the top of the head to the bottom of the buttock.

**Landmarks**    Measure from the top of the head to the posterior distal part of the thighs with legs extended at right angles at the hips (Fig. 4.15a).

**Instruments**    A recumbent measurement table or tape and table.

**Position**    The patient is lying on the side with the hips flexed to 90 degrees.

**Remarks**    Crown–rump length is a standard measurement to define fetal size (Chapter 15) and can be a useful measurement in the first few years of life. It can give valuable information to define disproportionate growth, especially in patients with reduction defects of the limbs or contractures (Figs. 4.16–4.18).

**Figure 4.15**    Measuring crown–rump length (a) and sitting height (b–d).

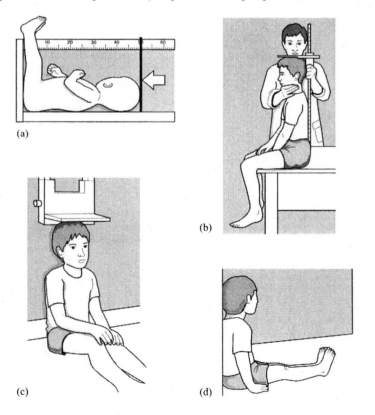

(a)

(b)

(c)

(d)

## Sitting Height

**Definition**  Sitting height is the distance from the top of the head to the buttocks when a sitting position.

**Landmarks**  Measure from the top of the head to the bottom of the thighs (surface on which the patient is sitting) (Fig. 4.15b,c).

**Instruments**  Sitting height table or stadiometer.

**Position**  The patients sits straight, eyes looking straight ahead (Frankfort horizontal plane). The back of the head, back, buttocks, and the shoulders are in contact with the vertical board. A moveable headboard is used to adjust the measurement (Fig. 4.15b,c).

**Alternatives**  The patient sits at the door jamb with the legs straight out in front, the back of the head, shoulders, and buttocks are in contact with the wall. A ruler or book can be used instead of a headboard. Measurements are taken with a tape from the floor to a marking on the door jamb (Fig. 4.15d).

**Remarks**  The charts from birth to 16 years are provided in Figs. 4.16–4.18.

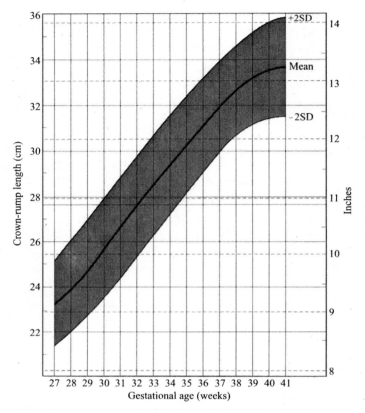

**Figure 4.16**  Crown–rump length at birth, both sexes. From Merlob et al. (1986), by permission.

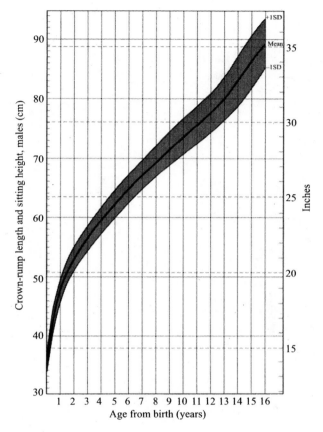

**Figure 4.17** Crown–rump length and sitting height, males, birth to 16 years. From Tanner (1978), by permission.

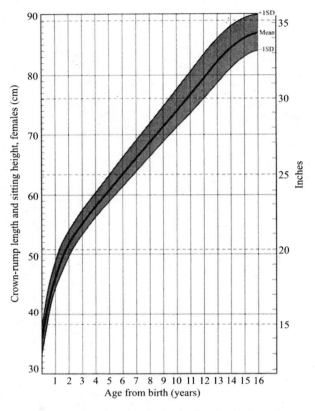

**Figure 4.18**  Crown–rump length and sitting height, females, birth to 16 years. From Tanner (1978), by permission.

## Mid-Parental Height (Used to Access Child's Growth Pattern)

**Definition**   Sum of parental heights divided by 2.

**Remarks**   Mid-parental height is an important parameter in children who appear to be smaller or taller than average. There is an almost linear correlation between height of children 2–9 years and the heights of their biological parents. Using mid-parental height, projections can be made of the child's growth centile using the combination curve of Tanner (Figs. 4.19, 4.20).

### How to Use the Combination Curve

Look up the child's height at the left margin (73–100 cm) or at the upper margin (101–150 cm).

- Follow the curved line from the left border of the chart until you cross the line for the child's age.
- Then draw a horizontal line to the second chart until you meet the vertical line coming from mid-parental height.
- Find the percentile of the child's height along the right-hand margin in relation to the parents' mid-parental height.

*Example*   A 6-year-old boy has a height of 110 cm, his parents (mother, 165 cm; father, 175 cm) have a mid-parental height of 170 cm. He is on the 10th percentile for expected height in view of his mid-parental height.

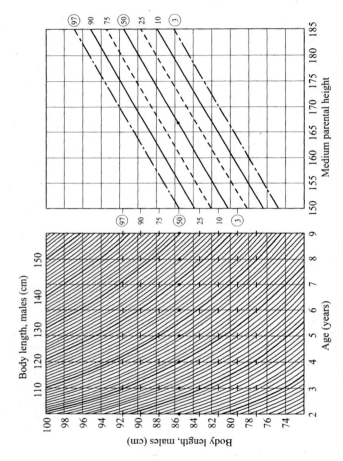

**Figure 4.19**  Mid-parental height, males, combination curve. From Tanner et al. (1970), by permission.

*Mid-Parental Height (Used to Access Child's Growth Pattern)*

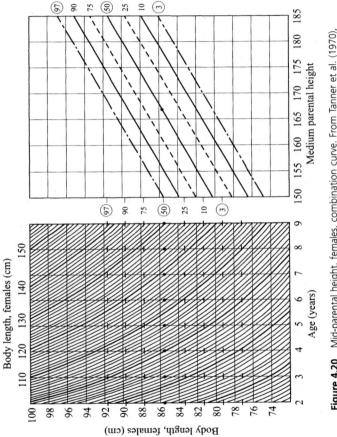

**Figure 4.20** Mid-parental height, females, combination curve. From Tanner et al. (1970), by permission.

39

## Prediction of Height

In normal children one can predict height with some accuracy after four years of age using height and assessment of bone age. Elaborate tables have been developed by Bayley and Pinneau (1952) which are said to be accurate within 2 inches of adult height (see references). However, the tables do not take into account parental height and velocity of puberty (although delayed and precocious puberty are taken into account by using the tables for delayed and advanced bone age). Many other methods to predict final adult height have been developed.

Garn has developed a "multiplier" for each age which can be used with the present height to predict ultimate height if bone age is normal. The tradition of doubling the height at two years to give predicted height was derived from this source (Fig. 4.21).

**Fig. 4.21** Multipliers for prediction of height of boys and girls of average parental stature

| Multiplier (boys) | Age | Multiplier (girls) |
|---|---|---|
| 2.46 | 1 | 2.30 |
| 2.06 | 2 | 2.01 |
| 1.86 | 3 | 1.76 |
| 1.73 | 4 | 1.62 |
| 1.62 | 5 | 1.51 |
| 1.54 | 6 | 1.43 |
| 1.47 | 7 | 1.35 |
| 1.40 | 8 | 1.29 |
| 1.35 | 9 | 1.23 |
| 1.29 | 10 | 1.17 |
| 1.24 | 11 | 1.12 |
| 1.19 | 12 | 1.07 |
| 1.14 | 13 | 1.03 |
| 1.09 | 14 | 1.01 |
| 1.04 | 15 | 1.002 |
| 1.02 | 16 | 1.001 |
| 1.01 | 17 | 1.001 |
| 1.00 | 18 | 1.00 |

From Garn (1966), by permission.

**Prospective Height**

When parents or children are at the lower or upper ends of the growth curve, prospective adult height may be of concern. There is a correlation between parental height and the final height of children. Formulas to calculate final height taking parental height into account are as follows.

*Height at maturity*

Boys = 0.545 height at 2 years + 0.544 parental height + 14.85 inches
Girls = 0.545 height at 2 years + 0.544 parental height + 10.09 inches

**Prediction of Adult Height for Females from Height at the Age of Menarche**

An alternative method for predicting height in females is the use of height at age of menarche. The data for females related to age of menarche are provided in Fig. 4.22.

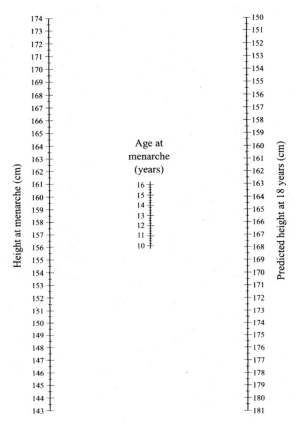

**Figure 4.22**  Nomogram for the prediction of adult height from the height and age at menarche. From Headings (1975), by permission.

## Height Velocity

Growth velocity is the rate of growth over a period of time (Figs. 4.23–4.25). It is most rapid immediately after birth and then, between the ages of 2 and 12 years in boys, or 2 and 10 years in girls, growth velocity slowly continuously decelerates. During adolescence, it increases again. The adolescence peak for girls is a approximately 12 years and boys, at approximately 14 years of age. It is useful to compare growth velocity with the normal yearly intervals: If a girl was 99 cm at 3 years 6 months and measured 106 cm at 4 years 4 months, she has grown 5 cm in 10 months (or presumably 6 cm per year). This rate is compared to her age at the middle of this time interval (3 years, 11 months) and gives the growth velocity for her at that age. In infancy, shorter time intervals are used to evaluate growth velocity.

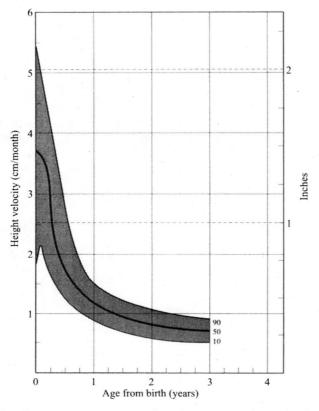

**Figure 4.23**  Height velocity, both sexes, birth to four years. From Brandt (1986), by permission.

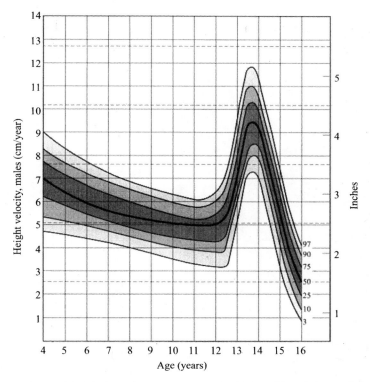

**Figure 4.24**   Height velocity, males. From Tanner and Whitehouse (1976), by permission.

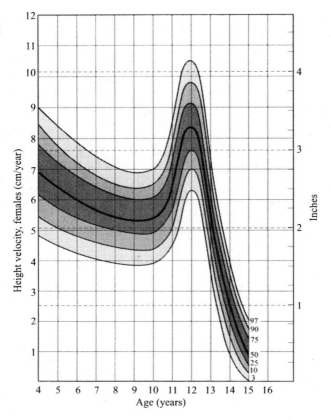

**Figure 4.25**   Height velocity, females. From Tanner and Whitehouse (1976), by permission.

## Expected Increments

There is a predictable height increase for each specific time interval. This increment changes with age. Males and females have the same incremental height increases for the first 48 months of life, then sex differences are noted. Expected height increase increment charts can be found in Fig. 4.26.

**Figure 4.26** Expected increments in height, both sexes, birth to 16 years. From Lowrey (1986), by permission.

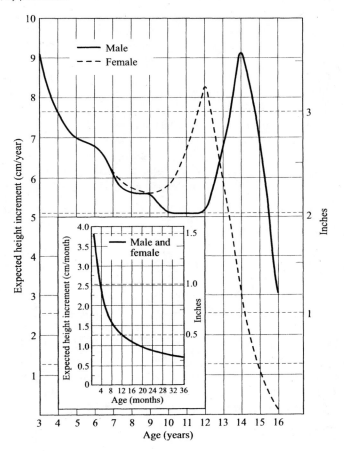

## Bibliography

Bayley, N. and Pinneau, S. R. (1952). Tables for predicting adult height from skeletal age: revised for use with the Greulich–Pyle hand standards. *Journal of Pediatrics*, 40, 423–44.

Brandt, I. (1986). Growth dynamics of low-birth-weight infants with emphasis on the prenatal period. In *Human Growth. A comprehensive treatise, Vol. 1* (ed. F. Falkner and J. M. Tanner), pp. 415–475. Plenum, New York.

Brooke, O. G., Butters, F., Wood, C., Bailay, P., and Tudkmachi, F. (1981). Size at birth from 31–41 weeks gestation: ethnic standards for British infants of both sexes. *Journal of Human Nutrition*, 35, 415–43

Garn, S. M. (1966). Body size and its implications. In *Review of child development research* (ed. L. W. Hoffman and M. L. Hoffman), *Vol. 2*, pp. 529–561. Russell Sage Foundation, New York.

Garn, S. M. and Rohmann, C. G. (1966). Interaction of nutrition and genetics in the timing of growth and development. *Pediatric Clinics of North America*, 13, 353–379.

Georgi, M., Schaefer, F., Wuehl, E., Schaerer, K. (1996). Heidelberger Wachstumskurven. *Monatsschrift Kinderheilkunde* 144, 813–824.

Hamill, P. V., Drizd, T. A., Johnson, C. L., Reed, R. B., Roche, A. F., and Moore, W. M. (1979). Physical growth: National Center for Health Statistics percentile. *American Journal of Clinical Nutrition*, 32, 607–629.

Headings, D. L. (ed.) (1975). *The Harriet Lane Handbook*. (7th ed). Year Book Medical Publishers, Chicago.

Hohenauer, L. (1980). Intrauterine Wachtumskurven fuer den Deutschen Sprachraum. *Zeitschrift fuer Geburtshilfe und Frauenheilkunde*, 184, 167–179.

Largo, R. H., Waelli, R., Duc, G., Fanconi, A., and Prader, A. (1980). Evaluation of perinatal growth. *Helvetia Paediatrica Acta*, 35, 419–436.

Lowrey, G. H. (1986). *Growth and development of children* (8th ed). Year Book Medical Publishers, Chicago.

Lubchenco, L. O., Hansmann, C., Dressler, M., and Boyd, E. (1963). Intrauterine growth as estimated from liveborn birthweight data at 24 to 42 weeks of gestation. *Pediatrics*, 32, 793–800.

Lubchenco, L. O., Hansmann, C., and Boyd, E. (1966). Intrauterine growth in length and head circumference as estimated from livebirth at gestational ages from 26 to 42 weeks. *Pediatrics*, 37, 403–407.

Merlob, P., Sivan, Y., and Reisner, S. H. (1986). Ratio of crown–rump distance to total length in preterm and term infants. *Journal of Medical Genetics*, **23**, 338–340.

Naeye, R. L., Benirschke, K., Hagstrom, J. W. C., and Marcus, C. C. (1966). Intrauterine growth of twins as estimated from liveborn birth-weight data. *Pediatrics*, **37**, 409–416.

Tanner, J. M. (1978). Physical growth and development. In *Textbook of pediatrics* (ed. J. O. Forfar and G. C. Arneil), pp. 253–303. Churchill Livingstone, Edinburgh.

Tanner, J. M. and Whitehouse, R. H. (1973). Height and weight charts from birth to 5 years allowing for length of gestation. *Archives of Disease in Childhood*, **48**, 786–789.

Tanner, J. M. and Whitehouse, R. H. (1976). Clinical longitudinal standards for height, weight, height velocity, weight velocity, and stages of puberty. *Archives of Disease in Childhood*, **51**, 170–179.

Tanner, J. M., Goldstein, H., and Whitehouse, R. H. (1970) Standards for children's height at ages 2–9 years allowing for height of parents. *Archives of Disease in Childhood*, **45**, 755–762.

Voigt M., Schneider, K. T. M. and Jahrig, K. (1996). Analyse des Geburtsgutes des Jahrgangs 1992 der Bundesrepublik Deutschland. Teil 1: Neue Perzentilwerte für die Körpermaße von Neugeborenen. *Geburtsh u. Frauenheilk*, **56**, 550–558.

Waelli, R., Stettler, T., Largo, R. H., Fanconi, A., Prader, A. (1980). Gewicht, Laenge und Kopfumfang neugeborener Kinder und ihre Abhaengigkeit von muetterlichen und kindlichen Faktoren. *Helvetia Paediatrica Acta*, **35**, 397–418.

# Weight

## Weight

**Definition**   Weight or heaviness of the individual.

**Instruments**   For infants and younger children, a scale in which the individual can lie or sit is used. For older children and adults, a standing scale is used.

**Position**   In a newborn infant or young child, weight is taken by laying the baby on the weighing table or infant scale (Fig. 5.1a); in older children and adults able to stand, a standing scale is used (Fig. 5.1b).

The individual should not be touching anything except the scale (wall, floor, scale upright, etc.) because that will affect the weight measurement. Most clothing is removed since it will affect the weight measurement.

**Alternative**   If no infant scales are available, a normal scale can be used, weighing an adult and child together, transferring the child to an assistant, and taking the adult's weight alone. The baby's weight will be calculated by the difference between the weight of the adult plus the child and the weight of the adult alone. In older individuals unable to stand, the weight of the bed or wheelchair is taken and subtracted.

**Remarks**   Weight measurement should be performed at least twice, preferably three times, to ensure accuracy. The patient should step on and off the scale between measurements.

As little clothing as possible should be worn for the weighing. In newborns and infants, the diaper is removed. A blanket may be used if the scale is cold, but its weight should be subtracted from the total. If weight is taken with the diaper on, the weight of the diaper should be subtracted from the baby's weight. In older patients, light underwear is usually worn (Fig. 5.1b). However, shoes, belts, regular clothing, and any jewelry should be removed.

In the absence of a limb, one has to adjust the expected weight in relationship to height. It is estimated that the upper limbs together account for approximately 11 percent of the total weight and the lower limbs together for approximately 20 percent of the total weight.

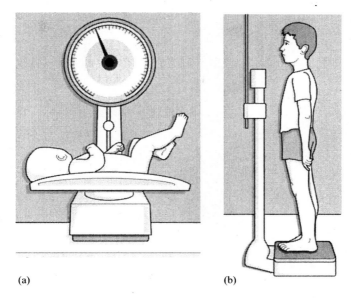

(a)                                         (b)

**Figure 5.1**   Measuring weight with an infant scale (a) and a standing scale (b).

During the first days of life a natural weight loss occurs. It usually is greatest at the third day of life, when it equals approximately 7 percent of the birthweight.

Weight for North European and North American children are shown in Figs. 5.2–5.9.

**Pitfalls**   In infants the effects of feeding and bowel movement can alter weight.

The weight should be recorded when the individual is quiet and still. Shifting weight and movement can change the measurement by several pounds.

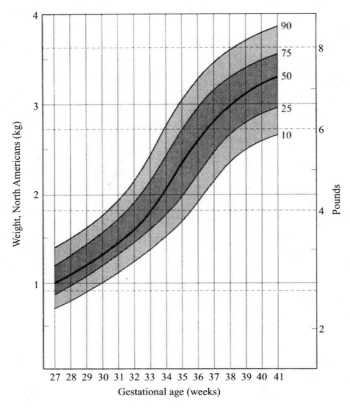

**Figure 5.2** Weight, North American infants at birth, both sexes. From Lubchenco et al. (1963), by permission.

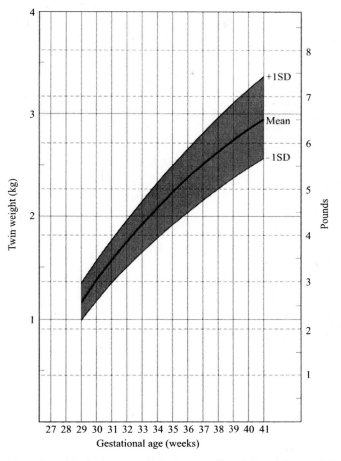

**Figure 5.3** Twin weight, both sexes at birth. From Waelli et al. (1980), by permission.

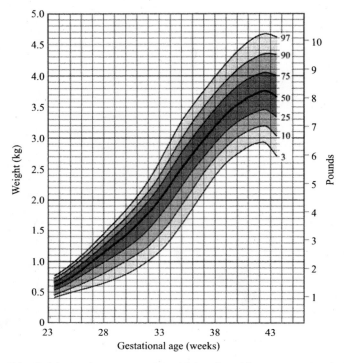

**Figure 5.4** Weight, North European males at birth. Adapted from Voigt et al. (1996).

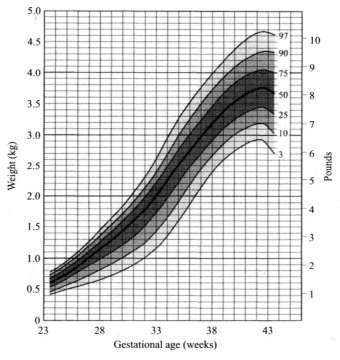

**Figure 5.5**   Weight, North European females at birth. Adapted from Voigt et al. (1996).

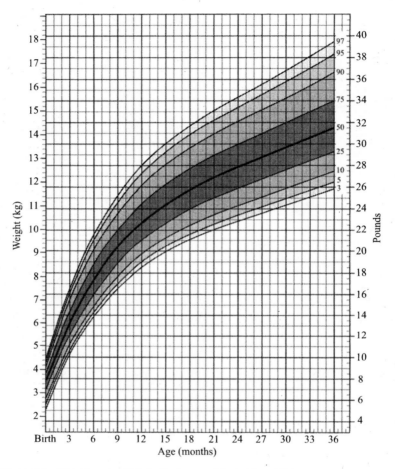

**Figure 5.6**  Weight, males, birth to three years. Adapted from CDC: http://www.gov/growthcharts.

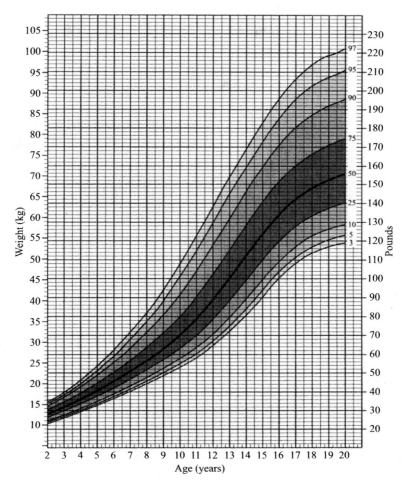

**Figure 5.7** Weight, males, 2 to 20 years. Adapted from CDC: http://www.gov/growthcharts.

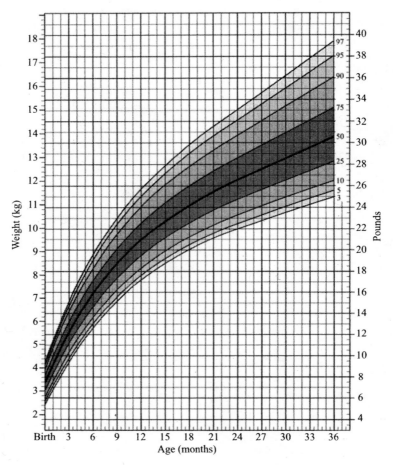

**Figure 5.8** Weight, females, birth to three years. Adapted from CDC: http://www.gov/growthcharts.

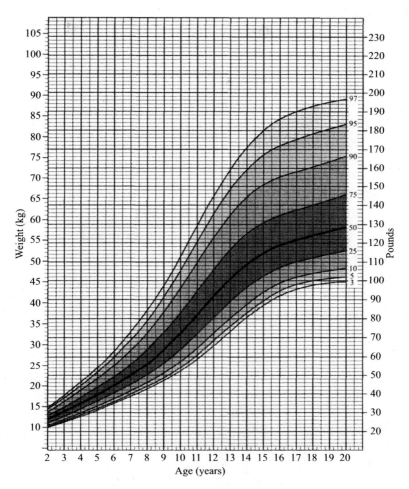

**Figure 5.9** Weight, females, 2 to 20 years. Adapted from CDC: http://www.gov/growthcharts.

## Body Mass Index

**Definition**   Body mass index (BMI) is defined as

$$BMI = \frac{\text{Weight in kg}}{(\text{Height in m})^2}$$

By definition, a person with a BMI greater than 25 is considered overweight; a BMI greater than 30 indicates obesity (Figs. 5.10–5.13).

**Figure 5.10**   Weight, North European males, 7 to 19 years. Adapted from Georgi et al. (1996).

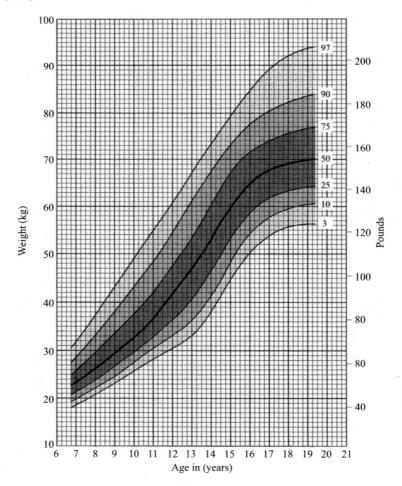

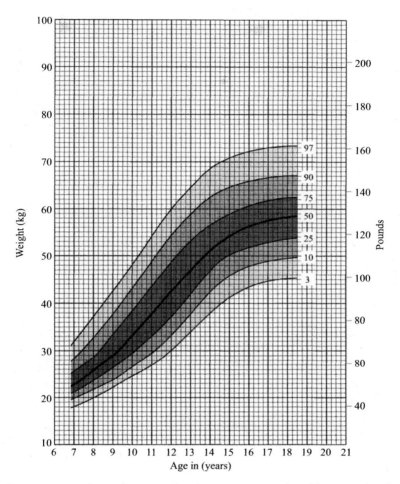

**Figure 5.11** Weight, North European females, 7 to 19 years. Adapted from Georgi et al. (1996).

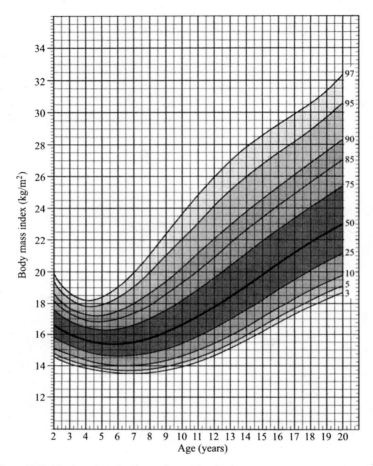

**Figure 5.12**  Body mass index for North American males, ages 2 to 20 years. Adapted from CDC: http://www.gov/growthcharts.

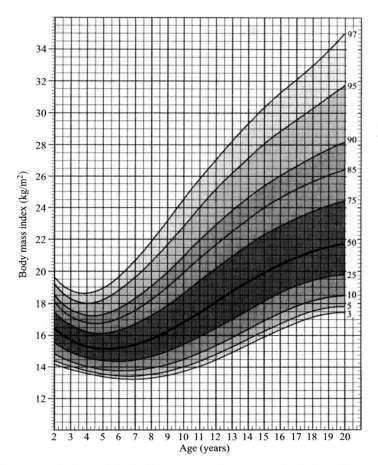

**Figure 5.13** Body mass index for North American females, ages 2 to 20 years. Adapted from CDC: http://www.gov/growthcharts.

## Weight Velocity

**Definition**   Weight velocity is the rate of weight gain or loss over a period of time (Figs. 5.14–5.16).

**Remarks**   As with other parameters of growth, weight gain is most rapid in the first months of life, and again between 12–16 years.

**Figure 5.14**   Weight velocity, both sexes, birth to four years. From Brandt (1986), by permission.

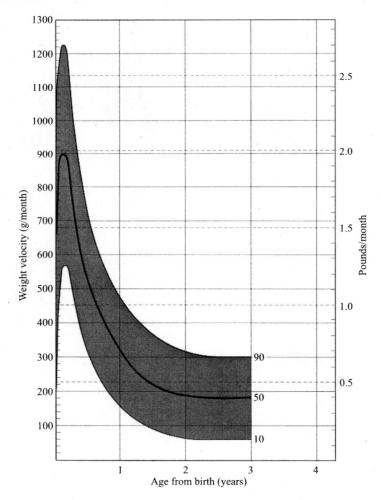

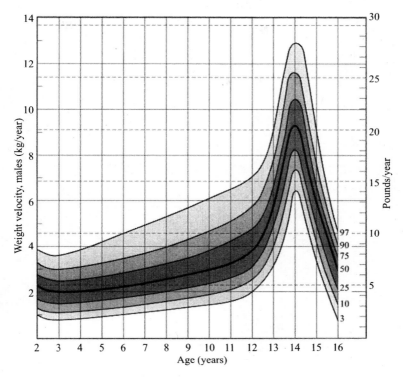

**Figure 5.15**   Weight velocity, males, 2 to 16 years. From Tanner and Whitehouse (1976), by permission.

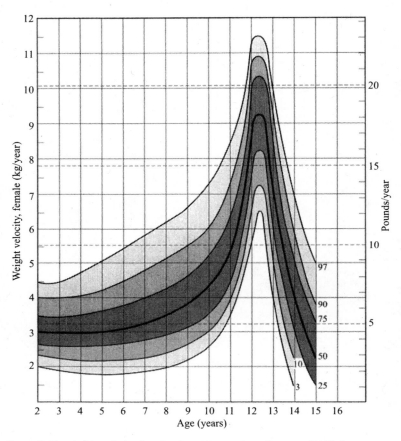

**Figure 5.16** Weight velocity, females, 2 to 16 years. From Tanner and Whitehouse (1976), by permission.

## Skinfold Thickness

**Definition**   Thickness of the skinfold.

**Landmarks**   Triceps and subscapular skinfold thickness are used. The left side of the body is usually chosen for these measurements. Triceps skinfold thickness is measured halfway down the left upper arm, while the arm is hanging relaxed at the patient's side (Fig. 5.17a).
The subscapular skinfold is measured laterally just below the angle of the left scapula (Fig. 5.17b).

**Position**   A skinfold is held between the investigator's thumb and index finger (subcutaneous fold without muscle). The caliper is placed about 1 mm below the left hand, perpendicular to the skinfold. The right hand holds the caliper and the measurement is read within 3 seconds (so that pressure does not compress the subcutaneous tissue).

**Instruments**   Special calipers are used for precise measurements. These are constructed to exert a constant pressure of 10 $g/mm^2$ at the opening and allow an accuracy up to 0.1 mm. Skinfold thickness is measured in millimeters (Figs. 5.18 and 5.19).

**Remarks**   The suprailiac skinfold can also be measured (just above the iliac crest in the mid-axillary line) and the sum of the three skinfold measurements (triceps skinfold + suprailiac skinfold + subscapular skinfold) is calculated to give an overall assessment (see Schlueter et al. (1976)).

**Pitfalls**   Too lengthy or too frequently repeated measurements at the same spot will result in compression of the tissue, leading to falsely low measurement.

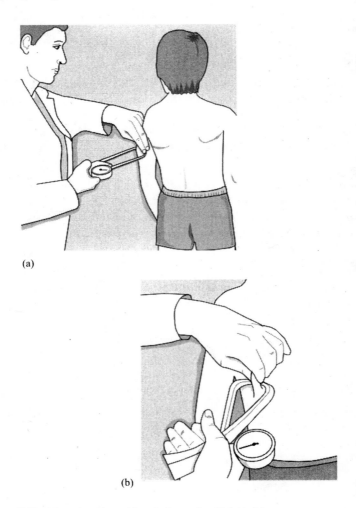

(a)

(b)

**Figure 5.17**  Measuring triceps (a) and subscapular skinfolds (b).

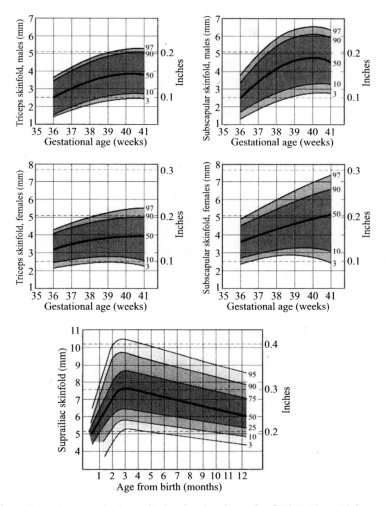

**Figure 5.18** Triceps and subscapular (newborn) and suprailiac (birth to 12 months) skinfolds. From Maaser et al. (1972) and Schlueter et al. (1976), by permission.

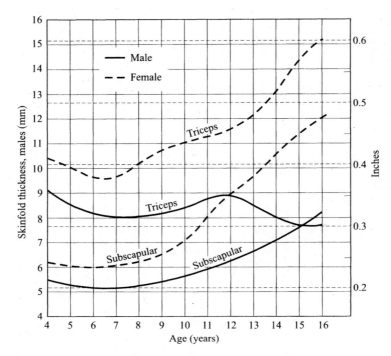

**Figure 5.19** Triceps and subscapular skinfolds, males and females, 4 to 16 years. From Maaser et al. (1972) and Schlueter et al. (1976), by permission.

## Bibliography

Brandt, I. (1986). Growth dynamics of low-birth-weight infants with emphasis on the prenatal period. In *Human growth. A comprehensive treatise, Vol. 1.* (ed. F. Falkner and J. M. Tanner), pp. 415–475. Plenum, New York.

Brooke, O. G., Butters, F., Wood, C., Bailay, P., and Tudkmachi, F. (1981). Size at birth from 31–41 weeks gestation: ethnic standards for British infants of both sexes. *Journal of Human Nutrition*, **35**, 415–430.

Georgi, M., Schaefer, F., Wuehi, E. and Schaerer, K. (1996). Heidelberger Wachstumskurven. *Monatsschrift Kinderheilkunde* **144**, 813–824.

Hamill, P. V., Drizd, T. A., Johnson, C. L., Reed, R. B., Roche, A. F., and Moore, W. M. (1979). Physical growth: National Center for Health Statistics percentile. *American Journal of Clinical Nutrition*, **32**, 607–629.

Hohenauer, L. (1980). Intrauterine Wachtumskurven fuer den Deutschen Sprachraum. *Zeitschrift fuer Geburtshilfe und Perinatologie*, **184**, 167–179.

Largo, R. H., Waelli, R., Duc, G., Fanconi, A., and Prader, A. (1980). Evaluation of perinatal growth. *Helvetia Paediatrica Acta*, **35**, 419–436.

Lubchenco, L. O., Hansmann, C., Dressler, M., and Boyd, E. (1963). Intrauterine growth as estimated from liveborn birthweight data at 24 to 42 weeks of gestation. *Pediatrics*, **32**, 793–800.

Lubchenco, L. O., Hansmann, C., and Boyd, E. (1966). Intrauterine growth in length and head circumference as estimated from livebirth at gestational ages from 26 to 42 weeks. *Pediatrics*, **37**, 403–408.

Maaser, R., Stolley, H., and Droese, W. (1972). Die Hautfettfaltenmessung mit dem Caliper-II. Standardwerte der subcutanen Fettgewebsdicke 2–14 jaehriger gesunder Kinder. *Monaitsschrift fuer Kinderheilkunde*, **120**, 350–353.

Schlueter, K., Funfack, W., Pachalay, J., and Weber, B. (1976). Development of subcutaneous fat in infancy. *European Journal of Pediatrics*, **123**, 255–267.

Tanner, J. M. (1978). Physical growth and development. In *Textbook of pediatrics* (ed. J. O. Forfar and G. C. Arneil), pp. 253–303. Churchill Livingstone, Edinburgh.

Tanner, J. M. and Whitehouse, R. H. (1973). Height and weight charts from birth to 5 years allowing for length of gestation. *Archives of Disease in Childhood*, **48**, 786–789.

Tanner, J. M. and Whitehouse, R. H. (1976). Clinical longitudinal standards for height, weight, height velocity, weight velocity, and stages of puberty. *Archives of Diseases in Childhood*, **51**, 170–179.

Voigt, M., Schneider, K. T. M. and Jaehrig, K. (1996) Analyse des Geburtsgutes des Jahrgangs 1992 der Bundesrepublik Deutschland. Teil 1: Neue Perzentilwerte fuer die Koerpermasse von Neugeborenen. *Geburtshilfe und Frauenheilkunde*, **56**, 550–558.

Waelli, R., Stettler, T., Largo, R. H., Fanconi, A., and Prader, A. (1980). Gewicht, Laenge und Kopfumfang neugeborener Kinder und ihre Abhaengigkeit von muetterlichen und kindlichen Faktoren. *Helvetia Paediatrica Acta*, **35**, 397–418.

# Head Circumference (Occipitofrontal Circumference, OFC)

6

## Introduction

The head circumference (distance around the head) is traditionally measured at the place where the largest measurement is obtained. This practice has given rise to the term occipitofrontal circumference (OFC), because these are usually the landmarks of the largest circumference. OFC has become synonymous with head circumference. Care should be taken to obtain the maximum circumference, which occasionally is not at the occiput.

## Head Circumference (OFC)

**Definition**   Maximum circumference of the head.

**Landmarks**   The maximum head circumference (usually horizontal just above the eyebrow ridges), is measured from just above the glabella area to the area near the top of the occipital bone (opisthocranion) (Fig. 6.1).

**Instruments**   Tape-measure.

**Position**   The patient should look straight ahead (Fig. 6.1).

**Alternative**   It is often easier, in young infants, to have them stay seated on an adult's lap while measuring the head circumference, and to do the measurement from behind.

**Remarks**   The head circumference measurement should be repeated after completely removing the tape from the head in order to ensure accuracy.

Although height and weight charts after birth are quite different for North American and North European populations, head circumference growth data after birth are not. Therefore, we have included only one figure for head circumference for each sex. We have added charts depicting neonatal head circumference size for North European males and females because these charts include earlier gestational ages compared to the data by Lubchenko et al. (Figs. 6.2–6.4)

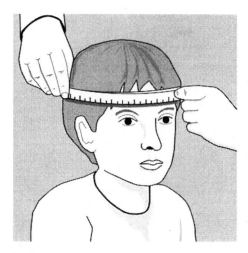

**Figure 6.1** Measuring head (OFC) circumference.

As more premature infants with very low birth weights survive, it is appropriate to use special curves for these infants. Most of the catch-up growth for OFC occurs during the first 6 months of life (Fig. 6.5).

Values for North American populations to age 16 years are given in Figs. 6.6–6.9.

*Microcephaly* is the term used for abnormal smallness of the head, usually as related to age; however, when the head is small it must be evaluated in the context of body size as well. Hence, a head can be described as microcephalic for age but relatively normocephalic for body size. *Microcranium* is the term used for an abnormally small skull. *Macrocephaly* (*megacephaly*) is the term for an abnormally large head (but does not imply the cause). Again, macrocephaly must be described in relationship to age and body size. *Macrocranium* is the term for an abnormally large skull.

**Pitfalls**   Thick hair, braids, or big ears can get in the way when measuring head circumference and can lead to falsely elevated OFC values. If the head is an unusual shape, it may be difficult to palpate the landmarks.

In the case of craniosynostosis or an unusual head shape, OFC measurements can give false impressions of micro- or macrocephaly. In those cases, the head width, length, and forehead height are useful parameters. X-rays should be taken for a more objective estimate of the actual space available for the brain.

**Figure 6.2**   Head circumference, both sexes, at birth. From Lubchenco et al. (1963), by permission.

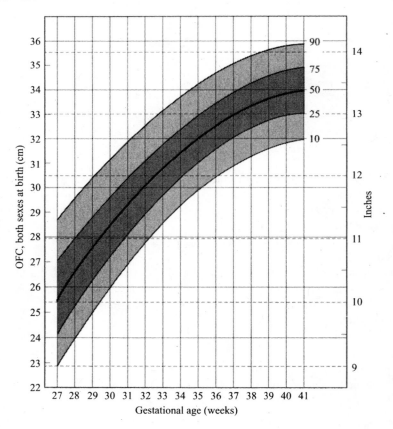

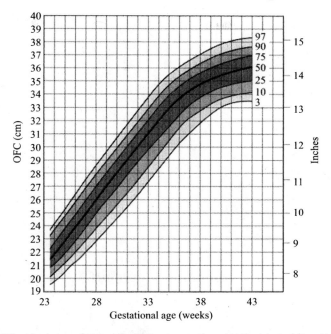

**Figure 6.3**    Head circumference, North European males, at birth. Adapted from Voigt et al. (1996).

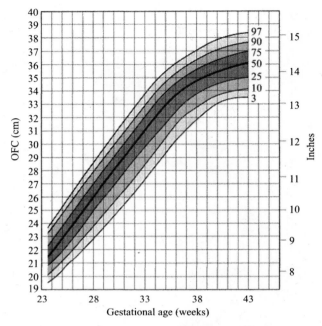

**Figure 6.4**  Head circumference, North European females, at birth. Adapted from Voigt et al. (1996).

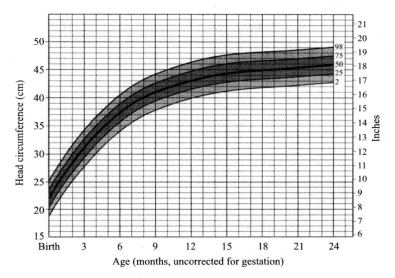

**Figure 6.5** Head circumference growth for infants with a birth weight of 501–1000 g, age birth to 24 months. Adapted from Shetu et al. (1995).

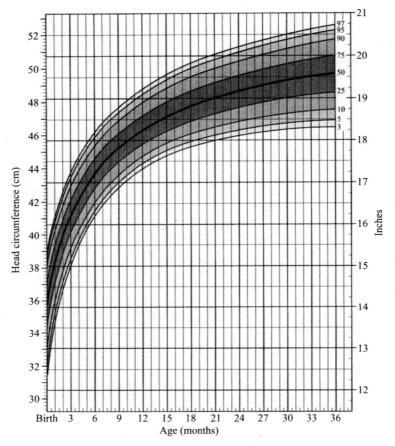

**Figure 6.6** Head circumference, males, birth to 36 months. Adapted from CDC: http://www.gov/growthcharts.

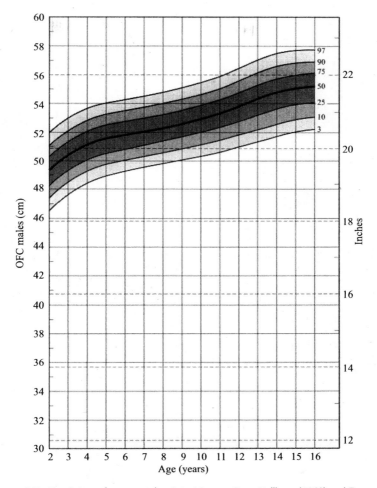

**Figure 6.7** Head circumference, males, 2 to 16 years. From Nellhaus (1968) and Tanner (1978), by permission.

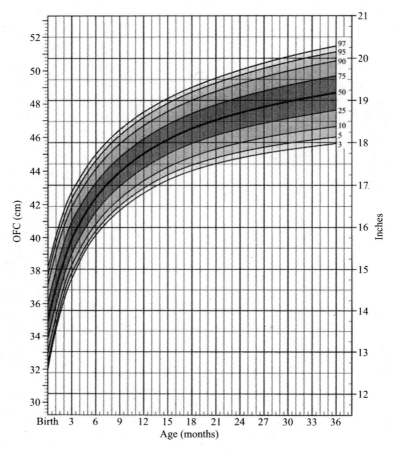

**Figure 6.8**  Head circumference, females, birth to 36 months. Adapted from CDC: http://www.gov/growthcharts.

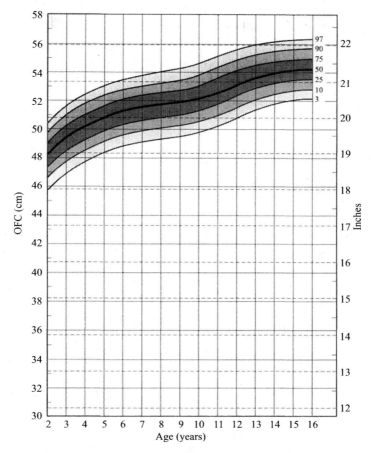

**Figure 6.9**   Head circumference, females, 2 to 16 years. From Nellhaus (1968) and Tanner (1978), by permission.

## Head Circumference (OFC) Velocity

The rate of head size growth decreases after birth. The deceleration is most dramatic in the first year, with the majority of head growth complete by 4 years of age.

**Figure 6.10** Head circumference velocity, both sexes, from 28 weeks to 1 year. From Brandt (1986), and Tanner (1978), by permission.

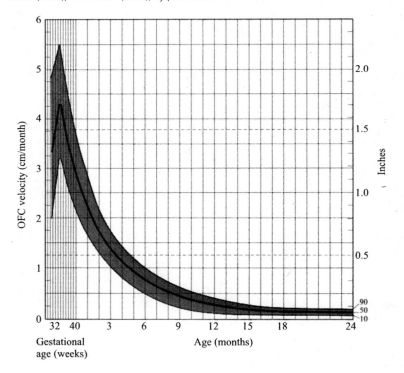

# Bibliography

Brandt, I. (1986). Growth dynamics of low-birth-weight infants with emphasis on the prenatal period. In *Human growth. A comprehensive treatise, Vol. 1*, (ed. F. Falkner and J. M. Tanner), pp. 415–475. Plenum, New York.

Brooke, O. G., Butters, F., Wood, C., Bailay, P., and Tudkmachi, F. (1981). Size at birth from 31–41 weeks gestation: ethnic standards for British infants of both sexes. *Journal of Human Nutrition*, **35**, 415–430.

Hohenauer, L. (1980). Intrauterine Wachtumskurven fuer den Deutschen Sprachraum. *Zeitschrift fuer Geburtshilfe und Perinatologie*, **184**, 167–179.

Lubchenco, L. O., Hansmann, C., Dressler, M., and Boyd, E. (1963). Intrauterine growth as estimated from liveborn birthweight data at 24 to 42 weeks of gestation. *Pediatrics*, **32**, 793–800.

Lubchenco, L. O., Hansmann, C., and Boyd, E. (1966). Intrauterine growth in length and head circumference as estimated from livebirth at gestational ages from 26 to 42 weeks. *Pediatrics*, **37**, 403–408.

Nellhaus, G. (1968). Head circumference from birth to eighteen years. Practical composite international and interracial graphs. *Pediatrics*, **41**, 106–114.

Sheth, R. D., Mullett, M. D., Bodensteiner, J. B., and Hobbs, G. R. (1995). Longitudinal head growth in developmentally normal preterm infants. *Archives of Pediatric and Adolescent Medicine*, **149**, 1358–1361.

Tanner, J. M. (1978). Physical growth and development. In *Textbook of pediatrics* (ed. J. O. Forfar and G. C. Arneil), pp. 253–303. Churchill Livingstone, Edinburgh.

Voigt, M., Schneider, K. T. M. and Jaehrig, K. (1996) Analyse des Geburtigutes des Jahrgangs 1992 der Bundesrepublik Deutschland. Teil 1: Neue Perzentilwerte fuer die Koerpermasse von Neugeborenen. *Geburtshilfe und Frauenheilkunde*, **56**, 550–558.

Waelli, R., Stettler, T., Largo, R. H., Fanconi, A., and Prader, A. (1980). Gewicht, Laenge und Kopfumfang neugeborener Kinder und ihre Abhaengigkeit von muetterlichen und kindlichen Faktoren. *Helvetia Paediatrica Acta*, **35**, 397–418.

# Craniofacies

7

## Introduction

The face is unique, both because of variability in size and shape and because of personal expression and emotion. Movements around the eyes and mouth contribute to the overall gestalt. Evaluation of the craniofacies is complex.

The development of the shape of the human head and face depends on a variety of interactive genetic and environmental factors. Intrinsic or extrinsic pressure and neuromuscular function contribute to the overall shape. Both nature and nurture should be considered when evaluating the individual with unusual craniofacial structures.

To define properly what is different in the individual with dysmorphic craniofacial features is a challenge. Comprehensive anthropometric descriptions have become available for many conditions for which data were previously lacking, and standards have been developed for several disorders so that affected children can be compared with their similarly affected peers and normal family members.

For practical purposes, in this text, we have limited the craniofacial measurements to those we find useful. The reader will find further details in references at the end of this chapter.

Development of the face from five facial primordia appearing around the stomodeum or primitive mouth occurs mainly between the fifth and eighth weeks of gestation. The five facial primordia consist of the frontonasal prominence, the paired maxillary prominences of the first branchial arch, and the paired mandibular prominences of the first branchial arch. The frontonasal prominence forms the forehead and the dorsum and apex of the nose. The alae nasi are derived from the lateral nasal prominences. The fleshy nasal septum and the philtrum are formed by the medial nasal prominences. The maxillary prominences form the upper cheek regions and most of the upper lip. The mandibular prominences give rise to the lower lip, the chin, and the lower cheek regions.

The primitive lips and cheeks are invaded by second branchial arch mesenchyme giving rise to the facial muscles. These muscles of facial expression are supplied by the facial nerve. The mesenchyme of the first pair of branchial arches gives rise to the muscles of mastication, which are innervated by the trigeminal nerve.

Maldevelopment of the components of the first branchial arch results in various congenital malformations of the eyes, ears, mandible, and palate. Maldevelopment is generally believed to be caused by insufficient migration or proliferation of cranial neural crest cells into the first branchial arch.

Development of the tongue, face, lips, jaws, palate pharynx, and neck largely involves transformation of the branchial apparatus into adult structures. Most congenital malformations of the head and neck originate during that transformation (e.g., branchial cysts, sinuses, fistulae). Because of the complicated development of the face and palate, congenital malformations resulting from an arrest of development and/or a failure of fusion of the prominences and processes are not uncommon.

There is also rapid growth of the face and jaws coinciding with the eruption of the deciduous teeth. These changes are even more marked after the permanent teeth erupt. There is concurrent enlargement of the frontal and facial regions associated with the increase in size of the perinasal air sinuses, which are generally rudimentary or absent at birth. Growth of the sinuses is important in altering the shape of the face.

Measurement of the craniofacies requires only a few standard instruments: sliding and spreading calipers and a tape-measure. In addition, a modified protractor and an instrument to determine ear location and rotation are useful but not essential. A general rule when measuring between two soft tissue landmarks is that the hard tips of the calipers touch but do not press on the skin surface. In contrast, when measuring between bony landmarks, the blunt pointers of the calipers are presented against the bony surface. When measuring the circumference, the length, or the width of the head, the examiner must be certain that the metric tape or the tips of the calipers are sufficiently pressed against the skull to eliminate the effect of thick hair cover. Accurate measurement requires correct use of the instrument and knowledge of the peculiarities of the landmark. For this reason, we have provided detailed explanations of measurement techniques and pitfalls for each particular parameter.

For measurement of the craniofacies, it is often easiest to have the head resting on a head support from a chair. However, this is not always possible in the field. If necessary, an assistant may gently hold the subject's head. Full exposure of the soft nose (alar shape, columella, nasal floor, nostrils) in the frontal plane is facilitated if the head is in the reclining position. Orbital measurements are most easily obtained when the patient's body is in a recumbent position with the eyes gazing straight up to the ceiling and the plane of the facial profile in the vertical.

The standard orientation of the head for craniofacial measurement is the Frankfort horizontal (FH). In this position, the line connecting the lowest point on the lower margin of each bony orbit (orbitale) and the highest point on the upper margin of the cutaneous external auditory meatus (porion) is horizontal. When the subject is recumbent, the FH becomes vertical.

An alternative head position (the rest position) is determined by the subject's own feeling of the natural head balance. In healthy persons, in the rest position, the inclination of the line connecting the orbitale and the porion (ear opening) is about 5 degrees higher than it is in the FH. Since the subject's head tends to return to the rest position during examination, head position must be rechecked before each measurement. Correct positioning techniques and use of standard landmarks are important, not only for the evaluation of the normal face, but particularly in the assessment of subjects with a cranial or facial anomaly. The most common palpable landmarks of the craniofacies are shown in Fig. 7.1, and a full definition of each of these landmarks is present in the Glossary.

An alternative approach to craniofacial measurement involves a photoanthropometric method using frontal and profile photographs. Photographs are standardized (one-fifth, one-fourth, one-third, one-half, or life-size) for quantification of surface features, to allow scientific, accurate documentations. Some centers prefer to have the patient free-standing, while other researchers have developed complex machinery to keep the patient in a fixed position at a defined distance from the camera. Details and sources of error are available in articles listed in the bibliography.

Another approach to craniofacial measurement involves craniofacial pattern profile analysis, which provides a simple and readily understandable method of classifying, illustrating, and comparing pattern deviations from the normal state. Measurements, from radiographs of the head and face are converted into normalized $z$ scores (standard deviation units). After conversion into $z$ scores, the pattern profile can be presented in simple graphic form. The reader is directed to the bibliography at the end of this chapter for further details.

A fourth approach to craniofacial measurement, cephalometry, employs radiography. For most analyses, only lateral cephalograms are taken. Most radiographic head films are still taken according to the standards of Holly Broadbent, who established them more than 50 years ago. His format for taking head films was quickly adopted by the scientific community because of the consensus that his instrumentaion, radiographs, and data were impeccable. Probably his major contribution was designing a cephalostat or orthodontic head-holder. Although the clinical

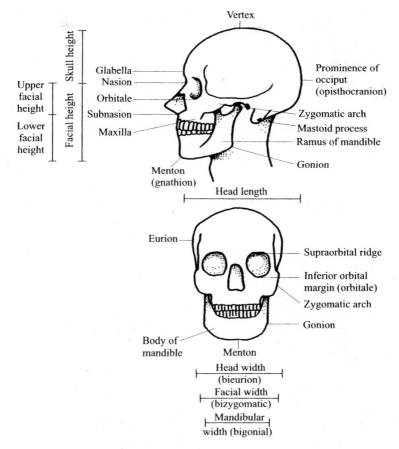

**Figure 7.1** Palpable landmarks of craniofacies.

cephalostats used today are much less obstructive and expensive than Broadbent's research instrument, the positioning of the head and the distance between the X-ray unit and the head-holder remain the same. The head is held in the cephalostat, which restrains the head in a precise manner. Adjustable ear rods fit into the external auditory meati, holding the head stable anteroposteriorly and preventing lateral rotation. The central beam of the X-ray is designed to pass through the ear rods. A 5 foot tube-to-film distance and a 52.4 inch tube-to-median plane distance are employed throughout. Further details may be found in the bibliography at the end of this chapter.

A new approach to document the three-dimensional surface of the face consists of multiple camera photography. Computerized programs merge the images into a single three-dimensional surface mesh. In addition to image documentation, this approach allows for identification of soft tissue landmarks, distance measurements between landmarks, and calculation of ratios. Software allowing computer image–driven syndrome identification is being developed.

Results of single measurements will indicate the patient's place within or outside the normal range. Repeated measurements allow calculation of changes and growth. Such changes affect the proportions of the face. In both sexes the vertical profile measurements increase more than horizontal measurements (maximum relative increments occurring earlier in girls than in boys). The upper face seems to grow more rapidly than the lower face up to about the 10th year. After that age, the reverse is apparent. The lower portion of the face, consisting of the mandible, manifests accelerated growth with the result that, at 21 years, the face has the same relative proportions as at three years. Growth is generally completed first in the skull, then in the width of the face, and last in the length and depth of the face. Peak growth occurs between 3–5 years, followed by continuous deceleration until the 13th year, and then a distinct adolescent acceleration. There is virtually complete cessation of growth of the craniofacies at age 21 years. However, many nasal dimensions, particularly nasal length, continue to increase. With increasing age, most craniofacial dimensions, with the exception of facial width and nasal length, are reduced. This can be ascribed mostly to soft tissue changes.

Normal growth and development of craniofacial structures also require movement of embryonic muscles during the prenatal period. Lack of movement during the fetal period, for any reason, particularly in the presence of neuromuscular disease, produces a characteristic facial appearance (fetal akinesia sequence)—for example, as seen in Pena Shokeir syndrome.

An approach to measurement of the craniofacies must include comparison with head circumference and height in addition to age. For example, inner and outer canthal distances on the 50th percentile, in the presence of microcephaly, would in fact be abnormal and relatively hyperteloric. Various indices comparing two craniofacial measurements are available in the dental and anthropological literature. Few have been included in this text, but references are found at the end of this chapter.

In addition to detailed individual measurements, an evaluation of the craniofacies requires an impression of the overall gestalt of the face both at rest and during movement such as crying, smiling, and frowning. It is important to remember that the shape of the face and its relative proportions change significantly with age, in both normal and dysmorphic individuals. For this reason, the overall gestalt may be quite different at different times during life. This change should be taken into account when a subject is evaluated.

The terminology used to describe the craniofacies is complex and somewhat confusing. A glossary of terms defining specific landmarks and anomalies is provided at the end of this book.

## Skull

### Introduction

The skull develops from mesenchyme around the developing brain. It consists of two parts—the neurocranium (the protection for the brain) and the viscerocranium (the main skeleton of the jaws). The neurocranium is further divided into cartilaginous and membranous portion. The cartilaginous neurocranium (or chondrocranium) consists initially of the cartilaginous base of the developing skull which forms by fusion of several cartilages. Later endochondral ossification of the chondrocranium forms the bones of the base of the skull. Intramembranous ossification occurs in the mesenchyme at the sides and top of the brain, forming the cranial vault or calvaria. During fetal life the flat bones of the vault are separated by dense connective tissue membranes called sutures. The seven large fibrous areas where several sutures meet are called fontanelles. The cartilaginous viscerocranium consists of the cartilaginous skeleton of the first two pairs of branchial arches which will ultimately form the middle ear ossicles, part of the hyoid bone, and the styloid process of the temporal bone. Intramembranous ossification occurs within the maxillary and mandibular prominences of the first branchial arch and subsequently forms the maxillary, zygomatic, and squamous temporal bones and the mandible.

Postnatal growth of the skull occurs because the fibrous sutures of the newborn calvaria permit the skull to enlarge during infancy and childhood. The increase in size is greatest during the first two years, the period of most rapid postnatal brain growth. The calvaria normally increases in capacity until 15 or 16 years of age. After this, a slight increase in size for three to four years is due to thickening of the bones.

The overall head shape is closely related to the bony structures of the skull and to the shape of the underlying brain. It is well established that alterations in head shape can be the result of unusual brain growth, but they may also reflect a number of other factors such as premature synostosis of cranial sutures or unusual intrauterine mechanical forces. Abnormal planes of muscle pull, as in torticollis, can cause asymmetric skull growth. The presentation of the individual during delivery also contributes to the shape of the head. Dolichocephaly or scaphocephaly (long narrow head) is a postural deformation of the head associated with intrauterine breech position or prematurity. It generally resolves during infancy with no apparent residual impairment.

Five major sutures are present in the calvaria (Fig. 7.2). Three—the coronal, lambdoidal, and squamosal—are paired, and two—the sagittal and metopic—are single. Cranial growth normally proceeds in a direction perpendicular to each of the major sutures. Increased length of the skull in comparison to width (dolichocephaly or scaphocephaly) and the converse (brachycephaly) can be normal variants. However, both can also occur because of premature synostosis of cranial sutures, where skull growth at right angles to the fused suture is inhibited with compensatory expansion at other patent sutural sites (Fig. 7.3). Head shape depends on which sutures are prematurely synostosed, the order in which they fuse, and the time at which they synostose. The earlier the synostosis occurs, the more dramatic the effect on subsequent cranial growth and development.

**Figure 7.2**  Normal fontanelle and suture landmarks. Adapted from Pruzansky (1973).

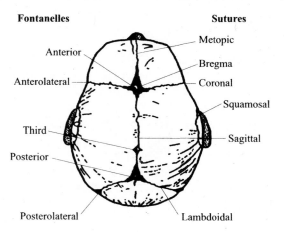

Fontanelles

Sutures

Anterior

Anterolateral

Third

Posterior

Posterolateral

Metopic

Bregma

Coronal

Squamosal

Sagittal

Lambdoidal

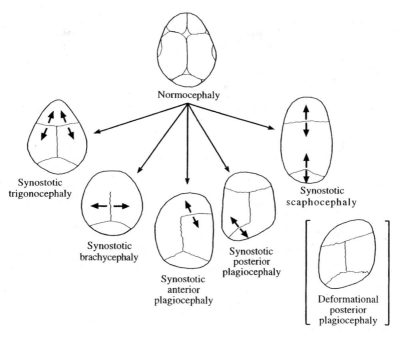

**Figure 7.3** Abnormal patterns of suture fusion. Adapted from Cohen and MacLean (2000).

Dolichocephaly can occur with early closure of the sagittal suture, producing a long, narrow cranium. When both sides of the coronal suture are prematurely fused, the head is brachycephalic (Fig. 7.3). Unilateral synostosis of the coronal suture results in asymmetry of head shape or plagiocephaly (Fig. 7.3). The frontal eminence on the fused side is flattened and the glabella region is underdeveloped. The eyebrows and orbit on the affected side appear elevated. Premature closure of one lambdoid suture can similarly result in plagiocephaly. In trigonocephaly, premature synostosis of the metopic suture results in a triangular prominence of the frontal bone, usually in association with ocular hypotelorism (Fig. 7.3.). Metopic ridging may occur.

When the major determinants of anteroposterior and lateral growth are impeded by coronal and sagittal synostosis, respectively, the cranial vault grows vertically rather than in its normal longitudinal and horizontal directions, resulting in acrocephaly. Acrocephaly is a tall or high skull (vertical index above 77), and the top of the head may be pointed, peaked, or conical in shape. It is also referred to as oxycephaly, turricephaly, steeplehead, or tower skull. A shortened length of the skull compared to its width is referred to as brachycephaly (cephalic index above 81.0); this is typically caused by premature fusion of both coronal sutures (bicoronal synostosis). An elongation of the skull with narrowing from side to side (cephalic index less than 76) is called dolichocephaly or scaphocephaly, and typically caused by premature fusion of the sagittal suture (see Fig. 7.3).

Premature closure of the cranial sutures can occur in isolation or as part of a syndrome, in association with other clinical anomalies.

In addition to describing the skull shape in terms of its length and width, we can also comment on the prominence of various parts of the skull. Bathrocephaly is a condition characterized by a step-like posterior projection of the skull, caused by external bulging of the squamous portion of the occipital bone. Various craniosynostoses can reduce the depth of the bony orbit, producing prominence of the globe, or proptosis.

Few individuals, if any, have true symmetry of the face. Differences in length and width of the palpebral fissures are common but are rarely significant. Frank asymmetry of any part of the face is an important observation and often will provide a clue to the underlying developmental anomaly.

### Head Length

**Definition**   Maximum dimension of the sagittal axis of the skull.

**Landmarks**   Measure between the glabella (the most prominent point on the frontal bone above the root of the nose, between the eyebrows) and the opisthocranion (the most prominent portion of the occiput, close to the midline on the posterior rim of the foramen magnum) (Figs 7.1 and 7.4). These landmarks are also critical for measurement of head circumference.

**Figure 7.4**   Measuring head length with calipers.

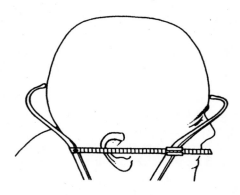

**Instruments**  Spreading calipers give the most precise measurement. A tape-measure can be used, stretched above or lateral to the head.

**Position**  The patient should be standing or sitting. The examiner views the skull in profile.

**Alternative**  The examiner may stand above the patient and look down on the skull.

**Remarks**  Charts of head length are presented in Figs. 7.5 and 7.6. Alterations in skull shape will produce marked variation in this measurement, and in head width. Dolichocephaly increases, while brachycephaly reduces, head length. X-ray measurements are more precise but do not take the skin thickness into account.

**Pitfalls**  A bulging forehead or cloverleaf deformity may make it difficult to define the landmarks. One should eliminate the effects of thick hair cover by applying the caliper tips firmly against the skull.

**Figure 7.5**  Head length, both sexes, at birth. From Merlob et al. (1984), by permission.

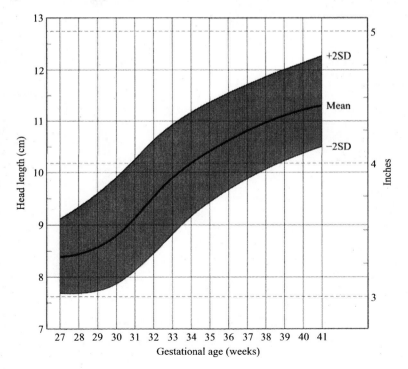

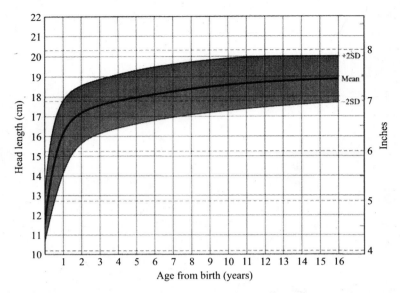

**Figure 7.6**   Head length, both sexes, birth to 16 years. From Feingold and Bossert (1974) and Farkas (1981), by permission.

## Head Width

**Definition**   Maximal biparietal diameter.

**Landmarks**   Measure between the most lateral points of the parietal bones (eurion) on each side of the head (Fig. 7.7).

**Figure 7.7**   Measuring head width with calipers.

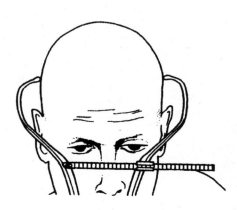

**Instruments**   Spreading calipers give most accurate measurements. A tape-measure held above the head, avoiding the natural curve of the cranial vault, may be substituted.

**Position**   The head should be held erect (in the resting position) with the eyes looking straight ahead.

**Alternative**   Viewing the skull from in front or behind may allow measurement, but the most lateral point of the parietal bone is best judged from above.

**Remarks**   Charts of head width are presented in Figs. 7.8 and 7.9. Alteration in skull shape will produce variation in this measurement; for example, dolichocephaly will reduce head width. X-ray measurements are more precise but do not take into account the thickness of soft tissues.

**Figure 7.8**   Head width, both sexes, at birth. From Merlob et al. (1984), by permission.

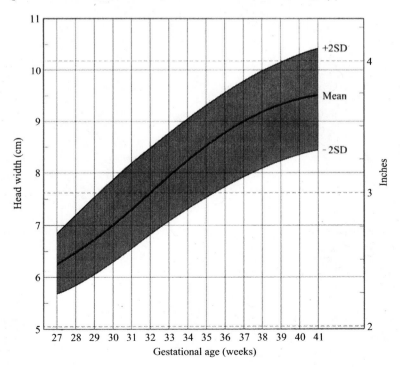

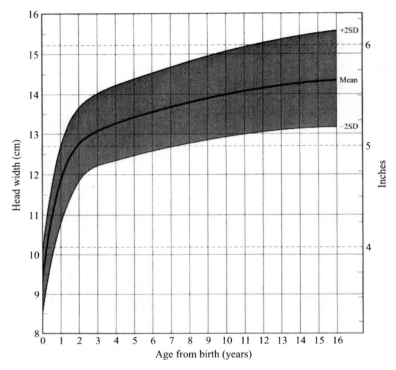

**Figure 7.9**  Head width, both sexes, birth to 16 years. From Feingold and Bossert (1974), by permission.

**Pitfalls**  Severe skull deformity and/or asymmetry may distort the measurement of head width. The calipers tips should be firmly applied to the skull to eliminate the effects of thick hair cover.

### Cephalic Index

**Definition**  This index is the ratio of head width, expressed as a percentage of head length (Fig. 7.10).

$$CI = \frac{\text{head width} \times 100}{\text{head length}}$$

**Remarks**  In the "normal" head, the *CI* is 76–80.9 percent. Dolichocephaly: *CI* < 76 percent. Brachycephaly: *CI* > 81 percent.

$$CI = \frac{\text{head width} \times 100}{\text{head length}}$$

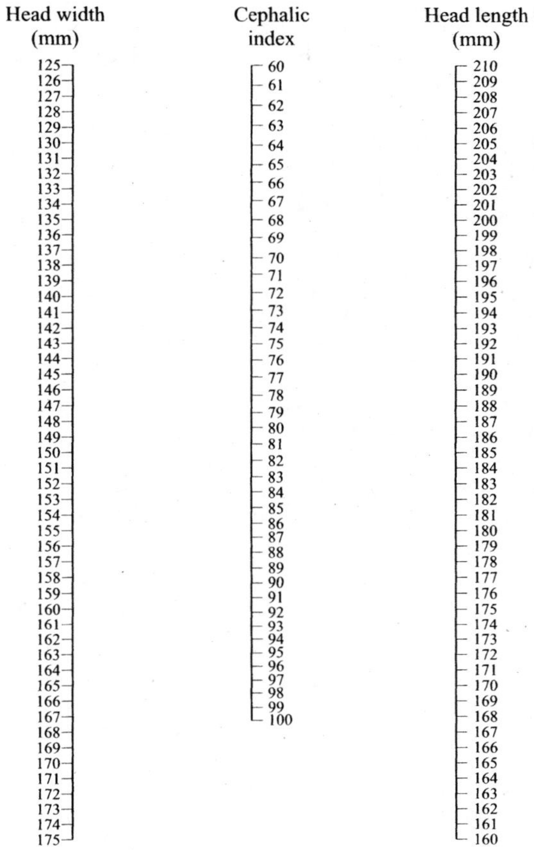

| Head width (mm) | Cephalic index | Head length (mm) |
|---|---|---|
| 125 | 60 | 210 |
| 126 | 61 | 209 |
| 127 | 62 | 208 |
| 128 | 63 | 207 |
| 129 | 64 | 206 |
| 130 | 65 | 205 |
| 131 | | 204 |
| 132 | 66 | 203 |
| 133 | 67 | 202 |
| 134 | | 201 |
| 135 | 68 | 200 |
| 136 | 69 | 199 |
| 137 | 70 | 198 |
| 138 | 71 | 197 |
| 139 | 72 | 196 |
| 140 | | 195 |
| 141 | 73 | 194 |
| 142 | 74 | 193 |
| 143 | 75 | 192 |
| 144 | 76 | 191 |
| 145 | 77 | 190 |
| 146 | 78 | 189 |
| 147 | 79 | 188 |
| 148 | 80 | 187 |
| 149 | 81 | 186 |
| 150 | 82 | 185 |
| 151 | 83 | 184 |
| 152 | 84 | 183 |
| 153 | 85 | 182 |
| 154 | 86 | 181 |
| 155 | 87 | 180 |
| 156 | 88 | 179 |
| 157 | 89 | 178 |
| 158 | 90 | 177 |
| 159 | 91 | 176 |
| 160 | 92 | 175 |
| 161 | 93 | 174 |
| 162 | 94 | 173 |
| 163 | 95 | 172 |
| 164 | 96 | 171 |
| 165 | 97 | 170 |
| 166 | 98 | 169 |
| 167 | 99 | 168 |
| 168 | 100 | 167 |
| 169 | | 166 |
| 170 | | 165 |
| 171 | | 164 |
| 172 | | 163 |
| 173 | | 162 |
| 174 | | 161 |
| 175 | | 160 |

**Figure 7.10** Cephalic index, nomogram, both sexes, birth to 16 years. From Lasker (1949), by permission.

## Skull Height (Forehead Height)

**Definition**  Distance from the root of the nose (nasion) to the highest point of the head (vertex).

**Landmarks**  Measure from the depth of the nasal root to the superior-most point of the skull in the vertical plane (Figs. 7.1 and 7.11).

**Instruments**  Spreading calipers are most accurate. A tape-measure could be used, being held vertically and avoiding the natural curve of the head.

**Position**  The head should be held erect (in the resting position) with the eyes looking straight forward. The patient should face the examiner.

**Alternative**  The patient may face perpendicular to the examiner.

**Remarks**  Charts of normal skull height are presented in Fig. 7.12. Alteration in skull shape will produce marked variation in this measurement. For example, turricephaly will increase the skull height. X-ray measurements are more precise.

**Pitfalls**  A prominent nasal root may make definition of the nasion difficult and reduce the accuracy of this measurement. If the nasion is poorly defined, measure from a point on the nose at the level of the inner canthi. The vertex is not identical to the bregma, the bony landmark in the middle of the top of the skull where the coronal and sagittal sutures cross.

**Figure 7.11**  Measuring skull height with calipers.

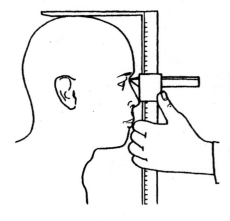

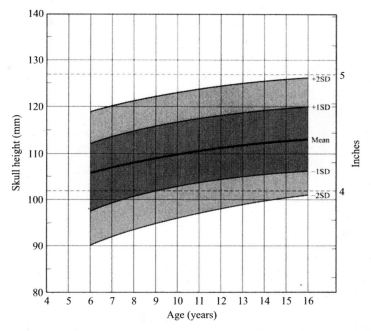

**Figure 7.12** Skull height, both sexes, 6 to 16 years. From Farkas (1981), by permission.

## Upper Facial Height (Nasal Height)

**Definition**   Distance from the root of the nose (nasion) to the base of the nose (subnasion).

**Landmarks**   Measure from the deepest part of the nasal root (nasion) to the deepest point of concavity at the base of the nose (subnasion), in a vertical plane (Figs 7.1 and 7.13).

**Instruments**   Sliding calipers are most accurate. A tape-measure could be used, avoiding the natural curve of the midface.

**Position**   Frankfort horizontal, with the facial profile in the vertical.

**Alternative**   If the nasal tip is long or pointed down, masking the subnasion, this measurement is best taken from the side.

**Remarks**   Upper facial height corresponds to nasal height (Fig. 7.14).

**Pitfalls**   A prominent nasal bridge may distort the position of the nasion and produce a less accurate measurement.

**Figure 7.13**   Measuring upper facial height with calipers.

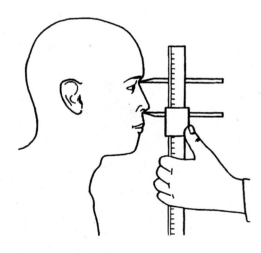

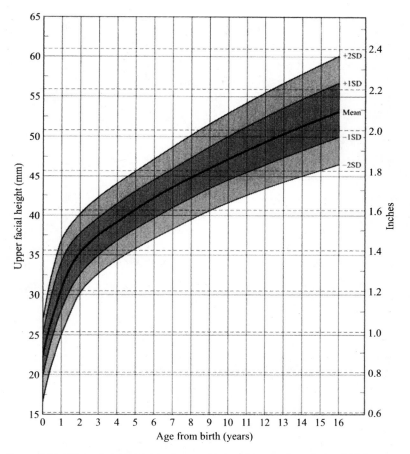

**Figure 7.14** Upper facial height, both sexes, birth to 16 years. From Farkas (1981) and Gorlin (1977), by permission.

## Lower Facial Height

**Definition**   Length of the lower one-third of the craniofacies (Fig. 7.15).

**Landmarks**   Measure from the base of the nose (subnasion) to the lowest median landmark on the lower border of the mandible (menton or gnathion). The menton is identified by palpation and is identical to the bony gnathion. (Figs 7.1 and 7.15a).

**Instruments**   Tape-measure or spreading calipers.

**Position**   Frankfort horizontal, with facial profile in the vertical. The mouth should be closed, with the teeth in occlusion.

**Remarks**   This measurement can also be obtained from a lateral radiograph. The measurement is then taken from the anterior nasal spine (the pointed process extending from the nasal floor, formed by the meeting of both nasal margins at the midline) to the bony gnathion. Spreading calipers are used to measure this distance on a radiograph (Fig. 7.15b).

**Pitfalls**   In comparing cephalometric with anthropometric data, one should remember that cephalometric data do not take into account soft tissue measurements. However, the data from both sources are surprisingly similar, and have been combined in Fig. 7.16.

In the presence of a mandibular abnormality such as a cleft, it may be difficult to obtain an accurate measurement of lower facial height. If the mouth is open, the lower facial height will be falsely increased.

**Figure 7.15**   Anthrometric (a) and cephalometric (b) measurement of lower facial height.

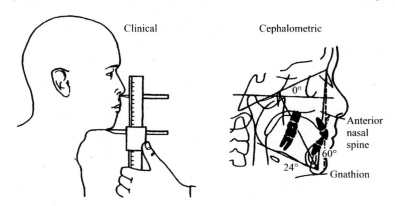

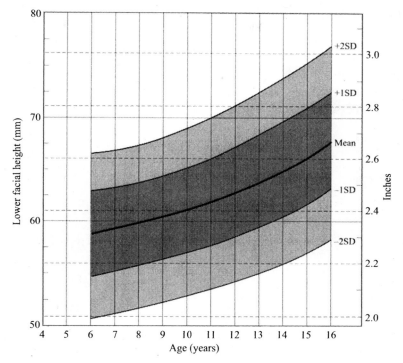

**Figure 7.16**   Lower facial height, both sexes, 6 to 16 years. From Saksena et al. (1987), McNamara (1984), and Farkas (1981), by permission.

## Facial Height

**Definition**   Distance from the root of the nose (nasion) to the lowest median landmark on the lower border of the mandible (menton or gnathion). Lower two-thirds of craniofacies (Fig. 7.17).

**Landmarks**   Measure from the root of the nose (nasion) to the inferior border of the mandible (menton or gnathion) in a vertical plane (Figs. 7.1 and 7.17).

**Instruments**   Spreading calipers give the most reliable measurements. A tape-measure can be used but should be held parallel to the sagittal axis of the face, in front of the tip of the nose.

**Position**   Frankfort horizontal, with the facial profile in the vertical. The mouth should be closed with the teeth in occlusion.

**Alternative**   Measurements may be obtained from lateral radiographs of the head.

**Remarks**   The facial height chart for children age 4–16 years is provided in Fig. 7.18. This measurement is used to calculate the length-to-width ratio of the head (facial index).

**Pitfalls**   Micrognathia or prognathism can make it difficult to find the lower landmark. Prominence of the nasal bridge with a high nasal root may alter the definition of the upper landmark.

**Figure 7.17**   Measuring facial height with calipers.

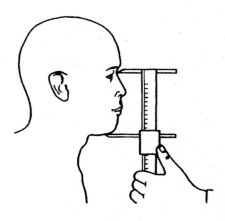

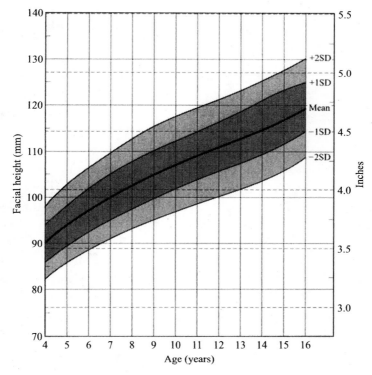

**Figure 7.18** Facial height, both sexes, 4 to 16 years. From Farkas (1981) and Saksena et al. (1987), by permission.

## Bizygomatic Distance (Facial Width)

**Definition**    The maximal distance between the most lateral points on the zygomatic arches (zygion) (Fig. 7.19).

**Landmarks**    Measure between the most lateral points of the zygomatic arches (zygion), localized by palpation (Figs 7.1 and 7.19).

**Instruments**    Spreading calipers will give the most precise results. A tape-measure can be used, but should be held in a straight line parallel to the zygomatic arches avoiding the curves of the zygomata.

**Position**    The head should be held erect (in the resting position) with the eyes looking straight forward.

**Remarks**    The most lateral point of each zygomatic arch is identified by trial measurement, not by anatomical relationship. X-ray measurements will give more exact results but will not take skin thickness into account. Once established, facial width does not change with age (Fig. 7.20).

**Pitfalls**    Conditions in which the first and second branchial arches are abnormal will produce distorted measurements. X-ray films are preferred in this situation.

**Figure 7.19**    Measuring facial width with calipers.

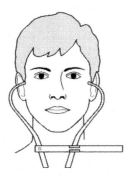

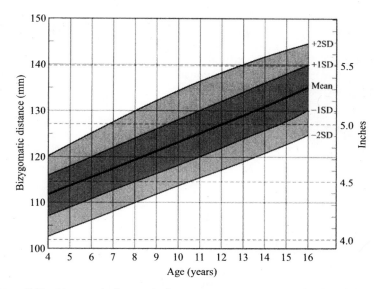

**Figure 7.20**  Bizygomatic distance, both sexes, 4 to 16 years. From Farkas (1981), by permission.

## Facial Index

**Definition**  This ratio utilizes the previous two measurements, facial height (nasion to menton) and bizygomatic distance (facial width), and provides a numerical estimate of facial height compared to width, in order to assess a long, narrow face as compared with a short, wide face (Fig. 7.21).

$$\text{Facial index} = \frac{\text{Facial height (mm)}}{\text{Facial width (mm)}} \times 100$$

**Figure 7.21**  Facial index, both sexes, birth to 16 years. From Feingold and Bossert (1974) and Farkas and Munro (1987), by permission.

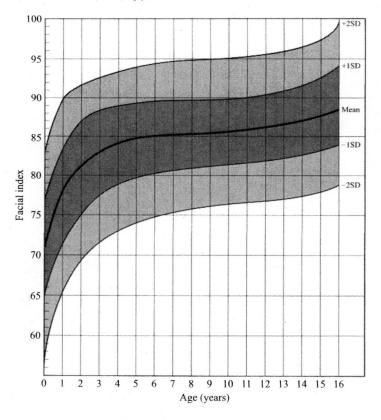

## Fontanelles

### Introduction

Examination of the fontanelles provides evidence of altered intracranial pressure and, less commonly, is an index of the rate of development and ossification of the calvaria, which may be altered in a wide variety of disorders. In order to utilize fontanelle size and patency as a clue to altered morphogenesis, it is necessary to have normal age-related standards.

Figs. 7.22 and 7.23 outline the constant and accessory fontanelles present at birth. The most common accessory fontanelle is the parietal (sagittal) fontanelle, otherwise known as a third fontanelle, which is found in 6.3 percent of infants and may be more common in infants with Down syndrome. The "metopic" fontanelle represents the extremely long anterior arm of the anterior fontanelle which, in the process of closure, becomes separated from the anterior fontanelle. A metopic fontanelle has been reported in association with craniofacial dysostosis, cleidocranial dysostosis, spina bifida occulta, and meningomyelocoele. It can also occur as an isolated finding. An increased incidence of open metopic fontanelles is found in infants with congenital rubella syndrome, Down syndrome, cleft lip with or without cleft palate, and widened sutures. The metopic fontanelle is easy to palpate, and the discovery of its presence during the examination of the newborn infant may be important clinically.

**Figure 7.22** Cranium at birth. From Caffey (1978), by permission.

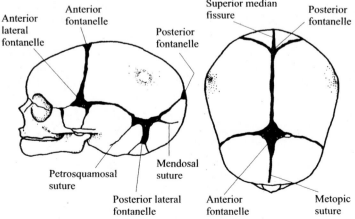

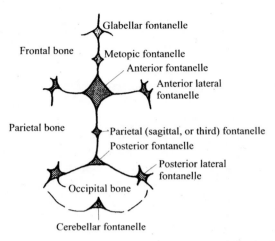

**Figure 7.23** Fontanelles at birth (constant and accessory). From Caffey (1978), by permission.

With increasing age, the fontanelles and sutures become smaller and narrower due to the ingrowth of bone into these remnants of the fetal membranous and cartilaginous skull. There is considerable variation in the velocity of this process in different individuals, and on the two sides of the same skull (Fig. 7.23). The anterior fontanelle usually is reduced to fingertip size by the first half of the second year. The posterior fontanelle may close during the last two months before birth or the first two months following birth. The anterolateral fontanelles disappear during the first three months of life, and the posterolateral fontanelles during the second year of life. The frontal (metopic) suture between the two halves of the frontal squamosa begins to close in the second year and is usually completely obliterated during the third year. It persists throughout life in about 10 percent of individuals. The great sutures of the vault (coronal, lambdoidal, sagittal) persist normally throughout infancy and childhood and do not completely close before the 30th year.

By comparing measurements with age-related fontanelle dimensions in normal persons, the clinician should be able to identify those individuals having either an abnormally large or small fontanelle for age. The presence of an unusually large fontanelle, without increased intracranial pressure, can be a valuable clue in the recognition of a variety of pathological disorders. An usually small anterior fontanelle for age may be a secondary feature in disorders that affect brain growth, such as primary microcephaly; it may be due to craniosynostosis, or it may be caused by accelerated osseous maturation secondary to maternal hyperthyroidism or hyperthyroidism in early life. Males have a slightly larger anterior fontanelle than females during the first six months of life.

Occasionally, numerous large and small accessory ossification centers may be seen within the sutures. These intrasutural or wormian bones can be mistaken for multiple fracture fragments but are present in the normal healthy individual. However, wormian bones can be associated with inherited disorders such as osteogenesis imperfecta.

## Anterior Fontanelle Size

**Definition**   The sum of the longitudinal and transverse diameters of the anterior fontanelle along the sagittal and coronal sutures (Figs. 7.24–7.28).

**Landmarks**   The index finger should be placed as far as possible into each of the four corners of the anterior fontanelle. These four positions may be marked with a dot immediately distal to the fingertip. The longitudinal and transverse diameters may be measured directly, or a piece of white paper can be firmly pressed over the fontanelle to transfer the marks (Fig. 7.25). The points are jointed to form a quadrilateral, and the sum of the longitudinal and transverse diameters along the sagittal and coronal sutures can be measured.

**Instruments**   Spreading calipers, tape-measure, or rule may be used.

**Position**   The head should be held erect with eyes looking straight forward. The examiner should look down on the skull vault from above.

**Fig. 7.24**   Closure of constant and accessory fontanelles and sutures

| Closure | Time |
|---|---|
| Anterior fontanelle | 1 year ± 4 months |
| Posterior fontanelle | Birth ± 2 months |
| Anterolateral fontanelle | By third month |
| Posterolateral fontanelle | During second year |
| Metopic suture | By third year (10%, never) |
| Clinical closure of sutures | 6–12 months |
| Anatomic closure of sutures | By 30th year |

*Adapted from Goodman and Gorlin (1977).*

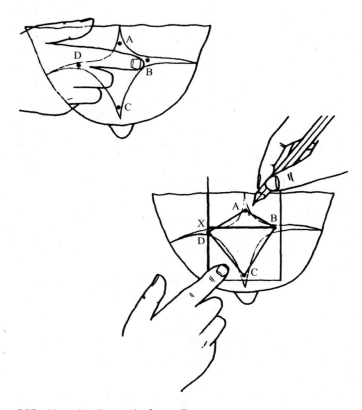

**Figure 7.25**   Measuring the anterior fontanelle.

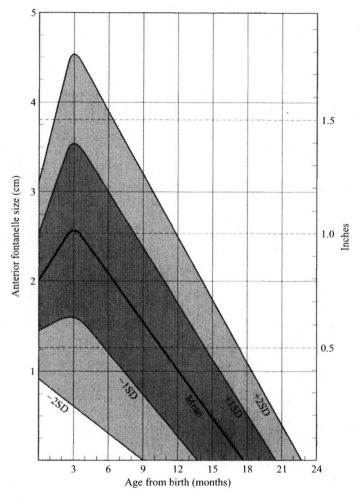

**Figure 7.26** Anterior fontanelle size (sum of longitudinal and transverse diameters). From Popich and Smith (1972), by permission.

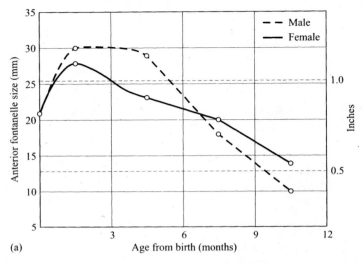

(a)

**Figure 7.27(a)** Anterior fontanelle, comparison of male vs. female. From Popich and Smith (1972), by permission.

**Figure 7.27(b)** Anterior fontanelle, comparison of length vs. width. From Popich and Smith (1972), by permission.

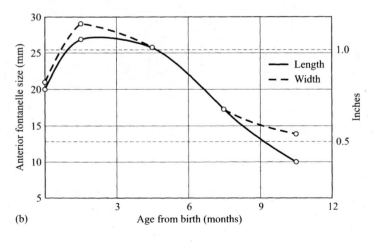

(b)

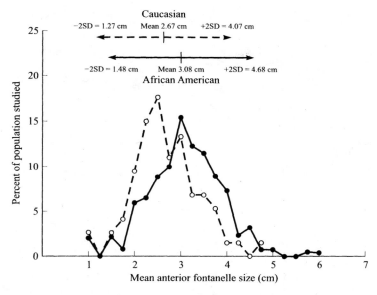

**Figure 7.28** Comparison of mean anterior fontanelle size in African American and Caucasian American populations, both sexes, at birth. From Faix (1982), by permission.

**Alternative**   The infant can be lying prone or supine with the skull again viewed from above.

**Remarks**   An alternative method for determining fontanelle size is to calculate the area of the fontanelle $(AC \times BX)/2$ in square millimeters (Fig. 7.25). An usually small anterior fontanelle may be caused by craniosynostosis involving the coronal and/or sagittal sutures. Males have a slightly larger anterior fontanelle than females for the first six months of life.

**Pitfalls**   Occasionally, in a young child, the sagittal suture is widely patent and communicates with the posterior fontanelle, making definition of the landmarks more difficult. The anterior fontanelle may extend anteriorly into an open metopic suture.

### Posterior Fontanelle Size

**Definition**   Length of the posterior fontanelle (Fig. 7.29).

**Landmarks**   The posterior fontanelle is a triangular structure. Measure from the anterior corner (A) to the midpoint (B) on a line connecting the two posterolateral margins created by the occipital bone (Fig. 7.29).

**Instruments**   Spreading calipers or a tape-measure can be used.

**Position**   The head should be held erect with the eyes facing forward.

**Alternative**   The neonate may lie prone.

**Remarks**   The posterior fontanelle is usually closed in neonates and only 3 percent of normal newborn infants have a posterior fontanelle that measures more than 2 cm. A third (or parietal) fontanelle may be found in about 5 percent of normal infants about 2 cm anterior to the posterior fontanelle. It occurs with greater frequency in Down syndrome and in congenital rubella syndrome. Fig. 7.30 shows normal values for posterior fontanelle size in African American and Caucasian American children at birth.

**Pitfalls**   If the sagittal suture is widely patent, the anterior border of the posterior fontanelle may be difficult to distinguish.

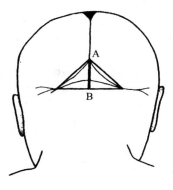

**Figure 7.29** Measuring posterior fontanelle size.

**Figure 7.30** Comparison of posterior fontanelle size in African American and Caucasian American populations, both sexes, at birth. From Faix (1982), by permission.

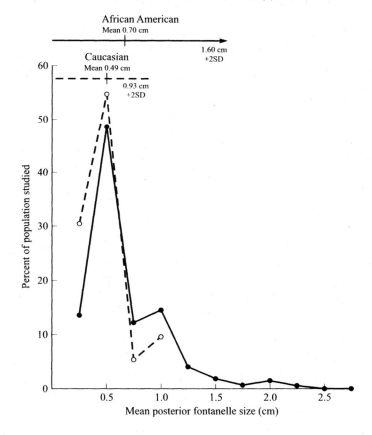

## Scalp and Facial Hair Patterning

Hair directional slope is secondary to the plane of stretch exerted on the skin by the growth of underlying tissues during the period of down-growth of the hair follicles at around 10–12 weeks gestation. The posterior parietal hair whorl is interpreted as the focal point from which the growth stretch is exerted by the dome-like out-growth of the brain during the time of hair follicle development. Malformations that antedate hair follicle development, such as encephalocele, produce aberrations in scalp patterning. Eighty-five percent of patients with primary microcephaly have altered scalp hair patterning, indicating an early onset of abnormal brain development. Aberrant scalp patterning is also found frequently in association with established syndromes including Down syndrome. Thus, aberrant scalp hair patterning may be utilized as an indicator of altered size and/or shape of the brain prior to 12 weeks gestation. Early anomalies in development of the eye and of the face can secondarily affect hair patterning over the eyebrow and frontal area, presumably related to altered growth tension on the skin during the period of hair follicle formation. Gross anomalies in development of the ear can also secondarily affect hair patterning, especially in the sideburn area.

Full details of hair patterning anomalies plus quantitative differences in hair are found in Chapters 11 and 12.

## Eyes

### Introduction

The eyes develop from three sources: the neural ectoderm of the forebrain, the surface ectoderm of the head, and the mesoderm between the two aforementioned layers. Eye formation is first evident at about 22 days gestation, when a pair of grooves called optic sulci appear in the neural folds at the cranial end of the embryo. Soon these sulci form a pair of optic vesicles on each side of the forebrain. The optic vesicles contact the surface ectoderm and induce development of the lens placodes, the primordia of the lenses. As the lens placodes invaginate to form lens vesicles, the optic vesicles invaginate to form optic cups. The retina forms from the two layers of the optic cup.

The retina, the optic nerve fibers, the iris muscles, and the epithelium of the iris and ciliary body are derived from neuroectoderm. Surface ectoderm gives rise to the lens, the epithelium of the lacrimal glands and ducts, the eyelids, the conjunctiva, and the cornea. The mesoderm gives rise to the eye muscles (except those of the iris) and to all connective and vascular tissues of the cornea, iris, ciliary body, choroid, and sclera. The sphincter and dilator muscles of the iris develop from the ectoderm of the optic cup.

The critical period of human eye formation is during developmental stages 10–20 (22–50 days). Because of the complexity of eye development, many congenital abnormalities can occur.

Examination of the eye should include a review of *periorbital* structures. Are the supraorbital brows prominent, pugilistic, heavy, or hypoplastic? Is there periorbital edema? Is there excessive pigmentation? Are the eyes deepset or prominent? Are there deep creases under the eyes?

The *spacing* of the eyes is discussed in greater detail in the measurement section. Although one might assume that the clinical impression concerning whether the eyes are too near or too far apart might be consonant with actual measurement, experience does not bear this out. The clinician may be misled by the width of the face, the form of the glabella area, the presence of epicanthal folds, and the width and shape of the nasal bridge. In addition, spacing of the eyes must be compared to the head circumference for valid interpretation. True ocular hypertelorism or wide spacing of the eyes occurs with an increased interpupillary distance or increased bony interobital distance. With lateral displacement of the inner canthi and lacrimal punctae (primary telecanthus), there may well be a false impression of widely spaced eyes. A rough clinical impression of whether there is lateral displacement of the lacrimal puncta can be obtained by seating the individual directly in front of the observer and drawing an imaginary vertical line through the inferior lacrimal point. If this line cuts the iris, there is lateral displacement of the inner canthus. The differences between telecanthus and pure hypertelorism are documented in Fig. 7.31. Soft tissue measurements of eye spacing are less precise than bony measurements obtained from a standard radiograph. The bony interorbital distance is discussed, in detail, in the measurement section.

The *eyelids* develop from two ectodermal folds containing cores of mesenchyme. The eyelids meet and adhere by about the 10th week and remain adherent until about the 26th week of pregnancy. A defect of the eyelid (a palpebral coloboma) is characterized by a notch in the upper or lower eyelid.

Evaluation of the eyelid includes an assessment of the length of the *palpebral fissure.* There may be a discrepancy in the length of the palpebral fissure between the two eyes, although this is generally minor. Palpebral fissure length may be reduced in several dysmorphic syndromes such as Dubowitz syndrome and fetal alcohol spectrum disorder. The width of the palpebral fissure, that is, the degree of opening of the eye, may also vary

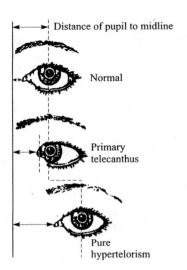

Distance of pupil to midline

Normal

Primary telecanthus

Pure hypertelorism

**Figure 7.31** Comparison of telecanthus and ocular hypertelorism. From Pashayen (1973), by permission.

and may be asymmetric. Frank ptosis or drooping of the eyelid is generally caused by weakness of levator palpebrae superioris. Ptosis is frequently found in association with dysmorphic syndromes such as Smith–Lemli–Opitz syndrome, Noonan syndrome, and Freeman–Sheldon syndrome. Obliquity of the palpebral fissures is discussed in detail in the measurement section. One refers to upward-slanting palpebral fissures if the lateral margin is superior to the medial margin, and downward-slanting palpebral fissures if the lateral margin is inferior to the medial margin.

An *epicanthal fold* is a lateral extension of the skin of the nasal bridge down over the inner canthus, covering the inner angle of the orbital fissure. The upper end of the fold can begin at the eyebrow, at the skin of the upper lid, or at the tarsal fold (Fig. 7.32). Approximately 30 percent of Caucasians under six months of age have epicanthal folds in association with normal depression of the nasal root. Only 3 percent of Caucasians between 12 and 25 years of age have epicanthal folds, as one might expect, because the root of the nose is less depressed in adulthood and the nasal bridge becomes more prominent. Epicanthal folds are more frequent in Asians. Epicanthus inverses refers to an epicanthal fold originating from the lower lid.

The thickness and length of the *eyelashes* should be evaluated. Eyelashes are ingrown in entropion and everted in ectropion. Distichiasis is the term for double rows of eyelashes–one row in the normal position, the other behind it and located at the site of the openings of the meibomian glands. These glands are hypoplastic or absent in such cases. All four lids can be affected.

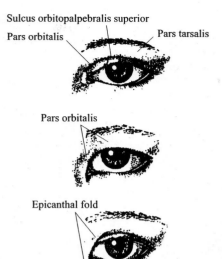

Sulcus orbitopalpebralis superior

Pars orbitalis

Pars tarsalis

Pars orbitalis

Epicanthal fold

**Figure 7.32** Epicanthal variations. From Goodman and Gorlin (1977), by permission.

The configuration of the *eyebrows* is useful in syndrome diagnosis. Evaluation should include position, shape, texture of hair, and distribution of the eyebrows. A medial flare is seen in association with Williams syndrome. A diamond shape with an arch laterally is seen in Noonan syndrome. Eyebrows which grow together over the nasal root are termed synophrys, and are seen in Cornelia de Lange syndrome. Fullness of the lateral aspect of the brow is seen in Noonan syndrome, Williams syndrome, and hypothyroidism.

Many anomalies of *iris* color and structure are found. Unilateral or patchy hypopigmentation can occur, producing heterochromia iridis. A prominent pattern of the iris stroma radiating out from the pupil is known as a stellate iris. Brushfield spots are elevated white, or light yellow, iris nodules. They are best seen in blue irides but are as frequent in brown irides. They are commonly present in the midzone of the iris in a ring, associated with peripheral iris hypoplasia in Down syndrome. They are seen more peripherally in normal individuals. Lisch nodules are small grey-tan hamartomata of the iris. Multiple Lisch nodules are seen in neurofibromatosis type 1. Careful slit-lamp examination is usually required to see them. Colobomas can also occur in the iris, giving the pupil a keyhole appearance. The gap or notch may be limited to the iris or may extend deeper and involve the ciliary body and retina.

Variation in size and shape of the *pupil* should be described. Pupil size varies under ordinary conditions in proportion to the amount of light let into the inner eye. Pupillary asymmetry or anisocoria may be congenital or may result from a disturbance either locally in the eye or in the neural pathways. Aniridia, congenital absence of the iris, may be an isolated finding or part of a syndrome (e.g., Wilms tumor–aniridia–genitourinary malformation [WAGR] syndrome).

The *cornea* may vary in size and shape. Microcornea consists of a reduction in size of the cornea to a diameter of 10 mm or less, in association with growth failure of the anterior part of the eye and incomplete development of the angle. Approximately 20 percent of patients with microcornea will develop glaucoma in later life. Megalocornea may occur as an isolated malformation, with a corneal diameter of 13–18 mm. If the anomaly is limited to the anterior portion of the globe, visual acuity can be normal. In association with megalocornea, there is frequently subluxation of the lens, cataract, enlargement of the ciliary ring, and noticeable iridodonesis. Iridodonesis is a shimmering of the iris when the eye is moved rapidly from side to side in the presence of a dislocated or absent lens. Keratoconus is an obtuse conical shape to the cornea, with the vertex in or near the corneal center. It produces abnormal refraction and is seen with an increased frequency in Down syndrome. It may be associated with retinitis pigmentosa and Alport syndrome. The cornea can appear cloudy in various storage disorders, particularly the mucopolysaccharidoses. Corneal clouding is best appreciated from the side of the eye or through a slit-lamp. Kayser–Fleischer rings are areas of greenish-yellow pigmentation in Descemet's membrane at the corneal periphery seen in Wilson's disease.

Abnormalities of the *conjunctiva* include telangiectasia, which are dilatations of capillary vessels and minute arteries forming a variety of angiomas, and pterygia, which are patches of thickened conjunctiva, usually fan-shaped, with the apex towards the pupil.

The *sclera* is generally white. It may be blue-grey in the neonate and in disorders such as osteogenesis imperfecta.

## Inner Canthal Distance

**Definition**   The distance between the inner canthi of the two eyes.

**Landmarks**   Measure from the innermost corner of one eye to the innermost corner of the other eye, in a straight line avoiding the curvature of the nose (Fig. 7.33).

**Instruments**   A graduated transparent ruler is most accurate; however, a tape-measure or blunt calipers can be used.

**Position**   The head should be held erect (in the resting position) with the eyes facing forward.

**Remarks**   Charts of inner canthal distance are provided in Figs. 7.34 and 7.35. Without accurate measurement, the distance between the eyes may appear greater or less than the mean, depending upon the width of the face, the form of the glabella area, the presence of epicanthal folds, and the width and shape of the nasal bridge. As with all other measurements, the inner canthal distance should be related to the head circumference for interpretation.

**Pitfalls**   In the presence of epicanthal folds, inner canthal distances are not easily ascertained.

**Figure 7.33**   Measuring inner canthal distance.

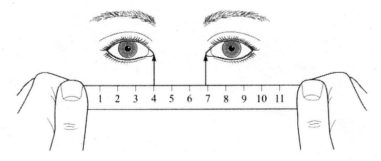

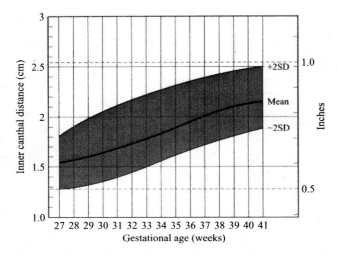

**Figure 7.34** Inner canthal distance, both sexes, at birth. From Merlob et al. (1984), by permission.

**Figure 7.35** Inner canthal distance, both sexes, birth to 16 years. From Laestadius et al. (1969) and Feingold and Bossert (1974), by permission.

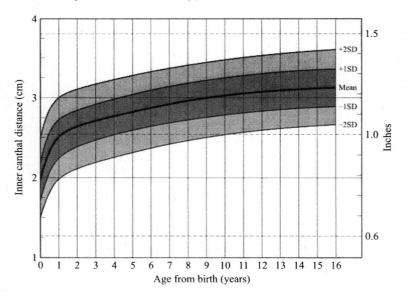

## Outer Canthal Distance

**Definition**   The distance between the outer canthi of the two eyes.

**Landmarks**   Measure from the most lateral corner of one eye to the most lateral corner of the other eye, in a straight line avoiding the curvature of the face (Fig. 7.36).

**Instruments**   A graduated transparent ruler is most accurate; however, a tape-measure or blunt calipers can be used.

**Position**   The head should be held erect (in the resting position) with the eyes open and facing forward.

**Remarks**   As with any other measurement, the outer canthal distance should be compared to the overall head circumference for interpretation.

**Pitfalls**   If the eyes are not fully open, or in the presence of ptosis, definition of the outer canthus may be difficult.

**Figure 7.36**   Measuring outer canthal distance.

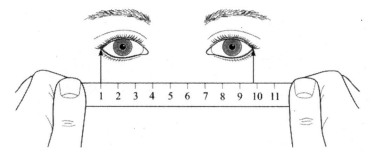

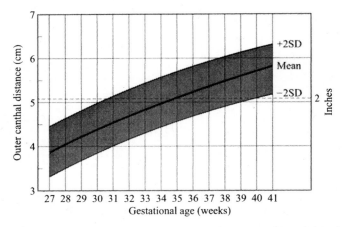

**Figure 7.37** Outer canthal distance, both sexes, at birth. From Merlob et al. (1984), by permission.

**Figure 7.38** Outer canthal distance, both sexes, birth to 16 years. From Feingold and Bossert (1974), by permission.

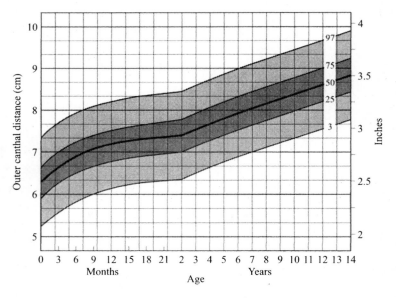

## Interpupillary Distance

**Definition**   The distance between the centers of the pupils of the two eyes.

**Landmarks**   Measure between the centers of both pupils (Fig. 7.39).

**Instruments**   A graduated transparent ruler is most accurate. A tape-measure can be used stretched in a straight line to avoid curvature of the face.

**Position**   The head should be held erect (in the resting position) with the eyes facing straight forward. This is easiest when the patient is reclining, the eye fissures are horizontal, and the eyes are gazing straight upward. A young child may need to be restrained for accurate measurement.

**Alternative**   The child or infant may lie supine.

**Remarks**   Charts of interpupillary distance are provided in Figs. 7.40 and 7.41. Since the measurement of interpupillary distance requires the eyes to be fixed, this is not an easy task in the infant or young child. Feingold and Bossert, by means of multiple linear regression techniques, have suggested the use of the following formula: $IP = 0.17 + 0.59IC + 0.41OC$, where $IP$ is the interpupillary distance, $IC$ is The inner canthal distance, and OC is the outer canthal distance (Fig. 7.42). The reason for distinguishing increased interpupillary distance from increased inner canthal distance is to distinguish between true hypertelorism and telecanthus or lateral displacement of the lacrimal punta. A rough clinical impression of whether there is lateral displacement of the lacrimal puncta can be obtained by seating the individual directly in front of the examiner and drawing an imaginary vertical line through the inferior lacrimal point. If this line cuts the iris, then there is lateral displacement of the inner canthus. If the inner canthal distance divided by the interpupillary distance is greater than 0.6, then lateral displacement of the inner canthus or dystopia canthorum is present.

**Figure 7.39**   Measuring interpupillary distance.

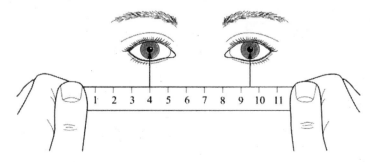

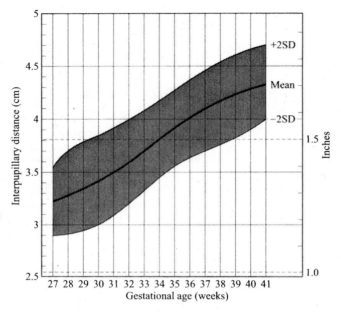

**Figure 7.40** Interpupillary distance, both sexes, at birth. From Merlob et al. (1984), by permission.

**Figure 7.41** Interpupillary distance, birth to 16 years. From Feingold and Bossert (1974), by permission.

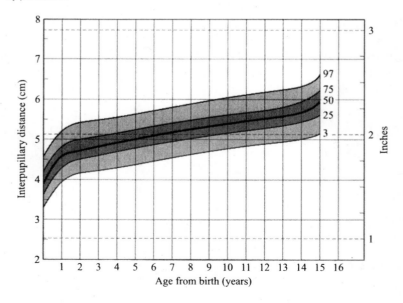

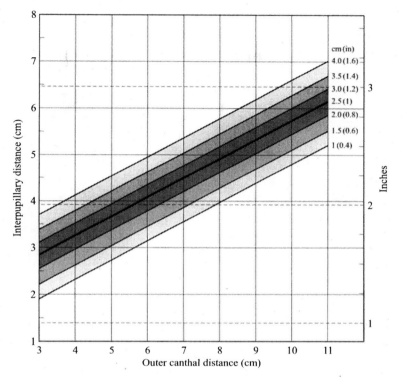

**Figure 7.42** Interpupillary distance calculated from inner and outer canthi. From Feingold and Bossert (1974), by permission.

**Pitfalls** Unless the individual can keep the eyes perfectly still, it is impossible to measure interpupillary distance. The formula outlined above can be used instead.

### Bony Interobital Distance: Cephalometric

**Definition** The distance between the medial margins of the bony orbit (Fig. 7.43).

**Landmarks** Measure between the medial walls of the orbits, at approximately the level of the junction between the medial angular process of the frontal bone and the maxillary and lacrimal bones (the dacrion).

**Instruments** Spreading calipers or a graduated ruler can be used.

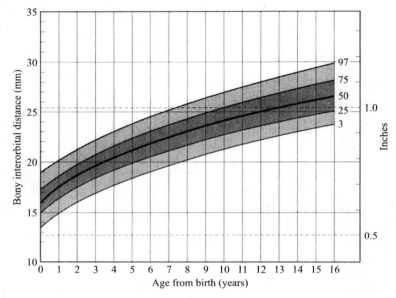

**Figure 7.43** Bony interorbital distance, birth to 16 years. From Hansman (1966) and Currarino and Silverman (1960), by permission.

**Position** The head is held in a cephalostat. Nonrotated, posteroanterior, Roentgen projections of the skull are used, exposed at a target–table-top distance of 100 cm, with a patient–film distance of 5 cm.

**Remarks** The dacrion is medial to the inner canthus. It is found at the junction of the nasal process of the frontal bone, the frontal process of the maxilla, and the lacrimal bone where the medial canthal ligament is attached. Since the interorbital space is occupied mainly by the ethmoid, it is probable that this bone is narrower than normal when the bony interorbital distance is small. This radiological measurement is more accurate than a soft tissue measurement.

**Pitfalls** If the skull film is rotated, the bony interorbital distance cannot be measured.

## Palpebral Fissure Length

**Definition** Distance between the inner and outer canthus of one eye.

**Landmarks** Measure from the inner to the outer canthus of the right eye. Repeat on the left eye (Fig. 7.44).

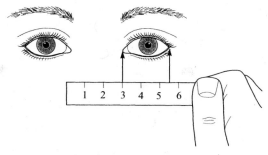

**Figure 7.44**   Measuring palpebral fissure length.

**Instruments**   A graduated transparent ruler or blunt calipers is most accurate; however, a tape-measure can be used.

**Position**   The head should be held erect (in the resting position) with the eyes open and facing forward.

**Alternative**   The infant or young child can lie supine.

**Remarks**   Charts of palpebral fissure length from birth to age 16 years are presented in Figs. 7.45 and 7.46. A difference in the length of the two

**Figure 7.45**   Palpebral fissure length, both sexes, at birth. From Mehes (1974) and Merlob et al. (1984), by permission.

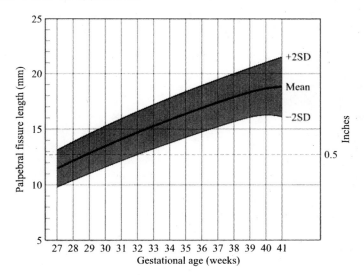

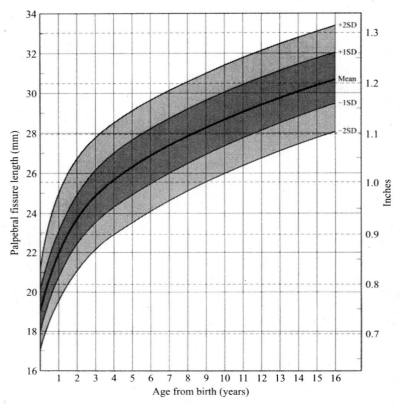

**Figure 7.46** Palpebral fissure length, both sexes, birth to 16 years. From Farkas (1981), Chouke (1929), Laestadius et al. (1969), and Thomas et al. (1987), by permission.

palpebral fissures occurs in about 30 percent of individuals, but it is rarely in excess of 1 mm. As a rough guide, the palpebral fissure length is approximately equivalent to the inner canthal distance. Blepharophimosis is a decrease in the width of the palpebral fissures without fusion of the eyelids. Ethnic variation occurs in palpebral fissure length (Fig. 7.47).

**Pitfalls** In the presence of epicanthal folds, the palpebral fissure length is not easily ascertained.

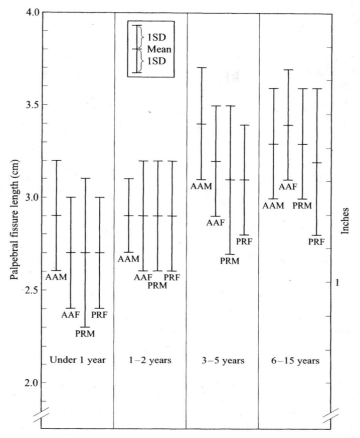

**Figure 7.47** Palpebral fissure length, ethnic differences in African American and Puerto Rican children (AAM, African American male; AAF, African American female; PRM, Puerto Rican male; PRF, Puerto Rican female). From Iosub et al. (1985), by permission.

## Obliquity (Inclination or Slant) of the Palpebral Fissure

**Definition**    Angle of slant of the palpebral fissure from the horizontal (Fig. 7.48).

**Landmarks**    A comparison between two lines is necessary. One line connects the inner canthus and outer canthus of the eye. The second line is defined by the Frankfort horizontal (FH), a line connecting the lowest point on the lower margin of each orbit, identified by palpation (the orbitale), and the highest point on the upper margin of the cutaneous

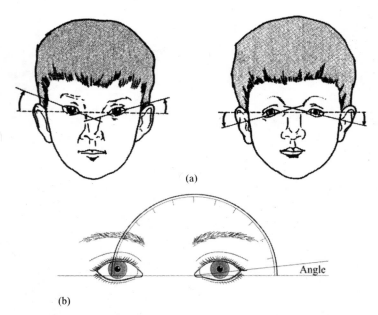

(a)

(b)

**Figure 7.48** The obliquity of the palpebral fissure (a) can be measures with a transparent protractor (b).

external auditory meatus (the porion) The slant of the palpebral fissure is the angle between the two lines (Fig. 7.48).

**Instruments** A commercial angle-meter, protractor, or goniometer is a useful instrument for this measurement. One edge is placed along the FH; the other straight side follows the line between the commissures of each eye.

**Position** The standard orientation of the head is the FH. The subject may be recumbent, in which case the FH becomes vertical.

**Alternative** A rough angle meter or protractor can easily be made on firm transparent material such as X-ray film. A horizontal line on this device is aligned with the FH in the patient and the angle of obliquity of the palpebral fissure is read according to the position of the outer canthus. A rough estimate of this horizontal can be made by joining a line between the two inner canthi and extending this laterally; however, the FH is more accurate.

**Remarks** This is a particularly difficult measurement unless the patient can be kept perfectly still. Palpebral fissure inclinations for ages 6–18 years are shown in Fig. 7.49.

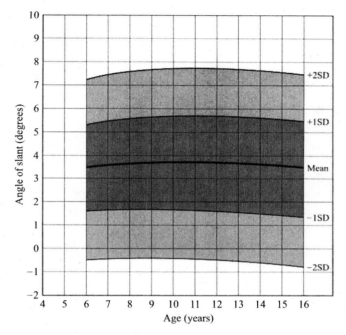

**Figure 7.49** Palpebral fissure inclination, both sexes, 6 to 18 years. From Farkas (1981), by permission.

**Pitfalls** The eyes should be open and relaxed, since the outer canthus is lower than the inner canthus when the eye is closed. The presence of epicanthal folds makes it difficult to locate the inner canthi. The presence of ectropion or lateral supraorbital fullness may create a false illusion of down-slanting palpebral fissures.

### Orbital Protrusion

**Definition** Degree of protrusion of the eye (exophthalmos).

**Landmarks** The calibrated end of a Luedde exophthalmometer is held firmly against the lateral margin of the orbit. The long axis of the instrument is held parallel to the long axis of the eyeball. The examiner sights the anterior margin of the cornea through the calibrated scale and reads the distance in millimeters (Fig. 7.50).

**Instruments** A Luedde exophthalmometer; for details, see Gerber et al. (1972). A transparent calibrated ruler could be substituted.

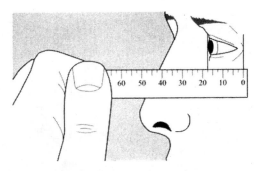

**Figure 7.50**   Measuring orbital protrusion.

**Position**   Frankfort horizontal, with the facial profile in the vertical. The patient should be viewed from the side.

**Remarks**   A Luedde ruler is easy to use and not frightening to children. Orbital protrusion will vary during puberty. Normal protrusion is between 13 and 22 mm for children and adults.

**Pitfalls**   In the presence of ptosis, it may be difficult to estimate the anterior margin of the cornea.

### Corneal Dimensions: Transverse Diameter

**Definition**   Transverse diameter of the cornea.

**Landmarks**   Measure between the medial and lateral borders of the right iris, which for practical purposes represent the edges of the cornea. Repeat measurements on the left eye (Fig. 7.51a).

**Instruments**   Spreading calipers, a transparent ruler, or tape-measure may be used.

**Position**   The standard orientation of the head is the Frankfort horizontal.

**Remarks**   The cornea is relatively large at birth and attains almost its adult size during the first and second years. Practically all its postnatal growth occurs in the second six months of life, although some increase in size may be evident up to the end of the second year. Although the eyeball as a whole increases its volume almost three times from birth to maturity, the corneal segment plays a relatively small part in this growth. The transverse diameter of the cornea increases roughly from 10 mm in the infant to a value slightly less than 12 mm in the adult. In the infant, values of less than 10 or more than 11 mm require further evaluation. Average values for the transverse diameter (external diameter of horizontal base) are found in Fig. 7.51b.

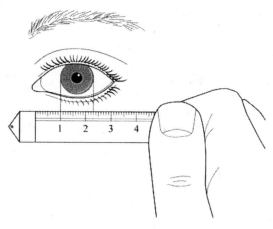

**Figure 7.51(a)** Measuring transverse diameter of the cornea.

**Fig. 7.51(b)** Corneal dimensions, both sexes, at birth and adult

| Transverse diameter | Newborn (mm) | Adult (mm) |
|---|---|---|
| External diameter of horizontal base | 10.0 | 11.8 |
| External diameter of corneal arc | 14.0 | 18.2 |
| Internal diameter of corneal arc | 11.0 | 16.4 |
| Mean thickness | 0.8 | 0.9 |
| Oblique thickness | 1.1 | 1.6 |
| External height | 3.0 | 3.4 |
| Internal height | 1.1 | 2.7 |

*From Duke–Elder (1963), by permission.*

# Ears

## Introduction

The ear consists of three anatomical parts–external, middle, and internal. The external and middle parts are concerned mainly with transferring sound waves from the exterior to the internal ear. The internal ear contains the vestibulocochlear organ, which is concerned with equilibrium and hearing.

The internal ear is the first of the three anatomical divisions of the ear to appear, early in the fourth week of gestation. At that time, surface ectoderm gives rise to the otic vesicle which becomes the membranous labyrinth of the internal ear. The otic vesicle divides into

1. a dorsal utricular portion that gives rise to the utricle, the semicircular ducts, and the endolymphatic duct;
2. a ventral, saccular portion that gives rise to the saccule and cochlear duct.

The organ of Corti develops from the cochlear duct. The bony labyrinth develops from the surrounding mesenchyme.

The epithelium lining the tympanic cavity, the mastoid antrum, the mastoid air cells, and the auditory tube are derived from the endoderm of the tubotympanic recess of the first pharyngeal pouch. The auditory ossicles (malleus, incus, and stapes) develop from the cartilages of the first two branchial arches.

The epithelium of the external acoustic meatus develops from ectoderm of the first branchial groove. The tympanic membrane is derived from

1. the endoderm of the first pharyngeal pouch;
2. the ectoderm of the first branchial groove;
3. the mesenchyme between these layers.

The external auricle develops from six swellings called auricular hillocks (Fig. 7.52), which arise around the margins of the first branchial groove. The swellings are produced by proliferation of mesenchyme from the first and second branchial arches. As the auricle grows, the contribution of the first branchial arch becomes relatively reduced. The lobule is the last part of the auricle to develop. The external ears begin to develop in the upper part of the future neck region but, as the mandible develops, the auricles move to the side of the head and ascend to the level of the eyes.

**Figure 7.52** Embryonic development of the ear.

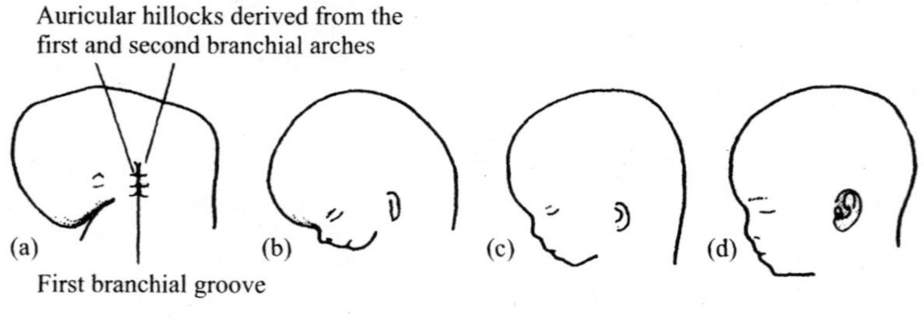

Auricular hillocks derived from the
first and second branchial arches

(a)   (b)   (c)   (d)

First branchial groove

The human usually has three external auricular muscles and six intrinsic muscles. A protruding or cupped auricle is usually the consequence of a defect in the posterior auricular muscle. A "lop ear" refers to a defect of the superior auricular muscle. Abnormalities of the intrinsic ear muscles may lead to abnormal ear creases and anatomy—for example, a prominent antihelix, or the crumpled ear of Beal syndrome. Absence of the superior crus is correlated with an increased risk for deafness.

Ears are almost as distinctive as fingerprints, and much has been written about their variation in form, size, and position. The main anatomical landmarks are noted in Fig. 7.53.

*Evaluation of the ears* should include an assessment of

1. both preauricular regions looking for skin appendages, fistulae, and pits;
2. the tragus, looking at the size in proportion to the size of the ear;
3. the external auditory meatus, whether normal, narrow, or atretic;
4. the shape of each ear and its symmetry, whether it has a free or attached ear lobe;
5. the anterior and posterior surface of each ear or helix;
6. the position and rotation of the ear;
7. the relative positions of the tragi, to see whether they are on the same level.

**Figure 7.53**   Landmarks of the external ear.

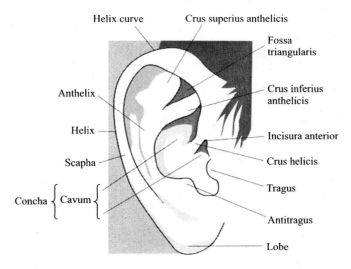

The right auricle is usually slightly larger than the left in both height and width. Discrepant growth can also occur secondary to pressure phenomena. In severe torticollis, compression of one ear against the ipsilateral shoulder will cause increased growth of the ear. The same situation can pertain *in utero*. The frequency of missing or attached ear lobes varies with the ethnic group studied but in Caucasians it averages about 20–25 percent. Clinically, any patient with a malformed external ear should be evaluated for hearing loss and abnormalities of the urinary tract.

Complete absence of the auricle, or anotia, is extremely rare. In microtia, vestiges of the external ear are present, and a graded classification is applied. Type I microtia (Fig. 7.54a) consists of a small external ear retaining the typical overall structure. Type II (Fig. 7.54b) describes a more severe anomaly with a longitudinal cartilaginous mass. In type III microtia (Fig. 7.54c) the rudimentary cartilaginous or soft tissue mass does not resemble a pinna. In type IV, or anotia (Fig. 7.54d), no soft tissue mass is present. In cryptotia, there is abnormal adherence of the upper part of the auricle to the head, as the skin of the postauricular region directly joins the skin of the upper portion of the auricle. Cryptotia (Fig. 7.54e) is attributed to the persistence of fetal attachment of the auricle to the underlying skin.

The Darwinian tubercle is a small projection arising from the descending part of the helix. Many variations in shape can be observed in this area. Anterior ear lobe creases are seen in Beckwith–Wiedemann

**Figure 7.54** Microtia classification type I (a), II (b), III (c), and IV (d), and cryptotia (e).

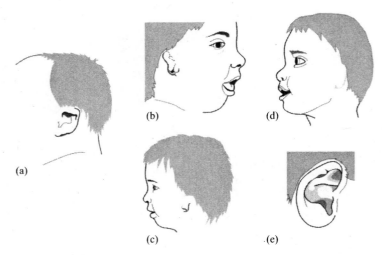

(b)

(d)

(a)

(c)

(e)

syndrome. In this condition, there may also be scored grooves or notches on the posterior aspect of the superior helix or lobe.

Variations in ear position and rotation are discussed in detail in the measurement section. Subjective assessment of ear position and rotation is extremely imprecise and is influenced by the position of the patient's head, the size of the cranial vault, and the size of the neck and mandible. There are several different methods for objective assessment of ear position and rotation, which are detailed below.

Auricular appendages or tags are relatively common and result from the development of accessory auricular hillocks. They are usually anterior to the auricle and more often unilateral than bilateral. The appendages consist of skin but may also contain cartilage. They vary greatly in size and may be sessile or pedunculated. The most frequent location is the line of junction of the mandibular and hyoid arches. Less frequently, they occur in the line of junction of the mandibular and maxillary processes, on the cheek, between the auricle and the angle of the mouth. Appendages in this area are more often associated with microtia or oblique facial fissures.

## Ear Length

**Definition**   Maximum distance from the superior aspect to the inferior aspect of the external ear (pinna).

**Landmarks**   Measure from the superior aspect of the outer rim of the helix to the most inferior border of the earlobe or pinna (Fig. 7.55).

**Instruments**   Tape-measure or transparent calibrated ruler.

**Position**   The head should be held erect (in the resting position) with the eyes facing forward. The head should not be tilted forward or backward. The facial profile should be vertical and the patient viewed from the side.

**Alternative**   A young infant or child can be held prone with the head turned to one side.

**Remarks**   Ear defects are important in syndrome diagnosis, particularly in the newborn infant. Small ears have been found to be a consistent clinical characteristic of Down syndrome and are the most clinically apparent malformation in Treacher Collins syndrome and hemifacial microsomia. External ear abnormalities are common in the 22q11.2 microdeletion syndrome. Ears are often protuberant in the presence of a myopathy. The ear is one of the few organs that continue to grow during adulthood. It is

**Figure 7.55** Measuring ear length.

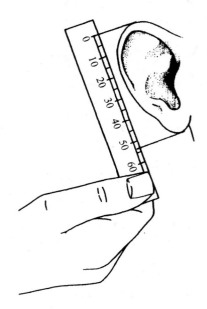

mainly an increase in length, since ear width changes little after 10 years of age. The ear is generally longer in males than in females. The sex difference increases with age. Charts of ear length from birth to 16 years of age are presented in Figs. 7.56 and 7.57.

**Pitfalls**  In the presence of a posteriorly rotated ear, the measurement should still be taken from the most superior portion of the helix to the inferior portion of the pinna, even though the axis of this measurement is not in the vertical plane. If the superior aspect of the helix is overfolded, do not unfold it to measure the length.

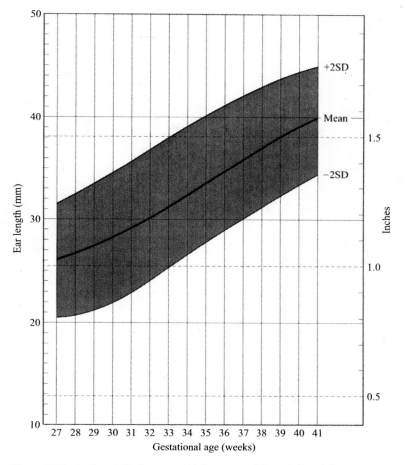

**Figure 7.56** Ear length, both sexes, at birth. From Merlob et al. (1984), by permission.

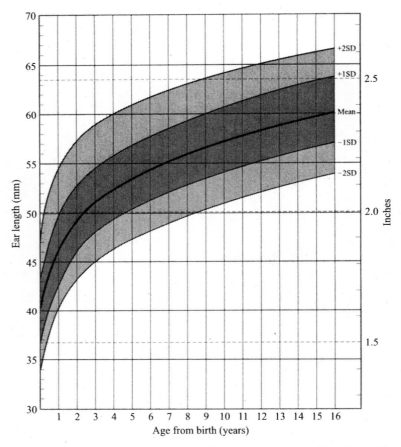

**Figure 7.57**    Ear length, both sexes, birth to 16 years. From Farkas (1981) and Feingold and Bossert (1974), by permission.

**Ear Width**

**Definition**   Width of external ear (pinna).

**Landmarks**   Measure transversely from the anterior base of the tragus, which can be palpated, through the region of the external auditory canal to the margin of the helical rim, at the widest point (Fig. 7.58).

**Instruments**   Tape-measure, calibrated transparent ruler, or calipers may be used.

**Position**   The head should be held erect (in the resting position) with the eyes facing forward.

**Alternative**   The infant or young child may be lying prone with the head tilted to one side.

**Remarks**   Normal ear width is shown in Chart 7.59. Ear width changes little after 10 years of age.

**Pitfalls**   The observer should be careful to take this measurement in the transverse dimension, otherwise, a falsely elevated value will be obtained. With cupped or protuberant ears, the most accurate measurement is obtained with the ear pressed firmly against the head.

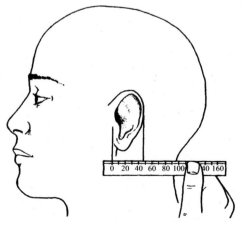

**Figure 7.58**   Measuring ear width.

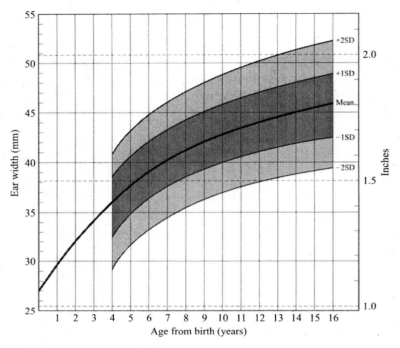

**Figure 7.59** Ear width, both sexes, birth to 16 years. From Goodman and Gorlin (1977) and Farkas (1981), by permission.

### Ear Protrusion

**Definition** Protrusion of each ear is measured as the angle subtended from the posterior aspect of the pinna to the mastoid plane of the skull.

**Landmarks** Measure between the posterior aspect of the pinna and the mastoid plane of the skull. The zero mark of the protractor is placed above the point of attachment of the helix in the temporal region, and its straight side is pressed against the subject's head. The extent of the protrusion is indicated on the curved side of the protractor (Fig. 7.60).

**Instruments** Transparent protractor.

**Position** The head should be held erect with eyes facing forward.

**Alternative** A linear measurement can be made with a tape-measure, calipers, or transparent ruler if a protractor is not available. If the greatest linear distance between the external ear and the temporal region of the

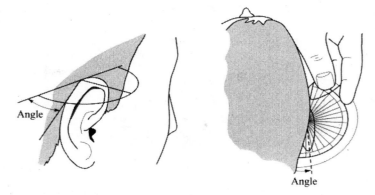

**Figure 7.60**   Measuring ear protrusion.

skull is more than 2 cm, then excessive protrusion of the ear is considered to be present.

**Remarks**   Ear protrusion values are shown in Fig. 7.61. Ear protrusion generally indicates weakness of the posterior auricular muscles, as in a myopathy. By contrast, a lop ear denotes weakness of the superior auricular muscles, and a cup ear generally reflects weakness of all three external auricular muscles.

**Pitfalls**   Several measurements should be taken in order to ascertain the maximum angle or maximum distance between the ear and the mastoid area.

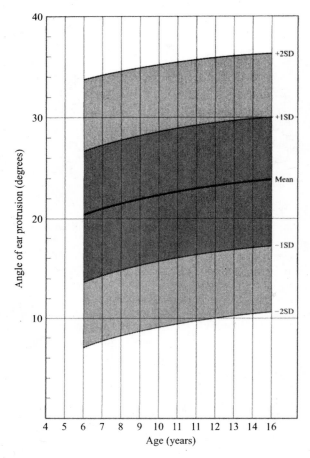

**Figure 7.61**  Ear protrusion angle, both sexes, 6 to 16 years. From Farkas (1981), by permission.

**Ear Position**

**Definition**  Location of the superior attachment of the pinna. Note: the size and rotation of the external ear are not relevant.

**Landmarks**  Four methods to determine the position of attachment of the ear are outlined.

  1. Draw an imaginary line between the outer canthus of the eye and the most prominent part of the occiput. The superior

attachment of the pinna should be on or above this line (Fig. 7.62a).

2. Draw an imaginary line through the inner and outer canthi and extend that line posteriorly. The superior attachment of the pinna should lie on or above that line (Fig. 7.62b).

3. Draw an imaginary line between both inner canthi and extend that line posteriorly. The superior attachment of the pinna should lie on or above that line (Fig. 7.62c).

4. Anthropologists determine the position of the ear according to a proposal by Leiber. The highest point on the upper margin of the cutaneous auditory meatus (porion) is the landmark used to determine position, rather than the superior attachment of the pinna. A profile line that touches the glabella and the most protruding point of the upper lip is imagined. A straight line is drawn from the porion to meet this profile line at 90 degrees (Fig. 7.62d). The area of the face between the free margin of the lower eyelid and the upper edge of the nasal ala must be crossed by the line drawn from the ear canal if it is to be considered at normal level. In a high-set ear, this line meets the profile line above the free margin of the lower eyelid, and in a low-set ear, this line meets the profile line below the upper edge of the nasal ala.

**Instruments**  A tape-mesure, flexible transparent ruler, or graduated piece of X-ray film can be used to define the horizontal plane for the first three methods outlined above. For Leiber's method, a special instrument that can be held along the facial profile line has a perpendicular arm that can be moved up and down until it touches the porion.

**Position**  The head should be held erect with eyes facing forward.

**Remarks**  The landmarks used to determine ear position are among the most controversial in clinical dysmorphology. None of them is perfect, and the reader is advised to become acquainted with one method that is comfortable and to use this method constantly. Although we prefer to use the superior attachment of the pinna as a landmark, other clinical dysmorphologists and anthropologists may assess ear position based on the level of the porion.

Photographs are useful to assess ear position only if all landmarks are shown.

**Pitfalls**  Subjective impression of ear placement seems to be influenced by the position of the person's head relative to that of the observer. In the frontal

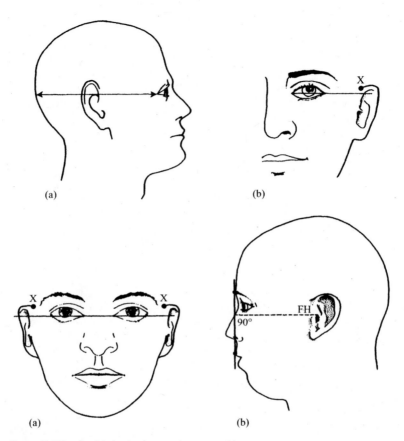

**Figure 7.62(a–d)** Methods of measuring ear position.

view, the ears are subject to parallax. If the neck is extended, they appear low. If it is flexed, they seem high. In the lateral view, ear position seems to be judged in relation to the vertex above, and the chin and level of the tip of the shoulder below. A high ratio between these distances gives the impression of low-set ears. This may explain why the ears of a small infant appear to be set lower than those of an older child. The infant's neck and mandible are relatively small compared to the cranium. The inclination of the auricle also affects the observer's impression of ear level. The ears book lower set when the auricles are tilted posteriorly. For this reason, ear length and position should be validated by quantitative criteria such as those outlined above.

## Ear Rotation

**Definition**   Angulation or rotation of the median longitudinal axis of the external auricle (pinna).

**Landmarks**   Inclination of the medial longitudinal axis of the ear from the vertical is measured by placing the long side of an angle-meter along the line connecting the two most remote points of the medial axis of the ear (see section on measurement of ear length). The vertical axis is then established in one of two ways.

1. The most accurate measurement of the vertical is a line perpendicular to the Frankfort horizontal plane (FH), which connects the highest point on the upper margin of the cutaneous auditory meatus (porion) and the lowest point on the bony lower margin of each orbit (orbitale). The angle between the median longitudinal axis of the ear and the Frankfort horizontal can be measured directly; however, this value can be estimated from the angle between the vertical axis and the median longitudinal axis of the ear (Fig. 7.63a).
2. The vertical axis can be estimated by imagining a line perpendicular to a line connecting the outer canthus of the eye and the most prominent point of the occiput. Once again the angle of rotation of the ear is that angle subtended between the median longitudinal axis of the ear and the vertical axis (Fig. 7.63b).

**Figure 7.63**   Methods of measuring ear rotation angulation.

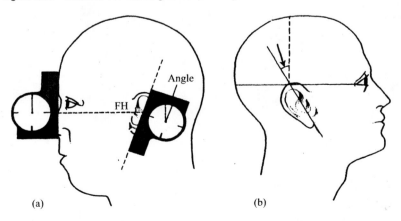

(a)                                    (b)

**Instruments** A special protractor with pointer is the ideal instrument. However, a tape-measure or transparent flexible ruler can be used to define landmarks, utilizing a protractor to measure the angle of rotation. Alternatively, graduated X-ray film can be used.

**Position** Frankfort horizontal, with the facial profile in the vertical.

**Remarks** As in the assessment of ear position, there is considerable controversy about the method of choice for defining ear rotation. Both of the above methods are practical. We recommend that the reader choose one method and become familiar with it.

Normal rotation is between 17 and 22 degrees (range 10–30 degrees) (Fig. 7.64).

**Figure 7.64** Ear rotation, both sexes, 6 to 16 years. From Farkas (1981), by permission.

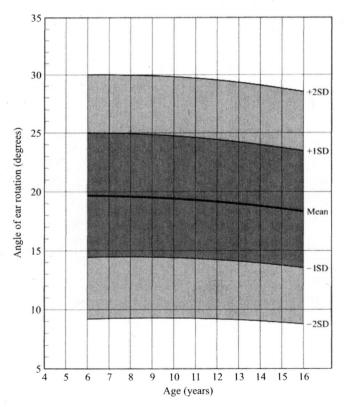

## Nose

### Introduction

The nose is remarkable in its variability, in profile, frontal plane, and from the undersurface. Details and definitions of the soft tissue and bony landmarks are available in references at the end of this chapter and are illustrated in Fig. 7.65a. A qualitative assessment of the nose should include:

1. the nasofrontal angle: is it normal, flat, or deep;
2. the nasal root protrusion: is it average, high, or low;
3. the nasal bridge: is it high, low, broad, beaky, or bulbous;
4. the nasal tip: is it normal, flat, or bifid;
5. the shape of each nasal ala: is it normal, slightly flat, markedly flat, slightly or markedly angled;
6. the nasal ala configuration: is it cleft, hypoplastic, hypertrophic, and is there a coloboma;
7. the type and size of the nostrils: are they symmetric, asymmetric, and what type are they according to the Topinard classification (Fig. 7.65b).

The Topinard classification describes seven types of nostrils, three of which are intermediate (Fig. 7.65b). Type 7 is characteristic of nostrils in patients with a repaired cleft lip. More than half of the general population have Type 2 nostrils; a quarter have Type 1 nostrils, the other types being less frequent. The Topinard classification outlines some of the variability in size and shape of the alae nasi, nares, and columella.

Common variations in nose shape are shown in Fig. 7.65c. Attempts to quantify changes in nose shape with age have rarely been documented. However, it is well known that the nasal root is depressed in the infant and young child, associated with a scooped-out nasal bridge. With increasing age, the nasal bridge rises, producing a more prominent root. Nostril type also varies with age. The prevalence of Topinard Type 4 decreases significantly after age 18.

Most nasal measurements are soft tissue measurements. However, many alternatives are available from radiographs. These will not be described in detail here, and the interested reader is referred to the literature cited at the end of this chapter.

The horizontal measurements of the nose, particularly the width of the nasal root and the interalar distance, provide information about midline development in the same way that the measurements of eye spacing reflect midline development. The nasal tip may be broad, grooved, cleft,

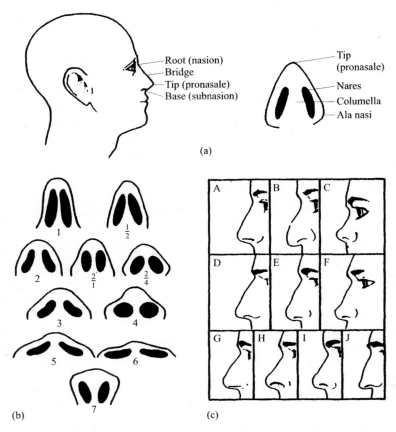

**Figure 7.65**   (a) Landmarks for measurements of the nose. (b) Topinard classification of nostrils. (c) Common variables in nose shape.

or actually bifid with increasing width of the nose. A bifid nose results when the medial nasal prominences do not merge completely. In this situation, the nostrils are widely separated and the nasal bridges is bifid. This type of malformation may be part of a spectrum known as frontonasal dysplasia.

Unlike most vertical facial dimensions, nasal length continues to increase throughout life.

**Nasal Height**

**Definition**   The distance from the nasal root (nasion) to the nasal base (subnasion).

**Landmarks**   Measure from the deepest depression at the root of the nose to the deepest concavity at the base of the nose, in a vertical axis (Fig. 7.66).

**Instruments**   Spreading calipers are most accurate. A tape-measure could be used if held straight in a vertical plane, avoiding the contours of the face.

**Position**   Frankfort horizontal, with the facial profile in the vertical. The patient can be observed from the front or from the side.

**Remarks**   Nasal height is the same as upper facial height, which has been documented in a previous section (Fig. 7.67).

**Pitfalls**   If the nasal root is high with a prominent nasal bridge, the actual position of the nasion may be difficult to place. If the nasal tip is pointed, long, and overhangs the upper lip, then the position of the subnasion may be difficult to place, particularly from an anterior view.

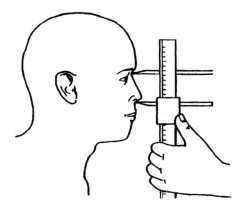

**Figure 7.66**   Measuring nasal length.

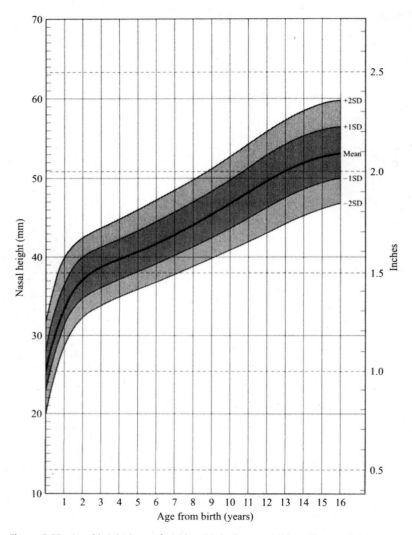

**Figure 7.67** Nasal height (upper facial length), both sexes, birth to 16 years. From Goodman and Gorlin (1977), Farkas (1981), and Saksena et al. (1987), by permission.

## Length of Columella

**Definition**  Length of the inferior-most aspect of the nasal septum.

**Landmarks**  Measure along the crest of the columella from the base of the nose (subnasion) to the most anterior point of the columella at the level of the tip of each nostril (Fig. 7.68).

**Instruments**  Tape-measure or sliding calipers.

**Position**  The patient should recline with the midfacial plane in the vertical.

**Remarks**  Normal columella length for children age 6–16 years is shown in Fig. 7.69. It is important to note that this measurement does not extend to the tip of the nose but only to the anterior-most part of the nostril. The measurement from the subnasion to the tip of the nose is that of nasal protrusion.

**Pitfalls**  The columella may be curved rather than linear. It is important that a tape-measure is used and worked along the skin surface of the columella in the presence of a curve, since a linear measurement with sliding calipers would falsely reduce this measurement.

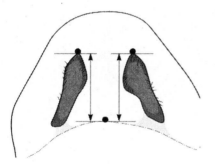

**Figure 7.68**  Measuring columella length.

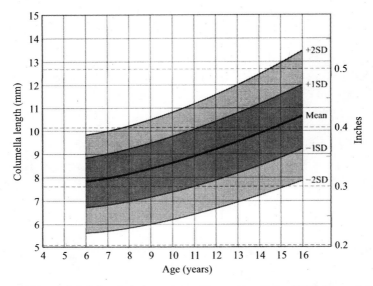

**Figure 7.69** Columella length, both sexes, 6 to 16 years. From Farkas (1981), by permission.

## Nasal Protrusion

**Definition**  Nasal protrusion or depth.

**Landmarks**  Measure from the tip of the nose (pronasale) to the deepest concavity at the base of the nose (subnasion) in a straight line (Fig. 7.70).

**Instruments**  Spreading calipers are most accurate. A transparent graduated ruler can be substituted.

**Figure 7.70**  Measuring nasal protrusion.

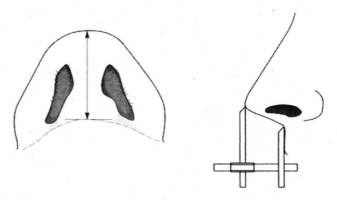

**Position**   The patient should be reclining in order that the nose is observed from its inferior aspect.

**Alternative**   Nasal protrusion can be assessed from the side with the patient perpendicular to the observer.

**Remarks**   The shape of the nose, seen from its inferior aspect, is tremendously variable both within and between ethnic groups. (Details are found in the introduction to this section.) Variability in the length of the columella accounts for part of the variability in protrusion of the nose (Fig. 7.71).

**Pitfalls**   Occasionally the columella and nasal septum protrude below the plane of the alae nasi. Measurement of nasal protrusion should not be made along the surface of the nasal septum following its curve to the nasal tip, but should be linear.

**Figure 7.71**   Nasal protrusion, both sexes, 6 to 16 years. From Farkas (1981), by permission.

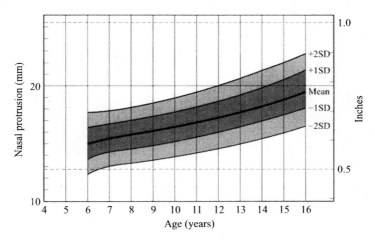

## Interalar Distance (Nasal Width)

**Definition**   Distance between the most lateral aspects of the alae nasi.

**Landmarks**   Measure from the lateral-most aspect of one ala nasi to the lateral-most aspect of the ala nasi (Fig. 7.72).

**Instruments**   Spreading calipers are the most accurate instruments, although a transparent calibrated ruler or tape-measure can be substituted.

**Position**   The patient should be reclining, with the vertical.

**Remarks**   Values for nasal width from birth to age 16 years are shown in Fig. 7.73. There is tremendous variation both within and between ethnic groups in the interalar distance. Nasal width, like most facial widths, continues to increase with age, mainly due to soft tissue changes.

**Pitfalls**   The nostrils should be held in the position of rest when this measurement is taken.

**Figure 7.72**   Measuring nasal width.

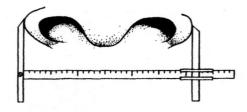

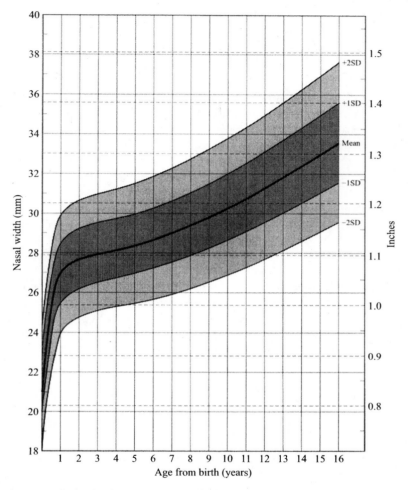

**Figure 7.73** Interalar distance (nasal width), both sexes, birth to 16 years. From Goodman and Gorlin (1977) and Farkas (1981), by permission.

## Philtrum

### Introduction

The philtrum, or vertical groove in the central part of the upper lip, extends from the base of the nose to the superior aspect of the vermilion border of the lip. In some individuals the philtrum is poorly demarcated, while in others the cutaneous elevations that mark its lateral borders or pillars are easily discernible. The enclosed area is usually depressed. The philtral margins or pillars may be parallel or divergent. Although adequate graphs are available for philtral length, normal philtral width has been of little concern to the clinician; however, increased width and flattening are subjectively established in fetal alcohol spectrum disorder and Cornelia de Lange syndrome.

Clefts involving the upper lip, with or without cleft palate, occur about once in 1000 births, but their frequency varies widely among ethnic groups. Sixty to 80 percent of affected infants are males. The clefts vary from small notches of the vermilion border of the lips to larger divisions that extend into the floor of the nostril and through the alveolar part of the maxilla. Cleft lip can be either unilateral or bilateral. Unilateral cleft lip results from failure of the maxillary prominence on the affected side to unite with merged medial nasal prominences. This is the consequence of failure of the mesenchymal masses to merge and of the mesenchyme to proliferate and push out the overlying endothelium. The result is a persistent labial groove. In addition, the epithelium in the labial groove becomes stretched, and then breakdown of tissues in the floor of the persistent groove leads to division of the lip into medial and lateral parts. Sometimes a bridge of tissue called Simonart's band joins the parts of the incomplete cleft lip.

*Bilateral cleft lip* results from failure of the mesenchymal masses of the maxillary prominences to meet and unite with the merged medial nasal prominences. The epithelium in both labial grooves becomes stretched and breaks down. In bilateral cases the defects may be similar or dissimilar with varying degrees of defect on each side. In complete bilateral cleft of the upper lip and alveolar processes, the intermaxillary segment hangs free and projects anteriorly. Such defects are especially deforming because of the loss of continuity of the orbicularis oris muscle, which closes the mouth and purses the lips as in whistling.

*Median cleft lip* is an extremely rare defect of the upper lip caused by a mesodermal deficiency that results in partial or complete failure of the medial nasal prominences to merge and form the intermaxillary segment. The presence of the median cleft lip should alert the observer to look for other midline abnormalities of the brain, including holoprosencephaly.

Other unusual types of facial cleft may occur, but each is individually rare. Oblique facial cleft are often bilateral and extend from the upper lip to the medial margin of the orbit. When this occurs, the nasolacrimal ducts are open grooves. Oblique facial clefts associated with cleft lip result from failure of the mesechymal masses of the maxillary prominences to merge with the lateral and medial nasal prominences. Lateral or transverse facial clefts run from the mouth toward the ear. This abnormality results from failure of the lateral mesechymal masses of the maxillary and mandibular prominences to merge. In severe cases, the cheek is cleft almost to the ear.

Clefts of the lower lip and mandible are also rare. The lip may be cleft superficially or, in severe cases, it may be split down to the chin, involving the mandible.

## Length of the Philtrum

**Definition**   Distance between the base of the nose and the border of the upper lip, in the midline.

**Landmarks**   Measure from the base of the nose (subnasion) to the superior aspect of the vermilion border of the lip, in the midline (Fig. 7.74).

**Instruments**   Ideally the philtral length is measured with spreading calipers; however, a calibrated transparent ruler could be used.

**Position**   The head should be held (in the resting position) erect with the eyes facing forward. The observer should be lateral to the patient so that the face is in profile.

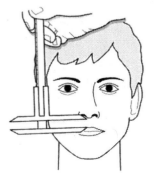

**Figure 7.74**   Measuring philtrum length.

**Alternative**  A young infant or child could lie supine with the head held.

**Remarks**  Variation in philtrum length is shown in Figs. 7.75 and 7.76. In some individuals the philtrum is poorly demarcated; in others the cutaneous elevations that mark its lateral borders are clearly discernible. The enclosed area is usually depressed. The philtral margins may be parallel or divergent.

**Pitfalls**  In the newborn with a cleft lip, either unilateral or bilateral, this measurement mat not be reliable. Facial expression, particularly smiling, will alter this measurement. Thus, the patient's facial expression should be neutral.

Philtrum smoothness and upper lip thinness are measured in five-point Likert pictorial scales by holding the lip-philtrum guide next to the patient's face and assigning each feature the Likert rank of the photograph that best matches each feature (Fig. 7.77).

**Figure 7.75**  Philtrum length, both sexes, at birth. From Merlob et al. (1984), by permission.

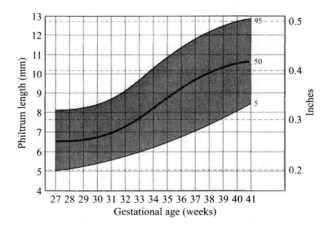

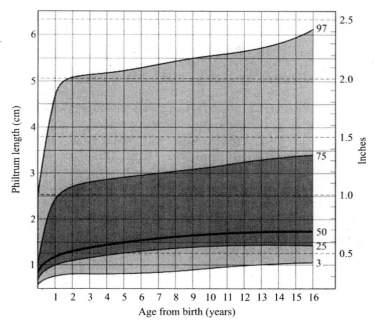

**Figure 7.76**   Philtrum length, both sexes, birth to 16 years. From Feingold and Bossert (1974), by permission.

**Figure 7.77**   Pictorial example of the five-point Likert scale. From Astley and Clarren (1995), by permission.

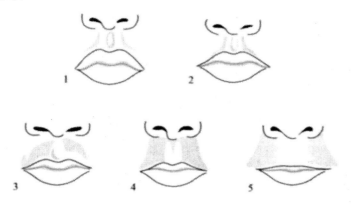

# Mouth

## Introduction

Variation in size of the mouth is well documented; detailed graphs are provided in the measurement section. It is far more difficult to evaluate the lips objectively. However, with the aid of calipers and a cooperative, relaxed patient, the visible vermilion of the upper lip, in Caucasians, when measured from the middle of the lip to the aperture, ranges from 3–3.5 mm in the newborn, to 4.7–4.8 mm in the one-year-old, to about 6 mm in the adult. Corresponding lower lip measurements are 3.6–4.7, 5.9–6.3, and 9–10 mm, respectively. Further variation in lip shape is associated with differences in philtral development. A well-formed, deeply grooved philtrum is usually associated with wide-spaced peaks to the vermilion border of the upper lip. Conversely, a poorly formed, flat philtrum is usually associated not with marked peaks, but with a relatively thin, even surface to the vermilion border. A tented upper lip often results from long-standing, bilateral, facial muscle weakness, such as that seen in congenital myotonic dystrophy.

Congenital pits or recesses of the lips are present in 2–3 percent of neonates. They usually occur in the lower lips, where they may be bilateral or unilateral, showing a well-defined circular depression on the vermilion border. In the upper lip, where they are rare, they are found lateral to the philtrum. They represent the orifices of mucous tracts that extend into the substance of the lip. A double lip is a deformity that consists of redundant tissue in the mucosal portion of the lip just inside its vermilion border. The anomaly, which can occur in the upper or in the lower lip, has been observed in both males and females and is individually rare. It is more conspicuous in the upper lip because the mucosal duplication, which shows a median notch, hangs down and partly covers the incisors. Double lip may be associated with relaxation of the supratarsal fold (blepharochalasis) and with thyroid enlargement.

Width of the mouth is a difficult soft tissue measurement to assess. Macrostomia, or large mouth, may be caused by lateral or transverse facial clefts running from the mouth toward the ear. This abnormality results from failure of the lateral mesenchymal masses of the maxillary and mandibular prominences to merge. Congenital microstomia (small mouth) results from excessive merging of the mesenchymal masses of the maxillary and mandibular prominences of the first branchial arch. In severe cases, it may be associated with mandibular hypoplasia. A small mouth, with pursed lips, may also result from perioral fibrosis.

Frenula are strands of tissue extending between the buccal and alveolar mucosae. Abnormal numbers of frenula may be associated with various craniofacial syndromes. An assessment of alveolar ridge thickness should be included in the evaluation of the mouth. Thickening may be congenital or acquired, for example, following prolonged therapy with antiepileptic medications.

The reader is referred to the references at the end of this chapter for further information.

## Intercommissural Distance (Mouth Width)

**Definition**   Mouth width at rest.

**Landmarks**   Measure from one cheilion (corner of the mouth) to the other cheilion (Fig. 7.78).

**Instruments**   Spreading calipers are best. A tape-measure held straight or a calibrated transparent ruler may be substituted.

**Position**   The head should be held erect (in the resting position) with the eyes facing forward and the mouth held close and in a neutral position.

**Alternative**   The young infant or child may lie supine.

**Remarks**   The intercommissural distance has been estimated by several authors in spite of the intrinsic difficulties in measuring soft tissue points (Figs. 7.79 and 7.80).

**Pitfalls**   The mouth should be at rest, as grimacing, crying, smiling, or any other facial expression will distort the measurement.

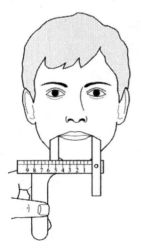

**Figure 7.78**   Measuring mouth width. Adapted from Garn et al. (1984).

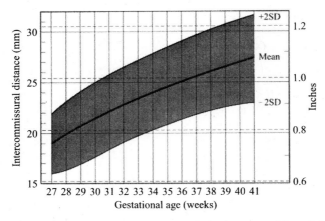

**Figure 7.79** Intercommissural distance, both sexes, at birth. From Merlob et al. (1984), by permission.

**Figure 7.80** Intercommissural distance, both sexes, birth to 16 years. From Feingold and Bossert (1974) and Farkas (1981), by permission.

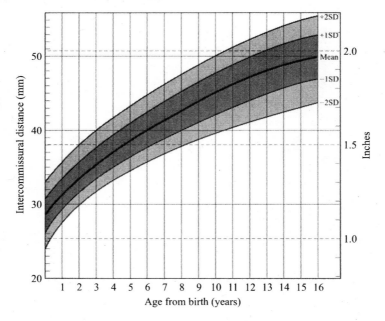

## Palate

### Introduction

Cleft palate, with or without cleft lip, occurs about once in every 2500 births and is more common in females than males. A cleft may involve only the uvula, giving a fishtail appearance. It may extend through the soft palate, or it may extend all the way forward to the hard palate. The cleft may be overt or submucous. In severe cases associated with cleft lip, the cleft in the palate extends through the alveolar process and lip on both sides. The embryological basis of cleft palate is failure of the mesenchymal masses of the lateral palatine processes to meet and fuse with each other, with the nasal septum, and/or with the posterior margin of the median palatine process or primary palate. Such clefts may be unilateral or bilateral and are classified into three groups:

1. clefts of the anterior or primary palate: clefts anterior to the incisive foramen resulting from failure of the mesenchymal masses of the lateral palatine processes to meet and fuse with the mesenchyme of the primary palate;
2. clefts of the anterior and posterior palate: cleft involving both the primary and secondary palates resulting from the failure of the mesenchymal masses of the lateral palatine processes to meet and fuse with the mesenchyme of the primary palate, with each other, and with the nasal septum;
3. clefts of the posterior or secondary palate: clefts posterior to the incisive foramen, resulting from failure of the mesenchymal masses of the lateral palatine processes to meet and fuse with each other and with the nasal septum.

The great majority of cases of cleft palate are associated with multifactorial inheritance. Others are part of single gene or chromosomal syndromes. A few cases appear to be caused by teratogenic agents, particularly anticonvulsants. The fact that the palatine processes fuse about a week later in females than in males may explain why isolated cleft palate is more common among females.

Simple devices have been designed to measure directly palatal height, width, and length. For detailed study, these data may be ascertained from plaster casts. Length of the palate can also be assessed from X-rays. The clinical dysmorphologist may find it easier to use a rough estimate of palate height in the "field." If the maximum height of the palate is greater than twice the height of the teeth, it can be considered abnormal.

Unususally prominent lateral palatine ridges are a nonspecific feature of a variety of disorders in which there is either neuromuscular dysfunction or an anatomic defect that prevents or limits tongue thrust into the palatal vault. The lateral palatine ridges are normally more prominent during prenatal life and infancy. With increasing age they become progressively flattened by the moulding forces of the tongue and usually disappear by five years of age. Prominent lateral palatine ridges may be misinterpreted as a true "narrow high arched palate," which is a much less common anomaly.

## Palate Length: Cephalometric

**Definition**   Length of the palate.

**Landmarks**   Measure from the anterior to the posterior nasal spine (Fig. 7.81).

**Instruments**   Spreading calipers are used to measure the distance on a radiograph taken with a "cephalostat."

**Position**   Standard cephalometry–see general introduction to Chapter 7 for details.

**Remarks**   Values for cephalometric measurement of the palate length are shown in Fig. 7.82. Soft tissue measurement of palate length is difficult and requires special instrumentation (Shapiro et al., 1963). With this instrument, palate length is defined as the distance from the labial point of the incisive papilla to the midline of the junction of the hard and soft palates (Fig. 7.83). The majority of clinical dysmorphologists will not have access to such instrumentation.

The palate is generally longer in males than females. This sex difference is accentuated with increasing age.

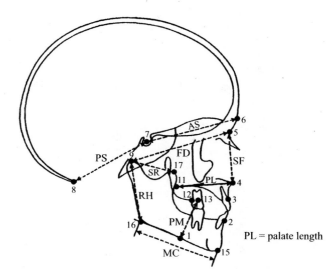

**Figure 7.81** Radiographic landmarks for measuring palate length (PL). Note: PS = posterior skull base length; AS = anterior skull base length; FD = facial depth; SR = superior ramus length; RH = ramus height; PM = palate-mandible height; SF = superior facial height. Adapted from Garn et al. (1984).

**Figure 7.82** Palate length (cephalometric), both sexes, 6 to 16 years. From Garn et al. (1984), by permission.

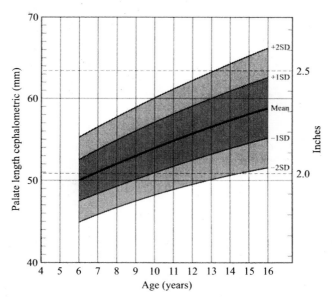

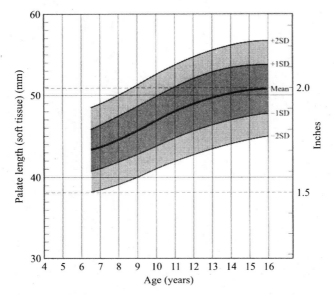

**Figure 7.83** Palate length (soft tissue), both sexes, 6 to 16 years. From Redman (1963), by permission.

## Palate Height

**Definition** Height of the palate.

**Landmarks** Measure the shortest distance between the midline of the junction of the hard and soft palates and the plane established by other reference points as outlined in palate length and palate width (Fig. 7.84).

**Instruments** A palatal measuring device is necessary (Shapiro et al., 1963).

**Figure 7.84** Measuring palate height.

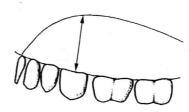

**Remarks**    Palate height for ages 6–16 years is shown in Fig. 7.85. This measurement point, the fovea palatinus, is not always the highest dimension of the palatal vault. Most clinical dysmorphologists will not have access to a palatal measuring device, but an assessment of the height of the palate is vital if deviation from normal palatal shape is to be defined. We suggest, as a rough guide, that when maximum palate height is greater than twice the height of the teeth, it should be considered abnormally high.

**Pitfalls**    Thickened palatine and alveolar ridges producing narrowness of the palate can give a false impression of increased palate height.

**Figure 7.85**    Palate height, both sexes, 6 to 16 years. From Redman (1963), by permission.

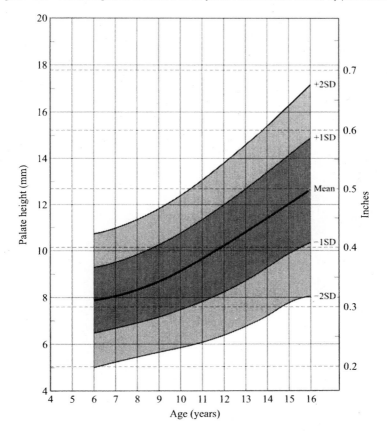

## Palate Width

**Definition**   Width of the palate.

**Landmarks**   Measure the distance between the maxillary first permanent molar on the right side and the maxillary first permanent molar on the left side at the lingual cervical line (Fig. 7.86).

**Remarks**   Palate width is once again measured with a specific device which is not generally available to the clinical dysmorphologist.

**Figure 7.86**   Measuring palate width.

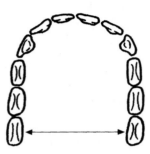

**Figure 7.87**   Palate width, both sexes, 6 to 16 years. From Redman (1963), by permission.

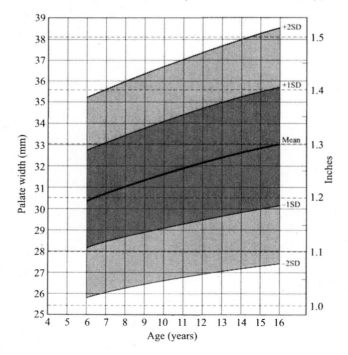

## Tongue

### Introduction and Landmarks

Around the end of the fourth week of gestation, a median, somewhat triangular elevation appears in the floor of the pharynx just rostral to the foramen caecum. This elevation, the median tongue bud, gives the first indication of tongue development. Soon, two oval distal tongue buds (lateral lingual swellings) develop on each side of the median tongue bud. These elevations result from proliferation of mesenchyme in the ventromedial parts of the first pair of branchial arches. The distal tongue buds rapidly increase in size, merge with each other, and overgrow the median tongue bud. The merged distal tongue buds form the anterior two thirds or oral part of the tongue. The posterior third or pharyngeal part of the tongue is initially indicated by two elevations that develop caudal to the foramen caecum, the copula from the second branchial arches, and the hypobranchial eminence from the third and fourth branchial arches. Branchial arch mesenchyme forms the connective tissue and the lymphatic and blood vessels of the tongue and probably some of its muscle fibers. Most of the tongue musculature, however, is derived from myoblasts that migrate from the myotomes of the cervical somites. The hypoglossal nerve accompanies the myoblasts during their migration and innervates the tongue musculature when it develops.

The papillae of the tongue appear at about 54 days of gestation. All the papillae will develop taste buds.

Tongue landmarks are outlined in Figure 7-88.

**Remarks** Congenital malformations of the tongue include congenital cysts and fistulae derived from remnants of the thyroglossal duct, ankyloglossia (tongue-tie), in which the frenulum from the inferior surface of the anterior part of the tongue extends to near the tip of the tongue and interferes with free protrusion; cleft tongue, caused by incomplete fusion of the distal tongue buds posteriorly; and bifid tongue, in which there is complete failure of fusion of the distal tongue buds.

There is variation in the size of the tongue among individuals, and no normal measurements have been established. Most pediatricians, however, have established their own norms for children. Detection of a large tongue or macroglossia is important, particularly in the neonatal and infantile periods, to allow early diagnosis of certain conditions such as congenital hypothyroidism. An illusion of a large tongue may be seen in a disorder

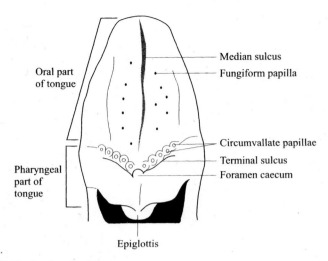

**Figure 7.88** Landmarks of the tongue.

that is characterized by a small oral cavity as in Beckwith–Wiedemann or Down syndrome. The tongue may be large if it is the site of a congenital vascular malformation. Acquired forms of macroglossia include trauma and allergic reactions, for example, angioneurotic edema. When considering the tongue in facial diagnosis, one should remember that largeness is not necessarily the same as protrusion.

Diminished bulk of the tongue may be associated with an atrophic process. Tongue atrophy is a very important clinical sign and usually indicates a lower motor neuron lesion or disturbance if the intrinsic tongue musculature. One should distinguish between bilateral atrophy and unilateral atrophy. The term aglossia refers to absence of the tongue, although usually some rudiments of the tongue are present. Aglossia may be seen in association with limb anomalies.

One should look for abnormal postures of the tongue or an inability to protrude the tongue. Topographic tongue abnormalities, such as a furrowed tongue or geographic tongue, should be noted.

# Teeth

## Introduction

The teeth develop from ectoderm and mesoderm. The enamel is produced by cells derived from oral ectoderm. All other dental tissues develop from mesenchyme. The mandibular teeth usually erupt before the maxillary teeth, and girls' teeth usually erupt sooner than boys' teeth. As the root of the tooth grows, the crown gradually erupts through the oral mucosa. The part of the oral mucosa around the erupted crown becomes the gum or gingiva.

Eruption of the deciduous teeth usually occurs between 6 and 24 months after birth (Fig. 7.89). The permanent teeth develop in a manner similar to that just described. As a permanent tooth grows, the root of the corresponding deciduous tooth is gradually resorbed by osteoclasts. Consequently, when the deciduous tooth is shed, it consists only of the crown and the uppermost portion of the root. The permanent teeth usually begin to erupt during the sixth year and continue to appear until early adulthood. They are often serrated initially and become smooth with time. The chronology of onset of prenatal and postnatal enamel formation is illustrated in Figure 7.90. Details of dental age are provided in Chapter 13.

**Remarks** Defective enamel formation results in grooves, pits, or fissures on the enamel surface. These defects result from temporary disturbances in enamel formation. Various factors may injure the ameloblasts, for example, nutritional deficiency, tetracycline therapy, and diseases such as

**Figure 7.89** Tooth eruption.

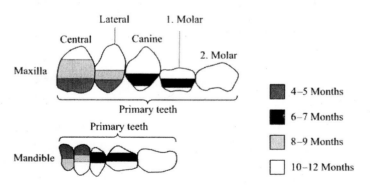

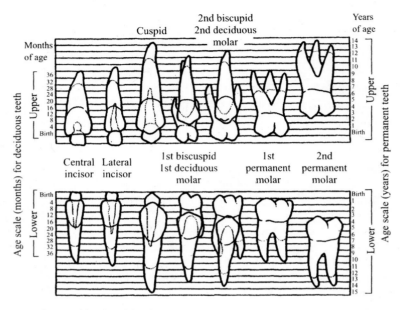

**Figure 7.90** Tooth enamel development.

measles. Rickets is probably the most common cause of enamel hypoplasia. In amelogenesis imperfecta, the enamel is soft and friable because of hypocalcification, and the teeth are yellow to brown in color. This genetic trait affects about one in every 20,000 children. In dentinogenesis imperfecta, a condition relatively common in Caucasian children, the teeth are brown to gray-blue with an opalescent sheen. The enamel tends to wear down rapidly, exposing the dentin. Foreign substances incorporated into the developing enamel will cause discoloration of the teeth. Hemolysis and tetracycline therapy are among the causes of tooth discoloration. The primary teeth are affected if tetracyclines are given from 18 weeks of gestation to 10 months postnatally, and the permanent teeth may be affected if exposure occurs between 18 weeks prenatally and 16 years of age.

Abnormally shaped teeth are relatively common. Occasionally, spherical masses of enamel called enamel pearls or drops are attached to the tooth. They are formed by aberrant groups of ameloblasts. The maxillary lateral incisor teeth may assume a slender tapering shape (peg-shaped lateral incisors). Congenital syphilis affects the differentiation of the permanent teeth, resulting in screwdriver-shaped incisors with central notches in their incisive edges, called Hutchinson teeth.

The most common dental anomaly present at birth is premature eruption of one or more of the deciduous teeth, usually the mandibular incisors. One or more supernumerary teeth may develop, or the normal number of teeth may fail to form. Supernumerary teeth usually appear in the area of the maxillary incisors, where they disrupt the position and eruption of normal teeth. The extra teeth commonly erupt posterior to the normal ones. In partial anodontia, one or more teeth are absent. In total anodontia, no teeth develop. This very rare condition is usually associated with an ectodermal dysplasia.

Disturbances during the differentiation of teeth may result in gross alterations in dental morphology, for example, macrodontia (large teeth) and microdontia (small teeth). Taurodontia is a variation in tooth form involving all or some of the primary and secondary molars, marked by elongation of the body of the tooth producing large pulp chambers and small roots. Taurodontia is found in association with several chromosomal abnormalities.

## Maxilla

### Introduction

The lateral parts of the upper lip, most of the maxilla, and the secondary palate form the maxillary prominences of the first branchial arch. These prominences merge laterally with the mandibular prominences.

Unilateral maxillary absence is a rare condition and is due to failure of development of one maxillary process. Absence of the premaxillary area is found in cyclopia when the frontonasal process does not form. Subtle hypoplasia of the maxilla is best appreciated on X-ray and is an important feature to be looked for in first-degree relatives of patients with Treacher Collins syndrome.

In the measurement section that follows, the maxilla is chiefly evaluated by cephalometric means. Clinical evaluation of the maxilla is extremely subjective and is best performed in profile, looking at the prominence of the maxilla in comparison to the prominence of the supraorbital ridges, malar area, and mandible. No objective clinical measurements appear to be available.

### Effective Midfacial Length: Cephalometric

**Definition**   Size and prominence of the maxilla (Fig 7.91).

**Fig. 7.91**  Effective midfacial length (mm), both sexes, 6 to 18 years

|  | 6 years | | 9 years | | 12 years | | 14 years | | Adults | |
|---|---|---|---|---|---|---|---|---|---|---|
|  | Mean | SD | Mean | SD | Mean | SD | Mean | SD | Mean | SD |
| Male | 81.7 | 3.4 | 87.7 | 4.1 | 92.1 | 4.1 | 95.2 | 3.2 | 98.8 | 4.3 |
|  | 81.7 | 3.4 | 87.7 | 4.1 | 92.1 | 4.1 | 95.2 | 3.2 | 99.8 | 6.0 |
|  | 80.5 | 2.4 | 84.9 | 2.5 | 90.3 | 3.6 | 93.9 | 4.6 |  |  |
| Female | 79.7 | 2.2 | 85.0 | 2.3 | 89.6 | 2.4 | 92.1 | 2.7 | 90.7 | 5.2 |
|  | 79.8 | 2.2 | 85.0 | 2.3 | 89.6 | 2.4 | 92.1 | 2.7 | 91.0 | 4.3 |
|  | 78.6 | 3.1 | 88.3 | 4.0 | 87.3 | 4.6 | 89.2 | 5.2 |  |  |

*From McNamara (1984) by permission.*

**Landmarks**  Measure from the condylion of the mandible (the most posterosuperior point of the condylar outline) to point A (the deepest midline point on the maxilla between the anterior nasal spine and the prosthion, which is the inferior labial termination of the cortical plate just above the maxillary incisors) (Fig 7.92).

**Instruments**  Spreading calipers are used to measure this distance on a radiograph taken with "cephalostat."

**Position**  Standard cephalometry—see introduction to Chapter 7.

**Figure 7.92**  Cephalometric measurement of effective midfacial length.

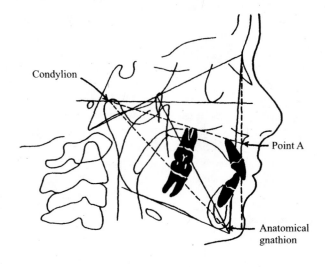

**Remarks**   Unfortunately, clinical evaluation of the maxilla and malar area is difficult and subjective. Relative prominence or flattening of the malar area is best appreciated in profile, relative to the prominence of supraorbital region. Similarly, prominence of the maxilla, in profile, should be relative to the mandible.

### Outer Canthal, Nasal, Outer Canthal (ONC) Angle

**Definition**   The angle subtended by the base of the nose in the midline to the outer canthi of the eyes.

**Landmarks**   Draw an imaginary line from the outer canthus of the right eye to the base of the nose (base of the columella) in the midline. Draw a second imaginary line from the outer canthus of the left eye to the same point at the base of the nose. Measure the angle between those two lines (Fig. 7.93).

**Instruments**   Two fixed measures such as a tape-measure or flexible ruler and protractor are necessary.

**Position**   The head should be held erect (in the resting position) with the patient facing forward.

**Alternative**   A young infant or child should be lying supine.

**Remarks**   This angle is best measured from a full frontal photograph taken at a fixed distance from the patient (Fig. 7.94). It provides an estimate of both the spacing of the eyes and the upper facial height, and thus it will vary in the presence of hypo- or hypertelorism or an increase or reduction in upper facial height. Although best appreciated from a photograph, it can still provide useful information during clinical evaluation.

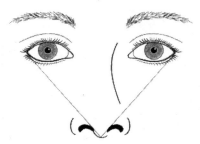

**Figure 7.93**   Measuring ONO angle.

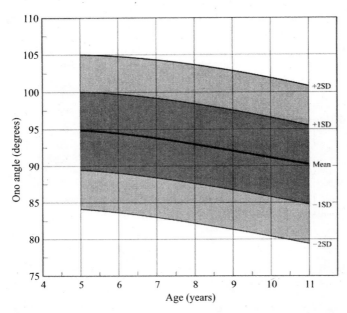

**Figure 7.94** ONO angle, both sexes, 5 to 11 years. From Patton (1987), by permission.

**Pitfalls** Depending on the prominence of the nose, it may be very difficult to draw a straight line between the outer canthus and the base of the nose in the midline. In this situation, photographic estimation is advised.

## Mandible

### Introduction

The mandible, or lower jaw, is the first part of the face to form, as the medial ends of the two mandibular prominences merge during the fourth week of gestation.

Agnathia, or absence of the mandible, is a developmental defect of the first branchial arch. The mandible may be missing on one side only, a condition sometimes associated with microtia or absence of the external or internal ear, or with unilateral congenital macrostomia. Micrognathia, or underdevelopment of the jaw may be severe enough to lead to cleft palate in the Pierre–Robin sequence. This can be seen as an isolated anomaly or in conjuction with other features as part of a syndrome diagnosis. Macrognathia, or a large jaw, is otherwise termed prognathism and is best appreciated in profile. The jaw is abnormally large or jutting forward. Various measurements of the jaw can be made from radiographs. The main clinical measurement, for which a graph is provided, is the mandibular width, or bigonial distance. The shape of the jaw can vary markedly depending on the relative proportions of the ramus and body of the mandible. The jaw articulates with the skull at the temporomandibular joint. Restricted movement at that joint may produce limited mouth opening or trismus.

A median cleft of the mandible is a deep cleft resulting from failure of the mesenchymal masses of the mandibular prominences of the first branchial arch to merge completely with each other. It is extremely rare. More superficial clefts of the lower lip may also occur. Clefts of the mandible are sometimes associated with cleft lip, cleft palate, or oblique facial clefts.

A simple dimple on the chin is a common feature inherited with an autosomal dominant pattern. A more complicated H-shaped groove of the chin is associated with Freeman–Sheldon syndrome. Mental spurs are bony spurs over the most prominent part of the jaw in the midline.

The shape and size of the chin contribute to the overall facial shape. A wide chin will tend to produce a round or square face, while a narrow, pointed chin promotes the appearance of an inverted triangular face because of the relative width of the forehead and cranial vault.

### Effective Mandibular Length: Cephalometric

**Definition**   Effective length and prominence of the mandible.

**Landmarks**   Measure from the condylion (the most posterosuperior point of the condylar outline) to the anatomic gnathion (determined by the intersection of the facial and mandibular planes) (Fig. 7.95). Typical values are shown in Fig. 7.96.

**Instruments**  Spreading calipers are used to measure this distance on a radiograph taken with "cephalostat."

**Position**  Standard cephalometry—see introduction to Chapter 7.

**Figure 7.95**  Cephalometric measurement of effective mandibular length

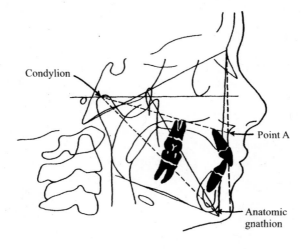

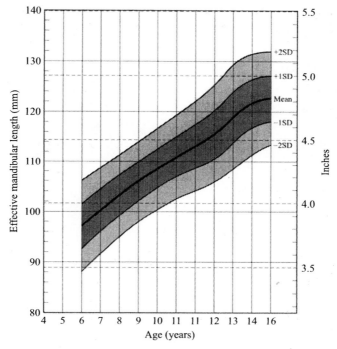

**Figure 7.96** Effective mandibular length, both sexes, 6 to 16 years. From McNamara (1984), by permission.

## Maxillomandibular Differential: Cephalometric

**Definition** This measurement is determined by subtracting the effective midfacial length from the effective mandibular length (Fig. 7.97).

**Landmarks** See sections on effective midfacial length and effective mandibular length for details.

## Mandible Width (Bigonial Distance)

**Definition** The bigonial width. The distance between the two most lateral aspects of the mandible.

**Landmarks** Measure from the most lateral aspect at the angle of the jaw (gonion) to the same point on the other side of the face (Fig. 7.98).

**Instruments** Spreading calipers.

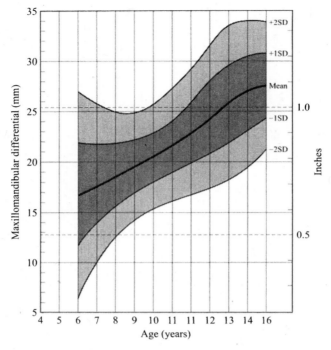

**Figure 7.97** Maxillo mandibular differential, both sexes, 6 to 16 years. From McNamara (1984), by permission.

**Figure 7.98** Measuring mandible width.

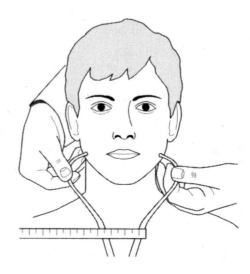

**Position**   The head should be held erect with the eyes facing forward.

**Alternative**   The infant or young child may lie supine.

**Remarks**   The mouth should be relaxed when this measurement is taken. Typical values for children age 4–16 years are shown in Fig. 7.99.

**Pitfalls**   Marked asymmetry of the mandible or malformation of the mandible may make it difficult to define the gonial points.

**Figure 7.99**   Mandibular width, both sexes, 4 to 16 years. From Farkas (1981), by permission.

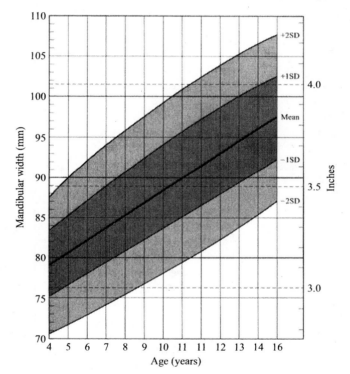

## The Neck

### Introduction

Most of the congenital malformations of the neck originate during trans-formation of the branchial apparatus into adult structures. Branchial cysts, sinuses, or fistulae may develop from parts of the second branchial groove, the cervical sinus, or the second pharyngeal pouch if they fail to regress. An ectopic thyroid gland results when the thyroid gland fails to descend completely from its site of origin in the tongue. The thyroglossal duct may persist, or remnants of it may give rise to thyroglossal duct cysts. These cysts, if infected, may form thyroglossal duct sinuses that open in the midline of the neck, in contrast to the branchial sinuses, which open off-center, close to the borders of the sternocleidomastoid muscle.

Torticollis (wry neck) usually is attributed to injury of the sterno-cleidomastoid muscle during delivery; however, prenatal onset of the anomaly cannot be ruled out. Torticollis can be caused by malformations of the cervical vertebrae. The right and left sides are affected equally with-out any sex predilection. The incidence is 0.6 per 1000 births. The presence of unequal muscle pull on the developing cranium by torticollis may lead to unequal growth of the skull, with resultant plagiocephaly. A contralat-eral epicanthal fold is frequently seen. In approximately one third of cases, torticollis is associated with congenital hip dislocation. Both are thought to be caused by cramped circumstances *in utero*, for example, due to abnormal uterine anatomy, a uterine fibroid, or oligohydramnios.

Estimation of the length and width of the neck is very subjective, and normal age-related charts are not available. The neck is generally short in the neonate and begins to elongate in the older child. The width of the neck obviously varies, increasing from a superior to an inferior aspect in general. A wide neck may be associated with marked skin folds or webs or with prominence of the trapezius muscle. Folds, webs, and prominent trapezius may be related to prenatal onset of lymphatic obstruction. An early clue in the newborn period is the presence of excess nuchal skin and posteriorly rotated auricles with an upturned lobule. The circumfer-ence of the neck may be quantified, and the charts are available in this section.

The neck should also be inspected for branchial arch remnants such as pits, sinuses, fistulae and tags.

## Neck Circumference

**Definition**   The distance around the neck.

**Landmarks**   Measure around the neck in a horizontal plane at the level of the most prominent portion of the thyroid cartilage (Fig. 7.100).

**Instruments**   Tape-measure.

**Position**   The head should be held erect (in the resting position) with the eyes facing forward.

**Remarks**   Normal values to age 12 years are presented in Fig. 7.101. The neck may be broad because of excessive prominence of the trapezius or secondary to skinfolds or webs. Both these anatomical differences can be associated with excess nuchal skin in the newborn period and with lymphatic obstruction during prenatal development.

**Pitfalls**   In the presence of prominent folds of skin or webs at the side of the neck, the tape-measure should carefully follow the surface of the skin to reflect circumference accurately. The horizontal plane at which measurement occurs should be carefully selected at the most prominent portion of the thyroid cartilage.

**Figure 7.100**   Measuring neck circumference.

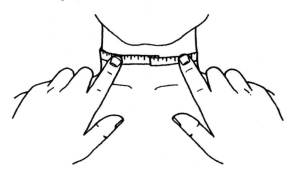

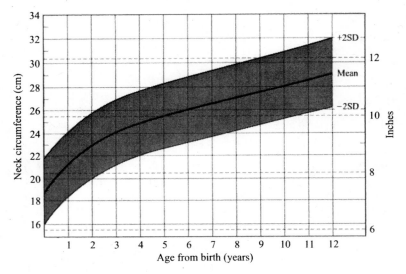

**Figure 7.101** Neck circumference, both sexes, birth to 12 years. From Feingold and Bossert (1974), by permission.

*Bibliography*

# Bibliography

Astley, S.J. and Clarren, S.K. (1995). A fetal alcohol syndrome screening tool. *Alcoholism: Clinical and Experimental Research*, **19**, 1565–1571.

Caffey, J. (1978). *J. Caffey's pediatric X ray diagnosis* (7th ed). Year Book Publishers, Chicago.

Chouke, K.S. (1929). The epicanthus or Mongolian fold in caucasian children. *American Journal of Physical Anthropology*, **13**, 255.

Cohen, M.M., and Maclean, R. (eds) (2000). *Craniosynostosis: Diagnosis, evaluations, and management*. New York: Oxford University Press.

Currarino, G. and Silverman, F.N. (1960). Orbital hypotelorism, arhinencephaly, and trigonocephaly, *Radiology*, **74**, 206–217.

Duke-Elder, S. (1963). *System of ophthalmology, Vol. 3*. C.V. Mosby, St Louis.

Faix, R.G. (1982). Fontanelle size in black and white term newborn infants. *Journal of Pediatrics*, **100**, 304–306

Farkas, L.G. (1981). *Anthropometry of the head and face in medicine*. Elsevier, New York.

Farkas, L.G. and Munro, I.R. (1987). *Anthropometric facial proportions in medicine*. Charles C. Thomas Springfield, Il.

Feingold, M. and Bossert, W.H. (1974). Normal values for selected physical parameters: an aid to syndrome delineation. *Birth Defects: Original Article Series*, **X(13)**, 1–15

Garn, S.M., Smith, B.H., and LaVelle, M. (1984). Applications of pattern profile analysis to malformations of the head and face. *Radiology*, **150**, 683–690.

Greber, F.R., Taylor, F.H., deLevie, M., Drash, A.L., and Kenny, F.M. (1972). Normal standards for exophthalmometry in children 10 to 14 years of age: relation to age, height, weight, and sexual maturation. *Journal of Pediatrics*, **81**, 327–329.

Goodman, R.M. and Gorlin, R.J. (1977). *Atlas of the face in genetic disorders* (2nd ed). C.V. Mosby, St Louis.

Hansman, C.F. (1966). Growth of interorbital distance and skull thickness as observed in roentgenographic measurements. *Radiology*, **86**, 87.

Iosub, S., Fuchs, M., Bingol, N., Stone, R.K., Gromisch, D.S., and Wasserman, E. (1985). Palpebral fissure length in Black and Hispanic children: correlation with head circumference. *Pediatrics*, **75**, 318–320.

Laestadius, N.D., Aase, J.M., and Smith, D.W. (1969). Normal inner canthal and outer orbital dimensions. *Journal of Pediatrics*, **74**, 465–468.

Lasker, G.W. (1949). *Yearbook of physical anthropology*.

Martin, R. and Saller, K. (1962). *Lehrbuch der Anthropologie, Vol. 3.* (ed. G. Fischer) pp. 2051–2084. Verlag, Stuttgart.

McNamara, J. A., Jr. (1984). A method of cephalometric evaluation. *American Journal of Orthodontics,* **86**, 449–469.

Mehes, K. (1974). Inner canthal and intermammary indices in the newborn infant. *Journal of Pediatrics,* **85**, 90.

Merlob, P., Sivan, Y., and Reisner, S.H. (1984). Anthropometric measurements of the newborn infant 27 to 41 gestational weeks. *Birth Defects: Original Article Series,* **20**, 7.

Moore, K.L. (1982). *The developing human* (3rd ed). W. B. Saunders, Philadelphia.

Pashayen, H. (1973). A family with blepharo-naso-facial malformations. *American Journal of Diseases in Children,* **125**, 389.

Patton, M. (1987). ONO angle. Personal communication.

Popich, G.A. and Smith, D.W. (1972). Fontanels: Range of normal size. *Journal of Pediatrics,* **80**, 749–752.

Pruzansky, S. (1973). Clinical investigation of the experiments of nature. *ASHA Reports,* **8**, 62–94

Ranly, D.M. (1980) A synopsis of craniofacial growth. Prentice Hall, New York.

Redman, R.S. (1963). Measurements of normal and reportedly malformed palatal vaults II: normal juvenile measurement. *Journal of Dental Research,* **45**, 266.

Robinow, M. and Roche, A.F. (1973). Low-set ears. *American Journal of Diseases in Children,* **125**, 482–483.

Saksena, S.S., Walker, G.F., Bixler, D., and Yu, P.-L. (1987). *A clinical atlas of roentgenocephalometry in norma lateralis.* Alan R. Liss, New York.

Shapiro, B.L., Redman, R.S., and Gorlin, R.J. (1963). Measurement of normal and reportedly malformed palatal vaults I: normal adult measurements. *Journal of Dental Research,* **42**, 1039.

Smith, D.W. and Gong, B.T. (1974). Scalp-hair patterning: its origin and significance relative to early brain and upper facial development. *Teratology,* **9**, 17–34.

Smith, D.W. and Takashima, H. (1980). Ear muscles and ear form. *Birth Defects: Original Article Series,* **XVI(4)**, 299–302.

Thomas, I.T., Gaitantzis, Y.A., and Frias, J.L. (1987). Palepebral fissure length from 29 weeks gestation to 14 years. *Journal of Paediatrics,* **III(2)**, 267–268.

# Limbs

## Introduction

Disturbance of limb growth generally leads to disproportion of the body, as the normal proportions of the body reflect changes in the relative size of the limbs at different ages.

The limb buds emerge as identifiable structures at about four weeks of embryonic development. Normal development depends on the interactions of developing vascular, nerve, muscle, and bony tissues. All are interdependent and have changing patterns and relationships during development. Initially, the limb is paddle shaped with a core of mesenchyme and a covering layer of epidermis. By six weeks, hand and foot plates can be seen and condensations of hyaline cartilage that will become bone are present. Normal limb structure is established by about the end of the eighth week, and ossification begins shortly thereafter. The arms develop more rapidly than the legs and the right side slightly ahead of the left. Intrauterine movement is essential for normal development and function of limbs at birth. Normal limb length measurements at various times in gestation and *in utero* limb movement patterns are presented in Chapter 15.

The relative proportions of bone, skin, fat, and muscle change with age, as does the ratio of limb-to-trunk length. At birth, span is less than height and the lower segment length is much less than the upper segment. By 10 years of age, the lower segment length approximately equals that of the upper segment. The limbs continue to grow disproportionately, and the lower segment becomes longer than the trunk, so that in the adult the upper-to-lower segment ratio is less than 1.0 (see Fig. 8.55). By about 10 years of age in boys and 12 years of age in girls, the span equals the height; thereafter, it exceeds height (see Fig. 8.3).

Many skeletal dysplasias result in disproportion of the limbs or some part of the limbs; the distal (acro), middle (meso) or proximal (rhizo) segments can be most severely affected, either prenatally or postnatally. A variety of disorders demonstrate asymmetry of the body. One limb can be larger (hemihyperplasia) or smaller (hemihypoplasia) than the other.

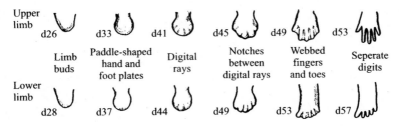

**Figure 8.1** Embryologic limb development.

An approach to limb evaluation must include assessment of relative proportions of various tissues (fat, muscle, etc.) and comparison with normal age-related measurements. Various indices for comparison are available but have not been included in this text.

The inspection of limbs should answer the following questions:

1. Is the general proportion of limb-to-trunk length normal?
2. Are the limbs symmetric in length?
3. Are the limbs symmetric in circumference?
4. If one arm/leg is longer than the other, which part of the limb is longer?
5. Is there evidence for muscular or vascular anomalies?
6. Is the muscle mass symmetric?
7. Are the hands and feet symmetric in size and shape?
8. Are there contractures?
9. Are the fingers and toes symmetric in length and proportionate to the rest of the limbs?
10. Are fingernails/toenails present?
11. Do the nails have anomalies in size or shape?

The evaluation of the hands and feet includes examination of nails, skin (see Chapter 11) and flexion creases (Chapter 12).

The presence of incomplete separation of finger- or toe-rays is called syndactyly and can affect the skin only (cutaneous syndactyly), or the bone can be also affected (bony syndactyly).

Supernumerary digits or toes (polydactyly) can be found on the ulnar side of the hand (postaxial), the fibular side of the foot (postaxial), the radial side of the hand (preaxial), or the tibial side of the foot (preaxial); supernumerary digits can also occur between the finger rays (mesoaxial polydactyly). They can be just an appendage of soft tissue or can contain bony parts. X-ray examinations will help to clarify how much of the underlying bony tissue is involved.

Bony prominences of the limbs provide good anatomical landmarks from which to measure, so that limb measurements have been well standardized.

Terminology to describe congenital limb anomalies has been confusing. A glossary of terms to define specific anomalies is at the end of this book. We have tried to avoid diagnostic entities but to include useful descriptive terms.

## Span

**Definition** Span is the distance between the fingertips of the middle fingers of each hand, the arms are stretched out horizontally from the body.

**Landmarks** With the arms completely extended horizontally from the body, measure between the tips of the middle fingers across the back or the front of the patient (Fig. 8.2).

**Instruments** Tape-measure.

**Position** The patient may be standing or lying down with the arms completely extended.

**Alternative** Place the patient adjacent to a wall or blackboard, make marks at the tips of the middle fingers, and measure between the markings.

In the case of a squirming infant, the child may be placed prone on a bed or table, with the arms out to the sides. Measure across the back.

**Remarks** If the individual has a span greater than the standard 150 cm tape-measure, simply bring the beginning end of the tape around and place it on the 150 cm point (be careful not to use the end of the tape) and continue the measurement, adding the additional distance to 150 cm.

**Figure 8.2** Measuring span.

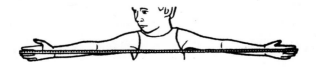

A normal span for age measurement is within 4.0 cm of the age-related median span (Fig. 8.3).

In infancy and early childhood, span is less than height. By about 10 years in males and 12 years in females, span equals height, thereafter, it exceeds height.

**Figure 8.3** Span measured in centimeters, with average difference from height shaded, both sexes, birth to 16 years. Adapted from Belt-Niedbala et al. (1986).

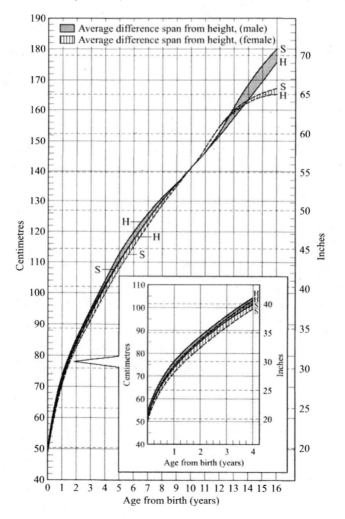

**Pitfalls**   The patient with contractures or limitations of full extension (as in achondroplasia) may give falsely low values unless the tape is worked along the contracture.

## Total Upper Limb (Hand and Arm) Length

**Definition**   Length of the whole arm (the arm and hand combined).

**Landmarks**   Measure between the acromion (the most prominent posterior lateral bony prominence of the shoulder joint) and the tip of the middle finger (Fig. 8.4).

**Instruments**   Tape-measure or calipers.

**Position**   Stand the patient erect with arms hanging loosely down at the side, parallel to the body.

**Alternative**   In patients who cannot stand, the arms can be measured while the patient lies down with the arms parallel to the body. Measurement of arm length by X-ray is more accurate, but the limb must be positioned properly.

**Remarks**   The arms account for approximately 11 percent of the total body weight in the age group 0.5–3.0 years in boys (10 percent in girls) and for 13 percent of total body weight in the age group 3–13 years in boys (16 percent in girls) (Figs. 8.5 and 8.6)

**Figure 8.4**   Measuring total upper limb length.

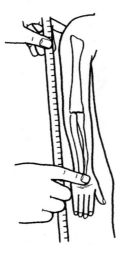
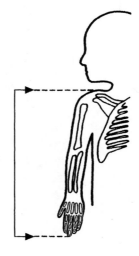

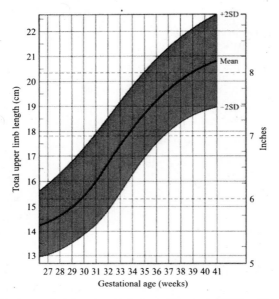

**Figure 8.5**  Total upper limb length at birth. From Sivan et al. (1983) and Merlob et al. (1984a), by permission.

**Figure 8.6**  Total upper limb length, both sexes, 4 to 16 years. From Martin and Saller (1962), by permission.

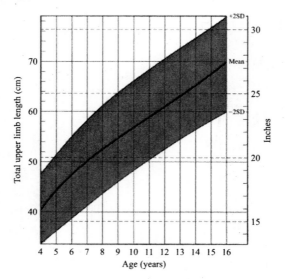

In individuals with contractures, a tape-measure should be worked along the limb.

Dislocated shoulders or hyperextensible joints can give abnormally long measurements.

## Upper Arm Length

**Definition**  Length of the upper arm or proximal (rhizomelic) segment of the arm.

**Landmarks**  Measure from the acromion (the most prominent posterior lateral bony prominence of the shoulder joint) along the posterior lateral aspect of the arm until reaching the distal medial border of the olecranon (Fig. 8.7).

**Instruments**  Tape-measure or calipers.

**Position** Stand the patient erect, with arms held loosely at the side and elbows slightly bent.

**Figure 8.7**  Measuring upper arm length.

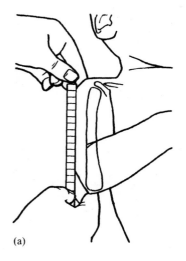
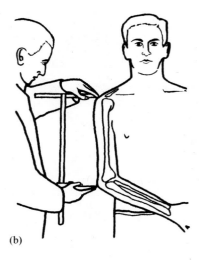

(a)

(b)

**Alternative**   The patient may lie in bed, supine, or prone, with the arms at the side of the body and elbow slightly bent. Measurement of upper arm length by X-ray is more accurate, but the limb must be positioned properly.

**Remarks**   Typical values per upper arm length from birth to age 16 years are presented in Figs. 8.8–8.10.

**Pitfalls**   A dislocated shoulder will give an abnormally long measurement.

**Figure 8.8**   Upper arm length, both sexes, at birth. From Merlob et al. 1984a), by permission.

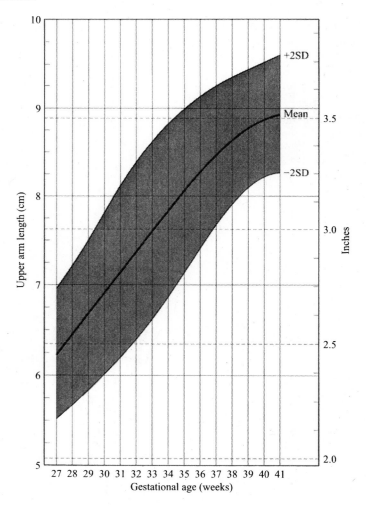

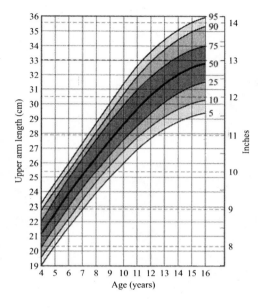

**Figure 8.9** Upper arm length, males, 4 to 16 years. From Malina et al. 1973), by permission.

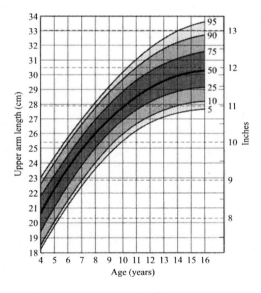

**Figure 8.10** Upper arm length, females, 4 to 16 years. From Malina et al. 1973), by permission.

## Forearm Length

**Definition**   Length of the forearm or middle (mesomelic) segment of the arm.

**Landmarks**   Measure the distance from the most prominent point of the olecranon to the distal lateral process of the radius along the lateral surface of the forearm (Fig. 8.11).

**Instruments**   Tape-measure or calipers.

**Position**   The patient stands or sits with the upper arm hanging at the side and the elbow bent at a 90 degree angle; the arm should be held in a neutral position (not in supination or pronation), with the hand in a vertical plane.

**Alternative**   Measurement by X-ray is more accurate, but the arm must be positioned properly with the forearm in neutral position.

**Remarks**   Forearm lengths are presented in Figs. 8.12–8.14. Although this may seem to be an awkward measurement, standards are available from anthropological studies. These distances obviously do not represent single bone lengths, but they do allow assessment of the different segments and proportions of the arm.

**Figure 8.11**   Measuring forearm length.

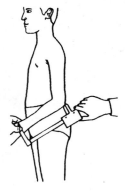 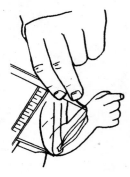

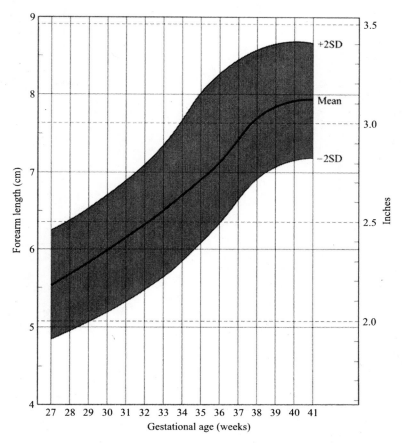

**Figure 8.12** Forearm length, both sexes, at birth. From Merlob et al. (1984a), by permission.

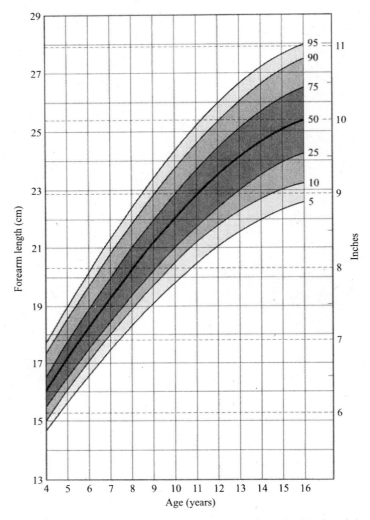

**Figure 8.13**  Forearm length, males, 4 to 16 years. From Roche and Malina (1983), by permission.

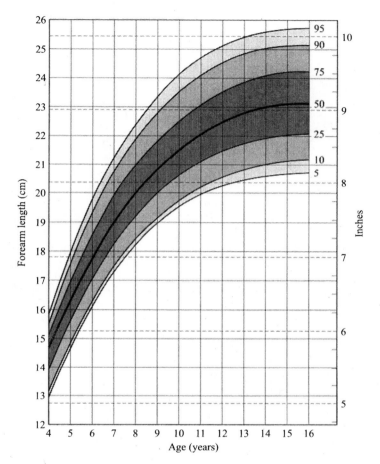

**Figure 8.14** Forearm length, females, 4 to 16 years. From Roche and Malina (1983), by permission.

## Carrying Angle

**Definition**   The carrying angle is the angle subtended by the forearm on the humerus (the deviation of the forearm relative to the humerus or the angle at the elbow joint).

**Landmarks**   Draw an imaginary line (A) through the axis of the upper arm extending down to a distance equivalent to the hand. Draw a second imaginary line (B) through the axis of the forearm and hand. The angle between these two lines, at the elbow, is the carrying angle (Fig. 8.15).

**Instruments**   A goniometer, or "eyeball estimate" of the angle between the two lines.

**Position**   Stand the patient with the shoulders hanging loosely, the palms facing anteriorly, the hands in the same plane as the body, and the arms fully extended. The elbow is extended and the forearm supinated.

**Alternative**   The patient may lie supine with the upper arm parallel to the body and the lower arm supinated, elbow extended, and the back of the hand against the bed. Photograph the patient in one of the above positions and measure the angle from the photograph.

**Remarks**   Normal values for carrying angle are shown in Fig 8.16. The carrying angle is usually greater in women than in men and increases slightly with age. The normal range is between 7 and 22 degrees with a mean of 14 degrees in the male and 16 degrees in the female. The carrying

**Figure 8.15**   Landmarks for measurement of carrying angle.

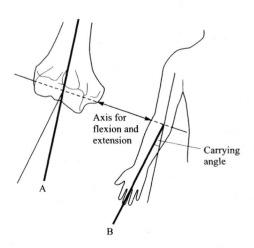

Axis for flexion and extension

Carrying angle

A

B

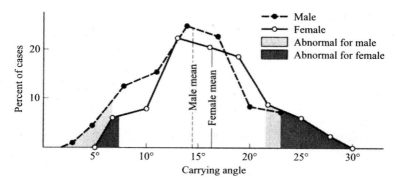

**Figure 8.16**   Carrying angle norms. From Atkinson and Elftman (1945), by permission.

angle may be altered by abnormalities of the elbow joint. Sex chromosome aneuploidy often affects the carrying angle.

**Pitfalls**   If there is limited extension of the elbow or if the arm cannot be fully supinated, the carrying angle will be difficult to assess. Radial head dislocation should not affect the carrying angle.

## Hand Length

**Definition**   Total length of the hand.

**Landmarks**   Measure from the distal crease at the wrist to the tip of the middle finger (Fig. 8.17).

**Instruments**   Tape-measure, calipers, or clear ruler.

**Figure 8.17**   Measuring hand length.

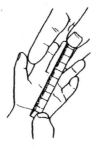
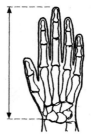

**Position**  The wrist is held in neutral position, and the fingers are fully extended. The measurement is taken on the palmar aspect of the hand.

**Alternative**  Draw a line around the hand and measure from an estimated point where the wrist begins.

**Remarks**  Some patients have multiple wrist creases; choose the most distal crease.

Normal values are shown in Fig 8.18–8.20. There are no significant differences in hand length between males and females.

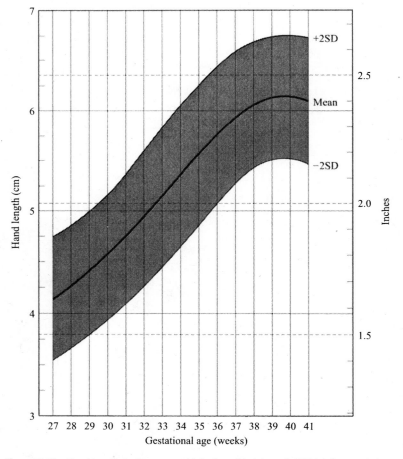

**Figure 8.18**  Hand length, both sexes, at birth. From Merlob et al. (1984a), by permission.

**Pitfalls** Individuals with disproportion within the hand will need to have the various segments of their hand separately evaluated.

In individuals with contractures of the wrist or hand the tape should be pressed along the palm of the hand, eliminating false reduction in length.

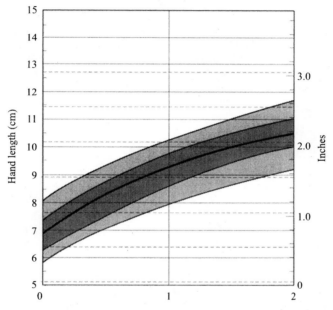

**Figure 8.19** Hand length, both sexes, birth to two years. From Feingold and Bossert (1974), by permission.

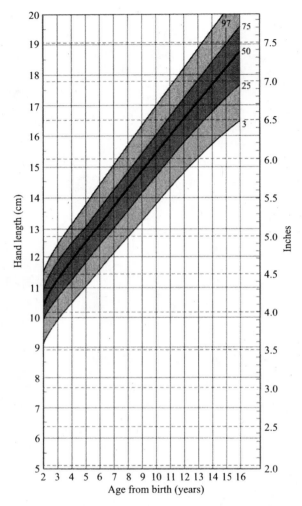

**Figure 8.20** Hand length, both sexes, 2 to 16 years. From Feingold and Bossert (1974), by permission.

## Middle Finger Length

**Definition**   Total length of middle finger.

**Landmarks**   Measure from the proximal flexion crease at the base of the middle finger to tip of the middle finger. The measurement is taken on the palmar aspect of the hand (Fig. 8.21).

**Instruments**   Tape-measure, calipers, or clear ruler.

**Position**   The wrist is in a neutral position and the hand is fully extended.

**Alternative**   Draw around hand and estimate where the proximal flexion crease of the middle finger would be, then measure from the paper.

**Remarks**   The proximal finger crease on the palmar aspect of the hand is about 1–2 cm distal to the knuckle on the dorsal aspect of the hand; therefore this measurement does not reflect the sum of the lengths of the phalanges of the middle finger. Middle finger lengths from birth to age 16 years are shown in 8.22–8.24.

**Pitfalls**   In various forms of brachydactyly, different finger lengths will be reduced. In some forms of brachydactyly, measurement of the middle finger will not reflect the lengths of the other digits.

In individuals with contractures, work the tape along the finger in order to get a measurement equivalent to total finger length.

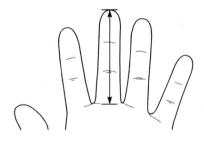

**Figure 8.21**   Measuring middle finger length.

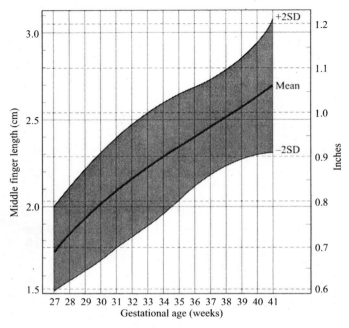

**Figure 8.22**  Middle finger length, both sexes, at birth. From Merlob et al. (1984), by permission.

**Figure 8.23(a)**  Middle finger length, both sexes, birth to two years. From Feingold and Bossert (1974), by permission.

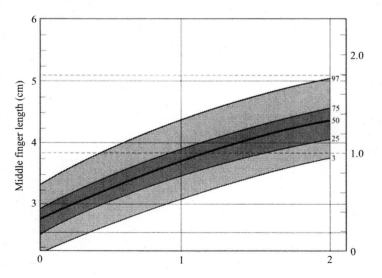

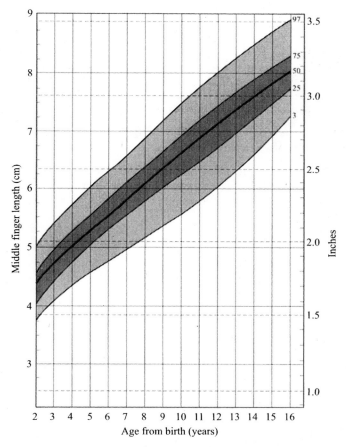

**Figure 8.23(b)** Middle finger length, both sexes, 2 to 16 years. From Feingold and Bossert (1974), by permission.

## Palm Length

**Definition** Total length of the palm.

**Landmarks** Measure between the distal flexion crease at the wrist and the proximal flexion crease of the middle finger (Fig. 8.24).

**Instruments** Tape-measure, calipers, or clear ruler.

**Position** The wrist is in a neutral position and the fingers are fully extended. The measurement is taken on the palmar aspect of the hand.

**Alternative** Subtract the middle finger length from the total hand length. Draw around the hand and then measure the palm length from the drawing, estimating the position of the creases.

**Remarks** Palm length from birth to age 16 years are shown in Figs. 8.25 and 8.26. A ratio of middle finger to total hand lenght (Fig. 8.27) is helpful in defining relative disproportion in the hand.

**Figure 8.24** Measuring palm length.

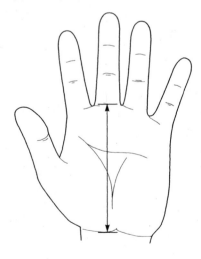

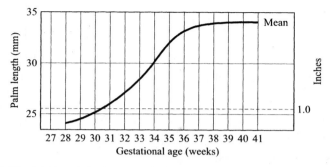

**Figure 8.25** Palm length, both sexes, at birth. From Sivan et al. (1983), by permission.

**Figure 8.26** Palm length, both sexes, birth to 16 years. From Feingold and Bossert (1974), by permission.

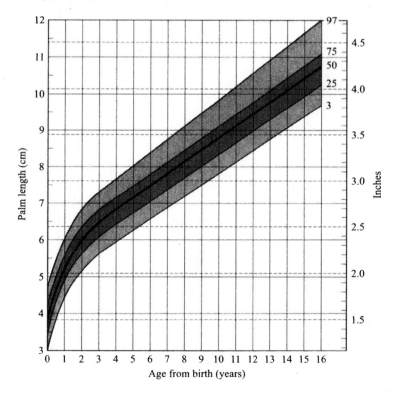

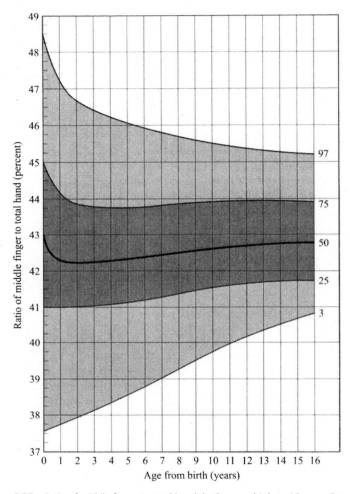

**Figure 8.27** Ratio of middle finger to total hand, both sexes, birth to 16 years. From Feingold and Bossert (1974), by permission.

## Palm Width

**Definition**   Width of the palm of the hand.

**Landmarks**   Measure from the edge of the hand on one side, across the palm to the edge of the hand on the other side, at the level of the metacarpophalangeal joints, with the fingers parallel and extended (Fig 8.28)

**Instruments**   Tape-measure, calipers, or clear ruler.

**Position**   The wrist is in a neutral position with the fingers fully extended. The measurement can be taken on either side of the hand but preferably is taken across the palm.

**Alternative**   Draw a line around the hand and measure between the markings at the level of the metacarpophalangeal joints.

**Remarks**   Palm widths are shown separately for males and females in Fig 8.29 and 8.30. In a hyperextensible hand, care must be taken not to squash the hand excessively, since this can alter the measurement.

The ratio of hand length to hand width changes considerably during intrauterine life. The hand form becomes relatively thinner and longer by the end of intrauterine life. This tendency continues until about 5 years of age. From then on hand length and width increase relatively proportionately (Fig. 8.31).

**Figure 8.28**   Measuring palm width.

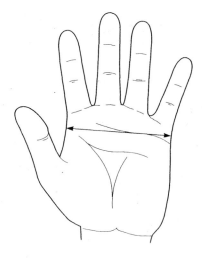

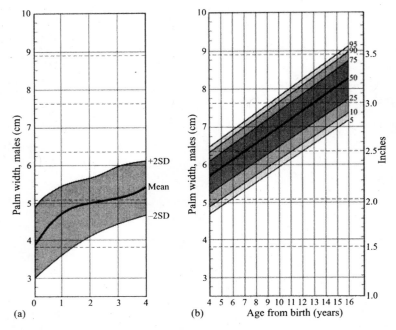

**Figure 8.29** (a) Palm width, males, birth to four years. From Snyder et al. (1975), and Malina et al. (1973), by permission. (b) Palm width, males, 4 to 16 years. From Snyder et al. (1975), and Malina et al. (1973), by permission.

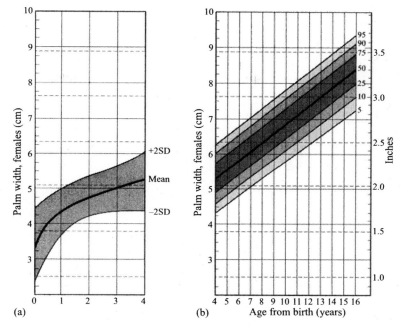

**Figure 8.30** (a) Palm width, females, birth to four years. From Snyder et al. (1975), and Malina et al. (1973), by permission. (b) Palm width, females, 4 to 16 years. From Snyder et al. (1975), and Malina et al. (1973), by permission.

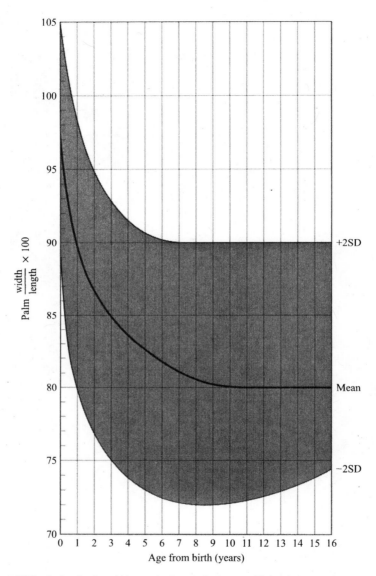

**Figure 8.31** Ratio of palm width to palm length, both sexes, birth to 16 years. From Snyder et al. (1975), and Malina et al. (1973), by permission.

## Thumb Position, Placement, and Range of Movement

### Introduction

The position, placement, and range of movement of the thumb may be unusual. Photographs often delineate deviation from the norm better than measurement; however, the two methods presented below have been established to describe unusual thumbs.

The size of the thumb should also be assessed. If the tip of the thumb is below the proximal crease at the base of the index finger when the thumb is held parallel to the hand, then the thumb is either hypoplastic or low set; if the tip of the thumb is above the interphalangeal joint of the index finger, it is too long or digitalized.

### Method 1. Thumb Placement Index

**Definition**   Ratio of the distance between

(1) the distance between the proximal flexion crease (A) at the base of the index finger and the distal insertion (B) of the thumb (Fig. 8.32a) and (2) the distance between the proximal crease (a) at the base of the index finger and the distal flexion crease (b) at the wrist (Fig 8.32b)

**Landmarks**   The first measurement (1) is taken on the lateral aspect of the index finger: Measure from the proximal crease at the base of the index finger to the basal crease of the thumb insertion. The second measurement (2) is taken from the proximal crease at the base of the index finger, on the palmar aspect, to the distal flexion crease at the wrist.

**Instruments**   Tape-measure, calipers, or clear ruler.

**Position**   Maintain the thumb in 90 degrees abduction.

$$\text{Thumb placement index} = \frac{(1)}{(2)} = 0.51 \pm 0.04$$

**Remarks**   If the thumb is digitalized, it may not be possible to abduct it to 90 degrees, but the creases will probably still be identifiable.

**Alternative**   Draw around the hand with the thumb held in 90 degrees abduction and measure between the points mentioned.

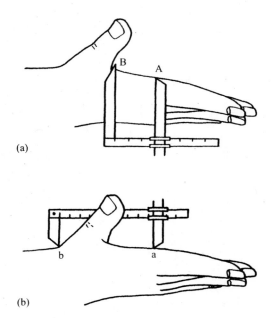

(a)

(b)

**Figure 8.32(a–b)** Measuring thumb placement.


## Method 2. Angle of Thumb Attachment

**Definition**   The angles of movement of the thumb (Fig. 8.33).

**Landmarks**   With the hand at rest on a flat surface, palm up, fingers parallel, and thumb extended and abducted away from the palm as far as possible comfortably, draw an imaginary line through the main axis of the index finger and another imaginary line through the main axis of the index finger and another imaginary line through the main axis of the thumb. Measure the angle made by the imaginary lines (Fig 8.33a). Keeping the same hand position with the palm up, pick the thumb up from the flat surface and, keeping the thumb fully extended, rotate the thumb toward the palm, and measure the angle made by the thumb from the flat surface (Fig 8.33b).

If either of the angles is greater than 90 degrees or less than 75 degrees, abnormal thumb joint movement is present.

**Instruments**   A goniometer, or "eyeball estimate" of the angle between the two lines.

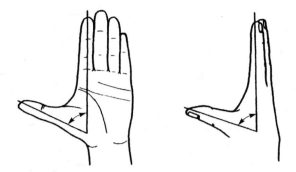

**Figure 8.33(a–b)**   Measuring the angles of thumb attachment.

**Position**   Keep hand palm up and flat against a hard surface with fingers parallel. Keep thumb fully extended as it moves through its range of motion.

**Remarks**   These measurements reflect thumb placement and flexibility.

## Total Lower Limb Length

**Definition**   Total length of the lower limb (including leg and foot).

**Landmarks**   In older children and adults, the total lower limb length is measured from the greater trochanter to the plane of the sole of the foot (floor) (Fig. 8.34). Traditionally, in infants, leg length has been measured

**Figure 8.34**   Measuring total lower limb length.

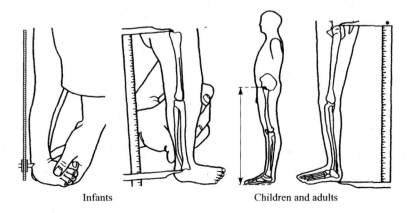

Infants                                   Children and adults

from the greater trochanter of the femur to the lateral malleolus of the ankle along the lateral aspect of the leg (total lower limb lengths are not available).

**Instruments**   Tape-measure or calipers.

**Position**   Infants may be measured lying supine or prone. Older children and adults are usually measured standing upright with the legs parallel.

**Alternative**   In Children and adults, lower limb length can be calculated from total body length by subtracting upper segment or sitting height, although this is not as accurate as direct measurement.

**Remarks**   By tradition leg length in infants is measured only to the ankle. The newborn graphs reflect that measurement rather than total lower limb length (Fig. 8.35). Values for older children are shown in Figs. 8.36 and 8.37.

In individuals with contractures or genu valgum or varum, the tape has to be worked along the leg to give an accurate estimate of total leg length.

X-ray measurements are more precise to assess bone length.

The highest point of the trochanter may be difficult to find in obese indi-, viduals. It then may be helpful to ask the patient to bend forward and thus estimate the trochanter point.

Lower limbs account for approximately one-third of length at birth; by five years, the lower limbs account for one-half of height, and by adulthood, more than one-half the total height.

**Pitfalls**   In infants the sum of the upper and lower leg measurements, as demonstrated in this book do not equal total limb measurement. Leg length is not equivalent to lower segment, which is measured from the pubis to the plane of the sole (i.e., floor).

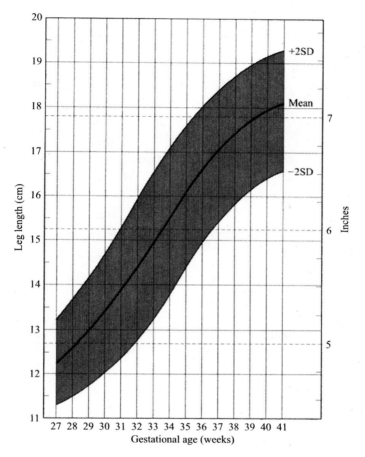

**Figure 8.35**  Leg length at birth. From Merlob et al. (1984b), by permission.

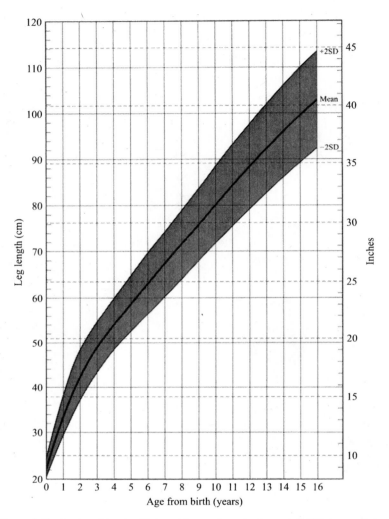

**Figure 8.36** Leg length, males, birth to 16 years. From Snyder et al. (1975), by permission.

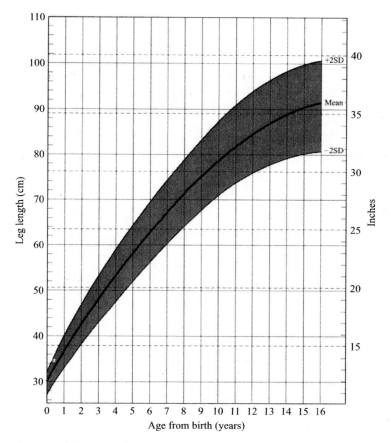

**Figure 8.37**    Leg length, females, birth to 16 years. From Snyder et al. (1975), by permission.

## Upper Leg (Thigh) Length

**Definition**   Total length of the upper leg.

**Landmarks**   Measure from the greater trochanter of the femur to the proximal lateral tibial condyle along the lateral aspect of the leg (Fig. 8.38).

**Instruments**   Tape-mesure or calipers.

**Position**   Patient can stand or be lying supine.

**Alternative**   X-ray measurements of the femur are more precise.

**Remarks**   When there is disproportion between the thighs, it is useful to measure circumference as well as length for documentation. X-ray measurements are more reliable when limb shortening or asymmetry is present. Normal values are presented in Figs. 8.39 and 8.40.

**Figure 8.38**   Measuring thigh length.

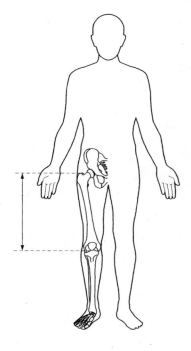

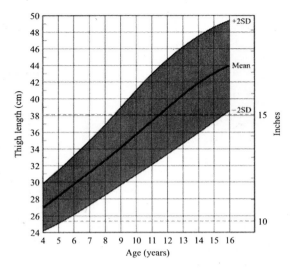

**Figure 8.39**  Upper leg length, males, 4 to 16 years. From Korgman (1970) and Roche and Malina (1983), by permission.

**Figure 8.40**  Upper leg length, females, 4 to 16 years. From Korgman (1970) and Roche and Malina (1983), by permission.

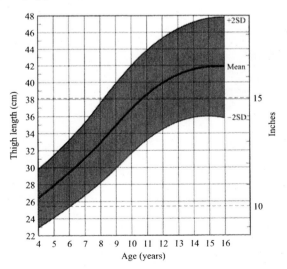

## Lower Leg (Calf) Length

**Definition**   Total length of the lower leg.

**Landmarks**   In children and adults, measure from the proximal lateral condyle of the tibia to a plane equivalent to the sole of the foot (floor) along the lateral aspect of the leg. In infants, the measurement is made from the lateral upper condyle of the tibia to the lateral malleolus of the ankle (Fig. 8.41).

**Instruments**   Tape-measure or calipers.

**Position**   Standing upright.

**Alternative**   The patient may be sitting or lying down.

**Remarks**   In individuals with contractures of the foot, it may be more accurate to use X-ray measurements. When there is discrepancy between the two legs, circumference should also be measured. Normal values are shown in Figs. 8.42–8.44.

**Figure 8.41**   Measuring calf length.

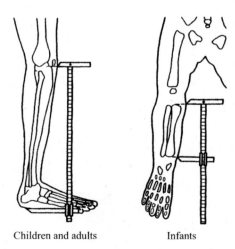

Children and adults          Infants

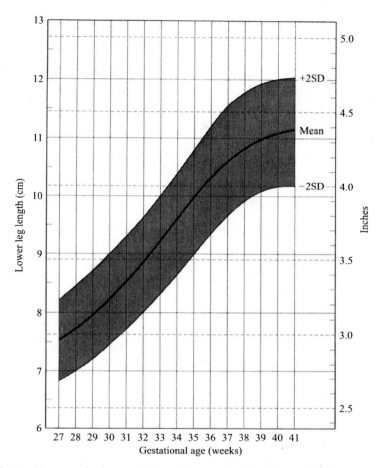

**Figure 8.42**    Lower leg length at birth, both sexes. From Merlob et al. (1984b), by permission.

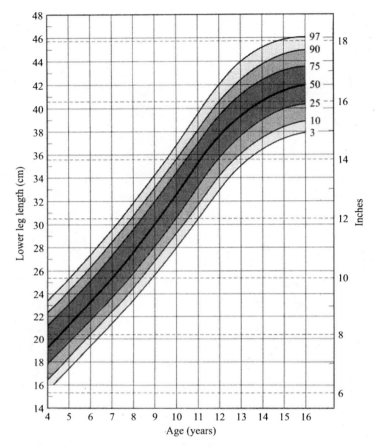

**Figure 8.43**  Lower leg length, males, 4 to 16 years. From Ròche and Malina (1983), by permission.

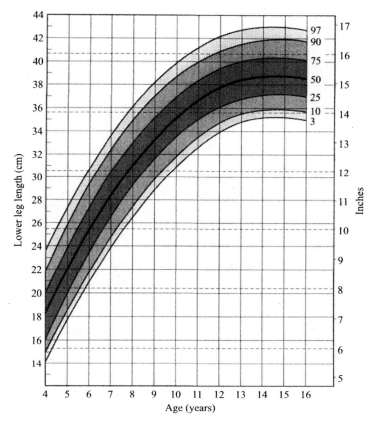

**Figure 8.44** Lower leg length, females, 4 to 16 years. From Roche and Malina (1983), by permission.

## Foot Length

**Definition**   Total length of foot.

**Landmarks**   Usually the foot length is the longest axis of the foot. It is measured from an imaginary vertical line drawn from the posterior prominence of the heel, to the tip of the longest toe, on the plantar aspect of the foot (in some people, the first toe is the longest; in other people, the second toe is the longest) (Fig. 8.45).

**Instruments**   Tape-measure or clear ruler.

**Position**   The length of the foot is easily and most accurately measured by standing the individual on a tape-measure.

**Alternative**   Measurement of the foot may also be taken with the patient in a relaxed sitting position or lying down. The ankle should be perpendicular to the foot. Draw around the foot and take the measurement between the tip of the longest toe and the edge of the prominence of the heel.

**Remarks**   In patients with contractures of the foot, the tape may be worked along the sole to give an estimate of the length. Values for foot length to age 16 years are presented in Figs. 8.46–8.48.

**Pitfalls**   In individuals with club-feet or very high arches, measurements may be distorted or difficult to obtain.

**Figure 8.45**   Measuring foot length.

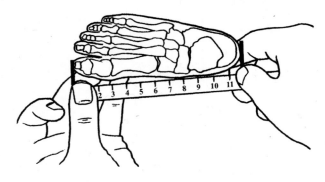

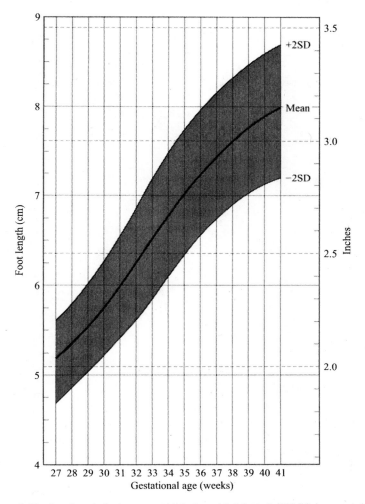

**Figure 8.46**   Foot length, both sexes, at birth. From Merlob et al. (1984b), by permission.

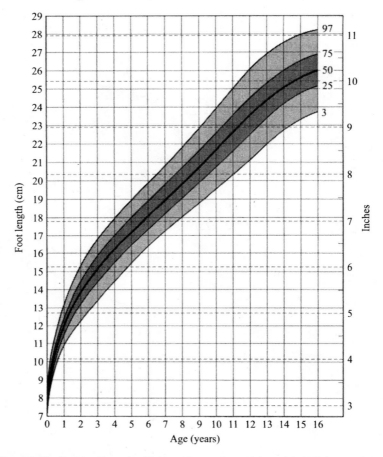

**Figure 8.47**  Foot length, males, birth to 16 years. From Blais et al. (1956), by permission.

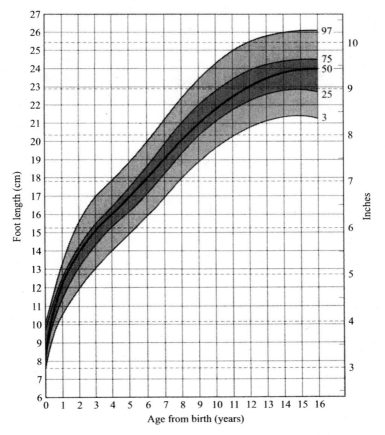

**Figure 8.48**  Foot length, females, birth to 16 years. From Blais et al. (1956), by permission.

## Foot Width

**Definition**   Total foot width at widest (broadest) point of the foot.

**Landmarks**   Measure between the medial prominence of the first metatarsophalangeal (MTP) joint and the lateral prominence of the fifth MTP joint of the foot. Measure on the plantar aspect (sole) of the foot (Fig. 8.49).

**Instruments**   Tape-measure, calipers, or clear ruler.

**Position**   Patients in a relaxed position, sitting, or lying down; however, foot width may be most easily measured with the individual standing on the tape-measure.

**Alternative**   Draw around the foot, marking the MTP joints, and measure between the markings.

**Remarks**   Normal values for males and females age 4–16 years are presented in Figs. 8.50 and 8.51.

**Figure 8.49**   Measuring foot width.

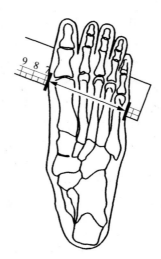

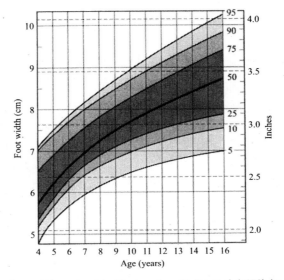

**Figure 8.50** Foot width, males, 4 to 16 years. From Malina et al. (1973), by permission.

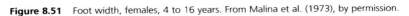

**Figure 8.51** Foot width, females, 4 to 16 years. From Malina et al. (1973), by permission.

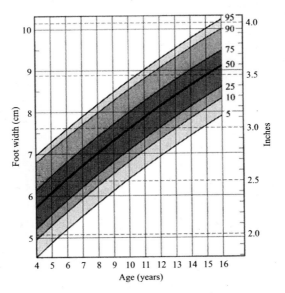

## Upper-to-Lower Segment Ratio

**Definition**   The ratio of the length of the upper part of the body to the length of the lower part of the body.

$$\frac{\text{Upper segment}}{\text{Lower segment}} = \frac{\text{Height} - \text{Lower segment}}{\text{Lower segment}}$$

**Landmarks**   The lower segment is measured from the top of the middle part of the public bone to the sole of the foot (Fig. 8.52). The upper segment is measured from the top of the middle part of the pubic bone to the top of the head. Upper segment and lower segment together equal total height.

**Instruments**   Tape-measure or calipers

**Position**   The individual is standing upright, and the top of the pubic bone is palpated.

**Remarks**   In infants the upper segment approximately equals the sitting height. In older children and adults, the lower segment can be measured and subtracted from the height to establish the upper segment length. Normal values for upper and lower segment lengths to age 16 years are shown in Figs. 8.53 and 8.54. The upper-to-lower segment ratio

**Figure 8.52**   Measuring the lower segment in infants (a) and adults (b).

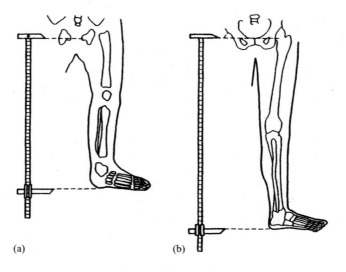

(a)                    (b)

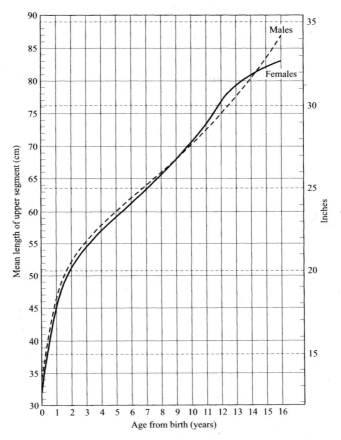

**Figure 8.53**  Upper segment length, both sexes, birth to 16 years. From Headings (1975), by permission.

decreases progressively during childhood. Adult males have smaller upper-to-lower segment ratios than females, since they generally have relatively longer legs.

Upper-to-lower segment ratios are useful in defining different forms of disproportionate growth and in distinguishing them from immaturity or retarded growth.

There are ethnic and family differences in the upper-to-lower segment ratio. As a generalization, the ratio is greater than 1.0 below age 10 years, 1.0 at 10 years at age, and less than 1.0 after age 10 years (Fig. 8.55).

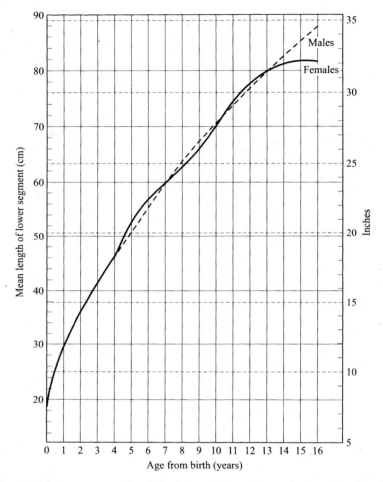

**Figure 8.54** Lower segment length, both sexes, birth to 16 years. From Headings (1975), by permission.

Asians have proportionately shorter legs, Caucasians intermediate lengths, and African Americans longer legs, in proportion to upper segment length (upper-to-lower segment ratio, 0.1–1.2 for Asians and 0.85–0.95 for African Americans). However, these data are not reflected in Fig. 8.56, because the lower segment was calculated as the difference between standing height and sitting height, rather than measured (Cheng et al. 1996).

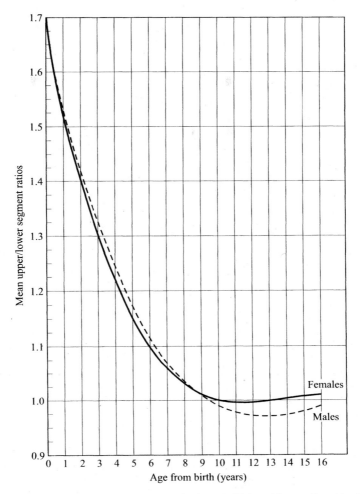

**Figure 8.55**   Upper-to-lower segment ratio, both sexes, birth to 16 years. From Headings (1975), by permission.

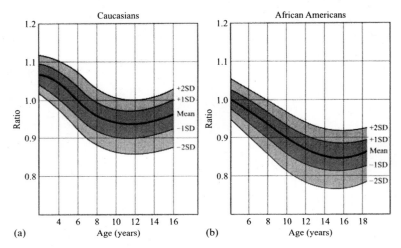

**Figure 8.56** Upper-to-lower segment ratios for Caucasians (a) and African Americans (b). Adapted from McKusick (1972).

*In the upper leg* (thigh) the widest point is usually just below the gluteal crease.

*In the lower leg* (calf) the widest point is in the mid-upper calf muscle.

**Pitfalls** If the individual bends forward to look at the measurement, this will result in falsely low measurements.

## Limb Circumference

**Definition** Circumference of a particular area of a limb, usually at the widest, largest, or maximum point.

**Landmarks** Circumference measurements are taken at the widest or largest diameter of the limb (Fig. 8.57) or from a fixed bony point (e.g., 10 cm distal to lower edge of the patella).

*In the upper arm* the widest point is at the middle of the biceps, just below the insertion of the deltoid.

**Instruments** Tape-measure.

**Position** When measuring for maximum circumference, the arm is slightly bent and the lower arm is supported so the muscle is not flexed. The tape-measure is moved up and down until it reaches the widest circumference.

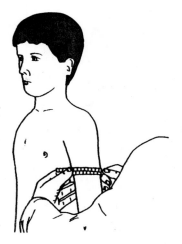 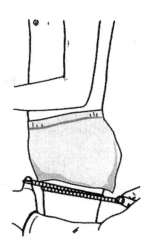

**Figure 8.57**  Measuring limb circumference.

Measurement of the leg for maximum circumference can be done with the patient either standing upright or lying down.

When measuring the circumference of a limb from a fixed point, palpate the point carefully or mark it with an ink pen, then record how far up or down from it the circumference measurement is taken in order to be consistent in subsequent measurements.

**Remarks**  Typical limb circumference values for ages 4–16 years are shown in Fig. 8.58. When limb length or circumference inequalities are present, it is particularly important to measure both sides in a reproducable way, since differential growth can be anticipated.

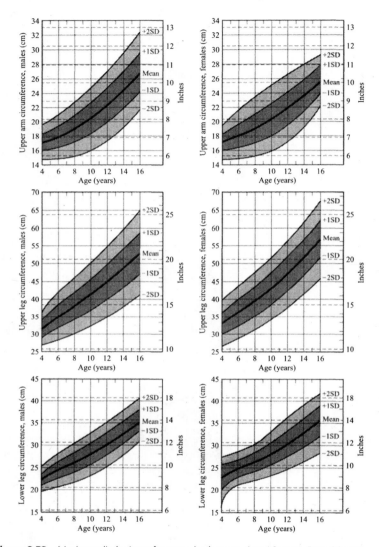

**Figure 8.58**  Maximum limb circumferences, both sexes, 4 to 16 years. From Maaser (1977), by permission.

## Range of Movement

### Introduction

Normal joints allow a range of purposeful movements as well as easy shifting from one position to another. They have active and passive ranges of movement or motion (ROM). In a healthy joint the active range of motion is almost as full as passive. If there are no major complaints or apparent limitations of movement, checking four important positions will provide rough estimates of the range of movement of the major joints (Fig. 8.59–8.62).

### Screening Positions

**Neutral position (general) (Fig. 8.59)**   The patient stands upright with the legs straight and parallel. The feet are together, the arms hanging down at the sides, with elbows, wrists, and fingers extended, and the palms of the hands facing forward. The back, knees, and trunk are straight. This position excludes limitation of full extension of the hips, knees, elbows, and wrists. It also indicates that the ankles, shoulders, and back can achieve a normal resting position.

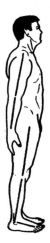

**Figure 8.59**   Range of movement—neutral position.

**Squatting position (Fig. 8.60)**   The patient is asked to sit on the calves and ankles, with hands folded behind the neck. This position excludes limitation of flexion of the knees or the ankle joints. It also demonstrates limitation of abduction or external rotation of the shoulder joint, limitation of flexion in the elbow joint, and limitation of pronation of the lower arms.

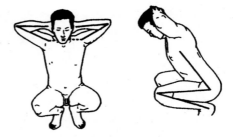

**Figure 8.60**   Range of motion—
squatting position.

**Shoulder and hip stretch position (Fig. 8.61)**   The patient is asked to stand with the legs apart and the backs of the hands held on the lower back. This position gives an estimate of abduction of the hips, internal rotation of the joints, and back flexibility.

**Figure 8.61**   Range of movement—shoulder
and hip stretch position.

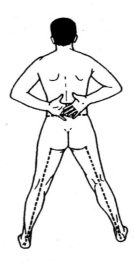

**Arm stretch position (Fig. 8.62)**   The patient is asked to stand with straight legs, turning toes inward, and to stretch the arms out to the side at shoulder level with the hands stretched out as far as possible, then to separate the fingers and rotate the hand into pronation, then to make a fist and rotate the forearm into supination. This position excludes forearm, wrist, and finger limitations. The position also evaluates hip adduction and internal rotation, and shoulder rotation. If the fingers easily reach the inner palm, there is no limitation of flexion in the finger joints.

**Figure 8.62**   Range of movement—arm stretch position.

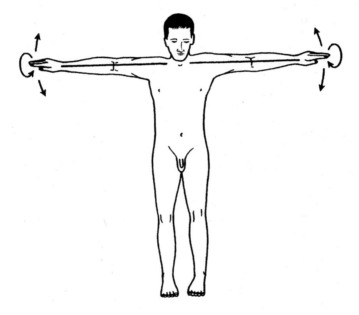

## Range of Movement

Measurements of ROM for specific joints are made from the neutral reference position. Obtain this position, then measure ROM of the various specific joints (Figs 8.63–8.68).

**Instruments**   A goniometer for measuring angles accurately (see Fig. 8.70).

**Remarks**   Newborns have mild limitation of ROM of most joints. Normally during infancy and childhood the ROM increases and is 5–10 degrees greater by puberty. With aging, the ROM of all joints decreases. Hyperextensible  joints are found in many conditions associated with connective tissue disturbances.

**Figure 8.63**   Normal range of motion of the shoulder joint.

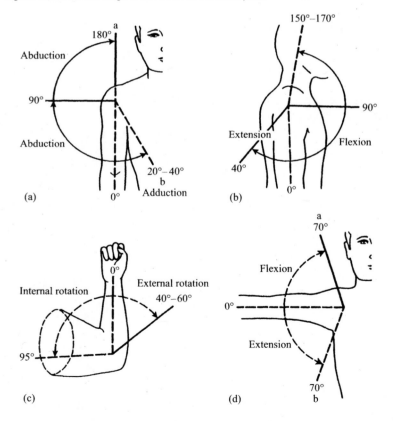

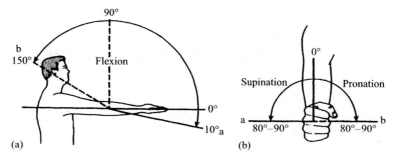

**Figure 8.64**  Normal range of motion of the elbow joint.

**Figure 8.65**  Normal range of motion of the wrist joint.

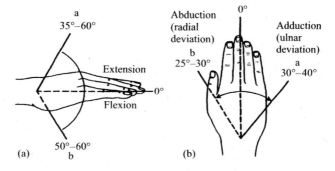

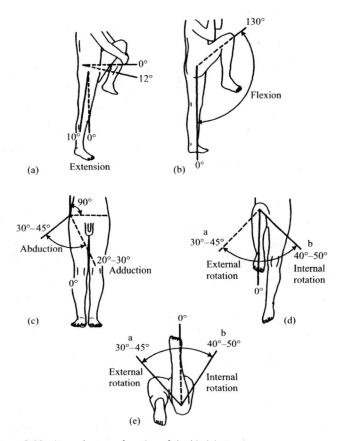

**Figure 8.66**   Normal range of motion of the hip joint.

**Figure 8.67**   Normal range of motion of the knee joint.

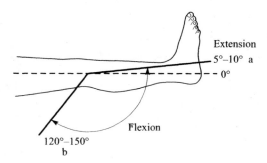

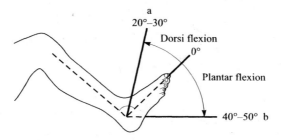

**Figure 8.68** Normal range of motion of the ankle joint.

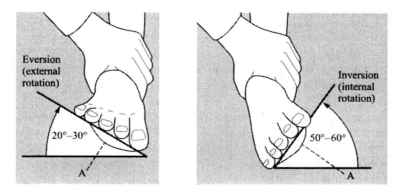

**Figure 8.69** Normal range of motion of the foot.

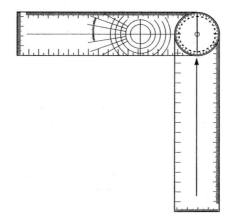

**Figure 8.70** Goniometer.

## Hyperextensibility

**Definition**   Greater range of motion of joints than normally seen for age.

**Diagnosis**   Determination of hypermobility in adults and adolescents can be assessed using the scale derived by Beighton and Wolf (Beighton et al., 1989). A score of 5/9 or greater defines hypermobility:

- Passive dorsiflexion of the little fingers beyond 90 degrees from the horizontal plane. One point for each hand.
- Passive apposition of the thumbs to the flexor aspect of the forearm. One point for each hand.
- Hyperextension of the elbows beyond 10 degrees. One point for each elbow.
- Hyperextension of the knees beyond 10 degrees. One point for each knee.
- Forward flexion of the trunk with knees fully extended so the palms of the hand rest flat on the floor. One point.

**Remarks**   Approximately 5 percent of the population is hyperextensible. More than twice as many females as males have increased range of motion of joints. Young children and adolescents seem particularly prone to hyperextensible joints and may develop arthralgias, particularly in the knees and fingers.

## Bibliography

Atkinson W.B. and Elftman, H. (1945). The carrying angle of the human arm as a secondary sex character. *Anatomical Record*, **91**, 49–52.

Baughman, F.A., Higgins, J.V., Wadsworth, T.G., and Demaray, M.J. (1974). The carrying angle in sex chromosome anomalies. *Journal of the American Medical Association*, **230**, 718–720.

Beals, R.K. (1976). The normal carrying angle of the elbow. *Clinical Orthopaedics and Related Research*, **119**, 194–196.

Beighton, P. Grahame, R. and Bird, H (1989). *Hypermobility of joints* (2nd ed.) London: Springer.

Belt-Niedbala, B.J., Ekvall, S., Cook, C.M., Oppenheimen, S., and Wessel, J. (1986). Linear measurement: A comparison of single arm-lengths and arm-span. *Develop Medicine and Child Neurology*, **28**, 319–324.

Bino, F., Gwanter, H.L., and Baum, J. (1983). The hypermobility syndrome. *Pediatrics*, **72**, 701–706.

Blais, M.M., Green, W.T., and Anderson, M. (1996). Length of the growing foot. *Journal of Bone and Joint Surgery*, **39A**, 998–1001.

Cheng, J.C.Y., Leung, S.S.F., and Lau, J. (1996) Anthropometric measurements and body proportions among Chinese children, *Clinical Orthopaedics and related Research*, **323**, 22–23.

Engelbach (1962). In *Growth and development of children* (4th ed). Year Book Medical Publishers, Chicago.

Feingold, M. and Bossert, W.H. (1974). Normal values for selected physical parameters: an aid to syndrome delineation. *Birth Defects: Original Article Series*, **X**, 13.

Frisancho, A.R. (1981). New norms of upper limb fat and muscle areas for assessment of nutritional status. *American Journal of Clinical Nutrition*, **34**, 2540–2545.

Headings, D.L. (ed.) (1975). *The Harriet Lane handbook* (7th ed). Year Book Medical Publishers, Chicago.

Krogman, W.M. (1983). In *Manual of physical status and performance in childhood, Vol. 1B* (ed. A.F. Roche and R.M. Malina), p.1010. Plenum Press, New York.

Maaser, R. (1977). In *Wachstum Atlas* (ed. R. Bergmann, K. Bergmann, F. Kollmann, F. Kollmann, R. Maaser, and O. Hoevels), pp. 67–71. Papillon, Wiesbaden,

Malina, R.M., Hamill, P.V.V., and Lemeshow, S. (1973). In *Manual of physical status and performance in childhood, Vol. 1B* (ed. A.F. Roche, and R.M. Malina), pp.1048–1056. Plenum Press, New York.

Martin, R. and Saller K. (1962). *Lehrbuch der Anthropologie*, Gustave Fischer, Stuttgart, Germany.

McKusick, V.A. (1972). *Heritable disorders of connective tissue* (4th ed). Mosby, St Louis.

Meredith, H.V. (1955). In *Manual of physical status and performance in childhood, Vol. 1B* (ed. A.R. Roche and R.M. Malina). Plenum Press, New York.

Merlob, P., Sivan, Y., and Reisner, S.H. (1984a). Anthropometric measurements of the newborn infant 27 to 41 gestational weeks. *Birth Defects: Original Article Series*, **20**, 7.

Merlop, P., Sivan, Y., and Reisner, S.H. (1984b). Lower limb standards in newborns. *American Journal of Diseases in childhood*, **138**, 140–142.

Merlob, P. Mimouni, F., Rosen, O., and Reisner, S.H. (1984c). Assessment of thumb placement. *Pediatrics*, **74**, 299–300.

Reinken, L., Stolley, H., Droese, W., and van Oost, G. (1980). Longitudinale Koerperentwicklung gesunder Kinder. *Klinische Paediatrie*, **192**, 551–558.

Roche, A.F. and Malina, R.M. (1983). *Manual of physical status and performance in childhood, Vol. 1B*, pp. 1008–1012. Plenum Press, New York.

Russe, H.O., Gerhard, J.J., and King, P.S. (1972). An atlas of examination. Standard measurements and diagnosis in ortopedics and traumatology (ed. O. Russe). Hans Huber Publishers, Bern, Switzerland.

Sivan, Y., Merlob, P., and Reisner, S.H. (1983). Upper limb standards in newborns. *American Journal of Diseases in Childhood*, **137**, 829–832.

Snyder, R.G., Spencer, M.L., Owings, C.L., and Schneider, L.W. (1975). In *Manual of physical status and performance in childhood, Vol. 1B* (ed. A.F. Roche, and R.M. Malina), pp. 999, 1105. Plenum Press, New York.

Usher, R. and McLean, F. (1969). Intrauterine growth of live-born Caucasian infants at sea level: standards obtained from measurements in 7 dimensions of infants born between 25 and 44 weeks of gestation. *Journal of Pediatrics*, **74**, 901–910.

# Chest and Trunk

## Introduction

Disturbance of growth of the chest and trunk may lead to disproportion of the body in much the same way as disproportion can be produced by disturbance of limb growth. In addition, disturbed growth of the chest may affect the relationship between the sternum and ribs (sternocostal relationship), producing a variety of pectus deformities and possibly compromising respiratory function.

The ribs develop from the mesenchymal costal processes of the thoracic vertebrae. They become cartilaginous during the embryonic period and later ossify. The original union of the costal process with the vertebra is replaced by a synovial joint. The sternum develops from a pair of mesenchymal sternal bands, which at first are widely separated, and develop ventrolaterally in the body wall, independently of the developing ribs. Chondrification occurs in these bands to form two sternal plates, one on each side of the median plane. The cranial six costal cartilages become attached to them. The plates gradually fuse craniocaudally in the median plane to form cartilaginous models of the manubrium, the sternebrae or segments of the sternal body, and the xiphoid process.

Centers of ossification appear craniocaudally before birth, except for the xiphoid process center of ossification, which appears during childhood.

The development of the vertebral column begins with a precartilaginous stage during the fourth week of gestation. Cells from the sclerotomes of the somites are found in three main areas. First, surrounding the notochord, some of the densely packed cells give rise to the intervertebral disc. The remaining densely packed cells fuse with the loosely arranged cells of the immediately caudal sclerotome to form the mesenchymal centrum of a vertebra. Thus, each centrum develops from two adjacent sclerotomes and becomes an intersegmental structure. The notochord degenerates and disappears where it is surrounded by the developing vertebral body. Between the vertebrae the notochord expands to form the gelatinous center of the intervertebral disc, called the nucleus pulposus. This nucleus is later surrounded by the circularly arranged fibers of the annulus fibrosus.

Second, cells of the sclerotomes of the somites surround the neural tube and later form the vertebral arch. Third, cells from the sclerotomes of the somites are found in the body wall and form the costal processes, which develop into ribs in the thoracic region. During the sixth week, chondrification centers appear in each mesenchymal vertebra. Ossification begins during the embryonic period and ends at about the 25th year. Malformations of the axial skeleton include spina bifida occulta, rachischisis, accessory or fused ribs, hemivertebrae, and cleft sternum.

Abnormalities of the back may result from congenital malformations of the spine, such as hemivertebrae, or from muscular imbalance, abnormalities of the pelvis, leg length discrepancy, or unusual posture, resulting in lordosis, kyphosis, scoliosis, or a combination of these three.

The appendicular skeleton consists of the pectoral and pelvic girdles and the limb bones. Details of limb bone embryology will not be presented here. The clavicle initially develops by intra-membranous ossification, but it later develops growth cartilages at both ends. The clavicles begin to ossify before any other bones in the body. Formation of the pectoral girdle and the pelvic girdle from the upper and lower limb buds respectively is detailed in Chapter 8.

At about 22 days of gestation, folding of the sides of the embryo produces right and left lateral folds. Each lateral body wall or somatopleure folds toward the midline, rolling the edges of the embryonic disk ventrally and forming a roughly cylindrical embryo. As the lateral and ventral body walls form, part of the yolk sac is incorporated into the embryo as the midgut. After folding, the region of attachment of the amnion to the embryo is reduced to the relatively narrow region—the umbilicus—on the ventral surface. Faulty closure of the lateral body folds during the fifth week produces a large defect in the anterior abdominal wall and results in most of the abdominal viscera developing outside the embryo in a transparent sac of amnion (an omphalocoele). Normally, after the intestines return from the umbilical cord, the rectus muscles approach each other and the linea alba, closing the circular defect. An umbilical hernia differs from an omphalocoele in that the protruding mass is covered by subcutaneous tissue and skin rather than a sac of amnion. The hernia usually does not reach its maximum size until the end of the first month after birth. The defect through which the hernia occurs is in the linea alba.

Gastroschisis is another abdominal wall defect; it is usually sporadic and present as an isolated birth defect. Gastroschisis is a congenital fissure of the abdominal wall. It is most likely caused by a vascular disruption, but primary incomplete folding and formation of the anterior abdominal wall or secondary rupture of the wall have also been proposed. It does not involve the site of insertion of the umbilical cord and usually is accompanied by protrusion of the small intestine and part of the large intestine.

Much information can be obtained about prenatal development by examination of the umbilical cord. The attachment of the umbilical cord is usually near the center of the placenta, but it may be found at any point. As the amniotic sac enlarges, the amnion ensheathes the umbilical cord, forming the cord's epithelial coverings. The umbilical cord usually contains two arteries and one vein surrounded by mucoid connective tissue often called Wharton's jelly. Because the umbilical vessels are longer than the cord, twisting and bending of the vessels is common. The vessels frequently form loops, producing so-called false knots that are of no significance. The umbilical cord is usually 1–2 cm in diameter and 30–90 cm in length (average 55 cm). Growth of the umbilical cord slows after the 28th week of gestation but does not stop before term.

**Figure 9.1** Trunk landmarks.

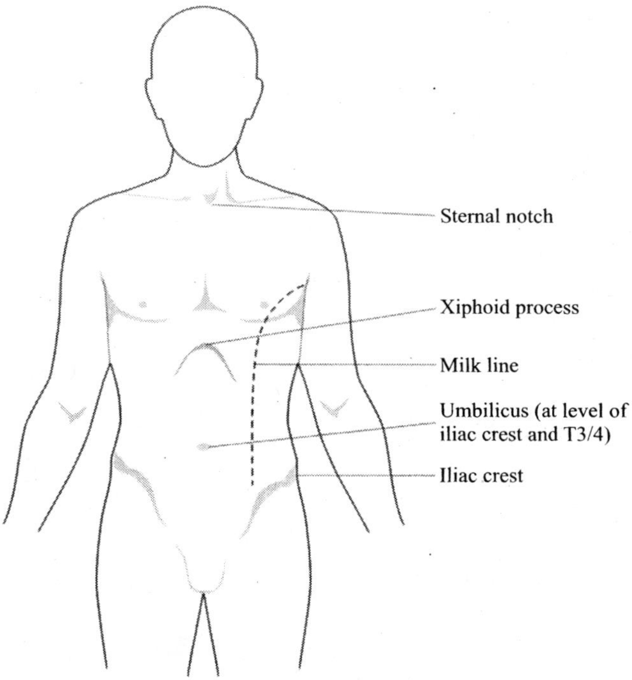
Sternal notch
Xiphoid process
Milk line
Umbilicus (at level of
iliac crest and T3/4)
Iliac crest

Cord length correlates positively with maternal height, pre-gravid weight, pregnancy weight gain, socioeconomic status, and a male fetus. The finding of a short umbilical cord suggests diminished fetal movement and may be associated with subsequent psychomotor abnormalities. A single umbilical artery is present in approximately 0.5 percent of placentas examined. The presence of a single umbilical artery is thought to correlate with an increased incidence of congenital anomalies. Further details of placental pathology are found in Chapter 16.

Breast development, variation, and measurements are discussed in Chapter 10.

Inspection of the chest should answer the following questions:

1. Is it symmetric?
2. Is one side flatter than the other?
3. What is the shape of the rib cage?
4. Is there evidence for pectus excavatum or pectus carinatum?
5. Is the scapula normal in size and position?
6. Is the scapula elevated (Sprengel's deformity)?
7. Is the spine straight?
8. Is there any evidence for kyphosis, scoliosis, or lordosis?
9. Are the nipples normal?
10. Are they inverted?
11. Are accessory nipples present?
12. Is the umbilicus normal in shape and position?

Examination of the breasts is discussed in Chapter 10. Examination of the genitalia is discussed in Chapter 10. Examination of the skin is described in Chapter 11. Examination of the umbilical cord and umbilical cord length in the newborn is described in Chapter 16.

Following inspection, detailed measurements using the charts in the following pages for comparison should be performed. A glossary of terms used to define specific anomalies of the chest and trunk is included at the end of the book.

## Chest Circumference

**Definition**   Circumference of chest.

**Landmarks**   Measure horizontally around the upper body at the level of the nipples or at the level just below the scapular angles Fig. 9.2. In the postpubertal female, measure just below the breasts.

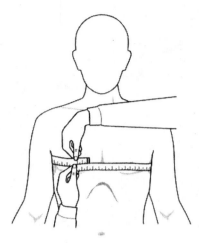

**Figure 9.2**   Measuring chest circumference.

**Instruments**   Tape-measure.

**Position**   The patient should stand upright with the arms down at the sides. The measurement should be made during mid-expiration. Infants should be measured lying supine, in mid-expiration.

**Alternative**   Measure at the nipple line, or in adults 10 cm down from the clavicles or 5 cm down from the apex of the axilla.

**Remarks**   Chest circumference values are presented in Figs. 9.3 and 9.4. With inhalation or exhalation, the chest circumference can change. There is some value in measuring at maximum inhalation in conditions with contractures in order to get some sense of the lung volume.

Between 2 and 16 years of age, the chest circumference increases as much as 40 cm; a "growth spurt" occurs between 12 and 15 years of ages.

**Pitfalls**   In females, it is important to make sure that the measurement excludes the breast tissue. In Noonan syndrome, the nipples tend to slip down, so the landmark for chest circumference needs to be related to a line 10 cm below clavicles, or at the fourth intercostal space.

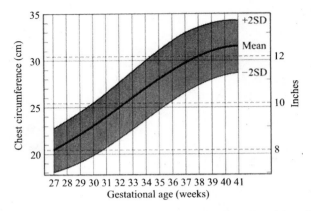

**Figure 9.3**   Chest circumference, both sexes, at birth. From Merlob et al. (1984), by permission.

**Figure 9.4**   Chest circumference, both sexes, birth to 16 years. From Feingold and Bossert (1974), by permission.

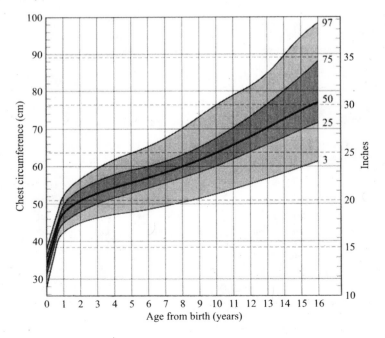

## Internipple Distance

**Definition**   Distance between the centers of both nipples.

**Landmarks**   Measure between the centers of both nipples (Fig. 9.5).

**Instruments**   Tape-measure.

**Position**   The patient stands upright, with the arms down at the sides; measure during mid-expiration. Infants should be measured lying supine during mid-expiration.

**Remarks**   Internipple distance cannot be measured from pictures. With inspiration and expiration the value will change, so two measurements, both taken during mid-expiration, are desirable. Values for children to age 16 years are shown in Figs. 9.6 and 9.7.

**Pitfalls**   In women with moderate to large breasts, the position of the nipples is variable, distorting this measurement.

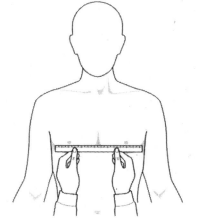

**Figure 9.5**   Measuring internipple distance.

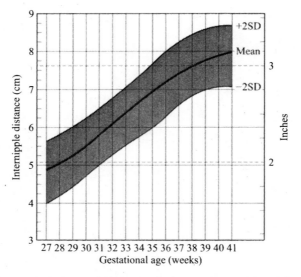

**Figure 9.6**  Internipple distance, both sexes, at birth. From Sivan et al. (1983), by permission.

**Figure 9.7**  Internipple distance, both sexes, birth to 16 years. From Feingold and Bossert (1974), by permission.

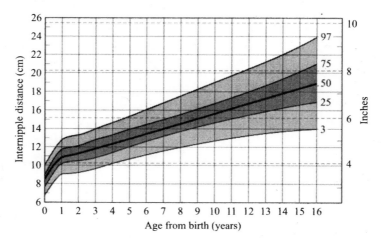

## Thoracic Index

**Definition**   Ratio of the anteroposterior diameter of the chest to the lateral diameter (chest width) multiplied by 100.

**Landmarks**   Anteroposterior diameter is measured (Fig. 9.8a) from the sternum, at the level of the nipples, to the vertebrae, at the same level, while at rest. Lateral diameter is measured between the midaxillary lines at the level of the nipples (Fig. 9.8b)

**Instruments**   Calipers.

**Position**   The patient should be standing with the arms hanging loosely at the sides; the measurement is made during mid-expiration.

**Alternative**   If calipers are not available, the patient can be placed against a wall, facing sideways and forward for each measurement, respectively, while the boundaries of the thoracic cage, at the nipple level, are marked on the wall. The marks are then measured with a measuring tape.

**Remarks**   Timing of respiration is important for accuracy of this measurement. Mid-expiration is the position of rest (prior to forced expiration). Ideally each measurement should be obtained twice. Thoracic diameters anteroposterior and lateral are shown in Fig 9.9, and values for the thoracic index in Fig. 9.10.

**Figure 9.8**   Measuring anteroposterior (a) and lateral (b) chest diameters.

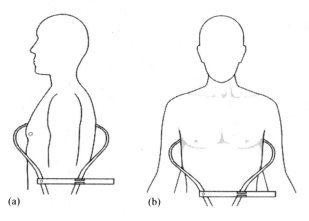

(a)                              (b)

**Pitfalls**  Variation in the body chest cage will distort the thoracic index. Pectus carinatum, or the barrel chest of an asthmatic, will lead to an increased value. Pectus excavatum will reduce the value. Hypotonia will also produce a reduced anteroposterior diameter.

In women the position of the nipples is extremely variable. This is less important in a ratio than in an absolute measurement. The fourth intercostal space can be used as an alternative landmark, or one can measure 10 cm down from the clavicles.

**Figure 9.9**  Thoracic diameters, both sexes, birth to 16 years. From Pryor (1966), by permission.

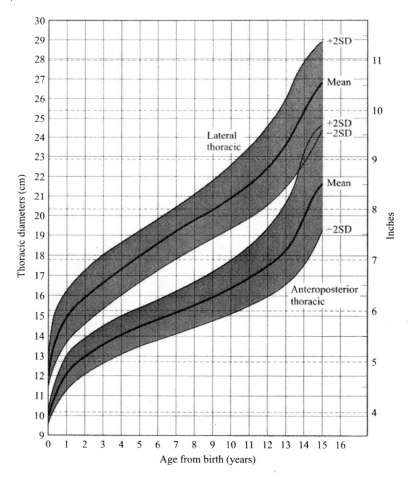

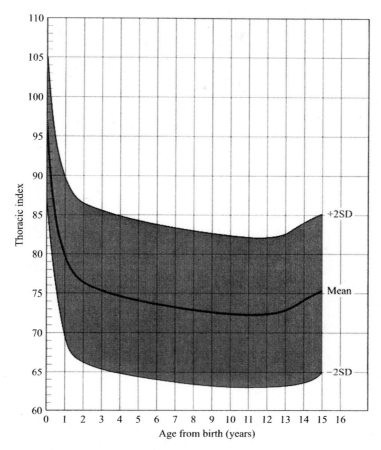

**Figure 9.10** Thoracic index, both sexes, birth to 16 years. From Feingold and Bossert (1974), by permission.

## Sternal Length

**Definition**  Length of the sternum.

**Landmarks**  Measure from the top of the manubrium to the lowest palpable edge of the sternum (Fig. 9.11).

**Instruments**  Tape-measure.

**Position**  Patient should be standing upright. Infants should be measured lying supine.

**Alternative**  Patient may be recumbent.

**Remarks**  Normal values are presented in Figs. 9.12 and 9.13. Longitudinal overgrowth of the ribs produces an anterior chest deformity, either depression (pectus excavatum) or protrusion (pectus carinatum). Both defects may be present in the same patient.

**Pitfalls**  The presence of a pectus deformity will distort the linear distance unless the tape is worked along the sternum in contact with the surface of the skin.

**Figure 9.11**  Measuring sternal length.

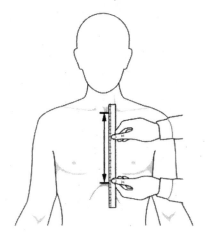

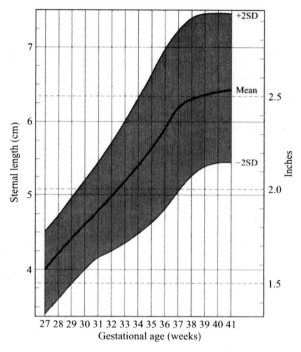

**Figure 9.12** Sternal length, both sexes, at birth. From Sivan et al. (1983), by permission.

**Figure 9.13** Sternal length, both sexes, birth to 13 years. From Feingold and Bossert (1974), by permission.

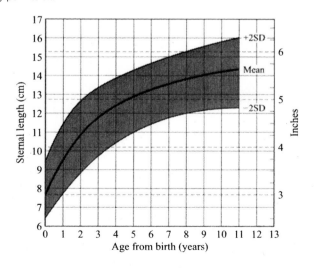

## Torso Length

**Definition**   Length from the top of the sternum to the top of the symphysis pubis.

**Landmarks**   Measure from the manubrial notch to the superior border of the symphysis pubis, defined by palpation, in the midsagittal plane (Fig. 9.14).

**Instruments**   Tape-measure.

**Position**   The patient should be standing upright, at rest, with the back straight and the shoulders back. The infant should be lying supine with legs extended.

**Alternative**   The patient may be supine, with legs extended.

**Remarks**   Spinal deformities, such as kyphosis or scoliosis, will reduce the torso length. Values for torso length at birth are presented in Fig. 9.15.

**Pitfalls**   The presence of sternal and vertebral anomalies should be disregarded in making this linear measurement. In contrast to measurement of the sternum, the tape should *not* be worked along the bony landmarks when pectus excavatum is present, but should be stretched between the two points of reference.

**Figure 9.14**   Measuring torso length.

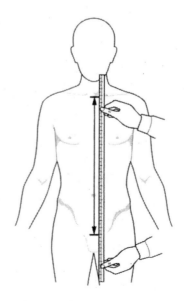

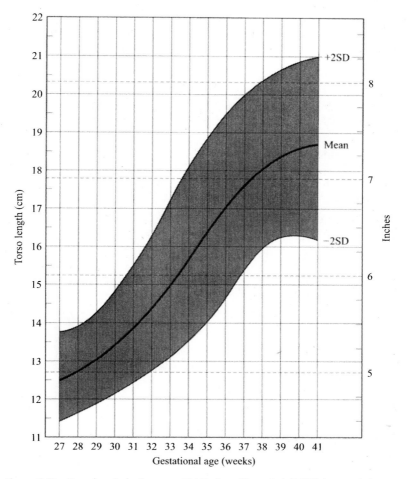

**Figure 9.15** Torso length, both sexes, at birth. From Sivan et al. (1983), by permission.

## Biacromial Distance

**Definition**  Maximum distance between the right and left acromion (shoulder width).

**Landmarks**  The spine of the scapula projects laterally and superiorly over the shoulder joint to form the acromion. The acromion articulates anteriorly with the clavicle. The acromion is the most lateral bony projection of the shoulder girdle and should be easily palpable. Measure between the right and left acromion across the back (Fig. 9.16).

**Instruments**  Tape-measure, or calipers.

**Position**  The patient should stand upright, hands at the sides, with the shoulders in a neutral position. The measurement is taken from behind. The infant can be seated, or lying face down, for measurement.

**Alternative**  The patient can sit or lie face down.

**Remarks**  The biacromial distance, like the bi-iliac distance, is a useful measurement of trunk width. However, there is greater variation in biacrominal distance than in bi-iliac distance between the sexes. Values for males and females to age 19 years are presented in Figs. 9.17 and 9.18.

**Pitfalls**  Abnormalities of the serratus anterior muscle causing a "winged scapula", or neuromuscular disease, may "round" the shoulders, increasing the biacromial distance. If the shoulders cannot be drawn back into a reasonable posture, the measurement should be made using calipers instead of a tape-measure.

**Figure 9.16**  Measuring biacromial distance.

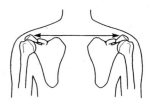 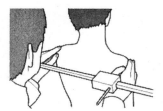

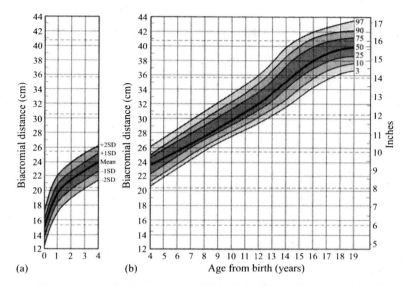

**Figure 9.17** (a) Biacromial distance, males, birth to 4 years. From Maaser (1977), Demirjian and Jenickek (1983), Roche and Malina (1983), and Feingold and Bossert (1974), by permission. (b) Biacromial distance, males, 4 to 19 years. From Maaser (1977), Demirjian and Jenickek (1983), Roche and Malina (1983), and Feingold and Bossert (1974), by permission.

**Figure 9.18** (a) Biacromial distance, females, birth to 4 years. From Maaser (1977), Demirjian and Jenickek (1983), Roche and Malina (1983), and Feingold and Bossert (1974), by permission. (b) Biacromial distance, females, 4 to 19 years. From Maaser (1977), Demirjian and Jenickek (1983), Roche and Malina (1983), and Feingold and Bossert (1974), by permission.

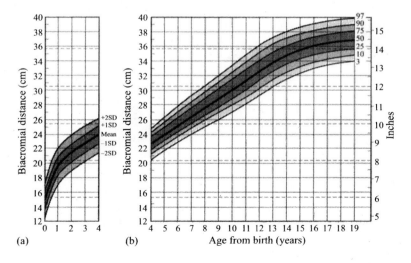

## Bi-Iliac Distance

**Definition** Distance between the most prominent lateral points of the iliac crest.

**Landmarks** Palpate the iliac crest to define its widest flare. Measure between the right and left points, from the front, using firm pressure to get as near as possible to a skeletal measurement (Fig. 9.19).

**Instruments** Calipers. A tape-measure may be used if calipers are unavailable, but the measurement is less accurate.

**Position** The patient should be standing upright. The infant should be lying supine with legs extended.

**Alternative** The patient may be lying supine with legs extended.

**Remarks** Normal values are presented in Figs. 9.20 and 9.21. In the patient with a skeletal dysplasis, pelvic anatomy may be distorted, and comparison with normal curves is less meaningful. The bi-iliac distance is considered the most important of the transverse distances because it is the best indicator of the width of the trunk, it is not variable with posture or respiration, and the land-marks are very definite. The bi-iliac distance is similar in males and females at any given age. Variation in hip width reflects soft tissue, not bony, differences between the sexes.

**Pitfalls** The most prominent lateral point of the iliac crest must be located precisely. If a tape-measure is used, the measurement may be distorted by abdominal protrusion.

**Figure 9.19** Measuring bi-iliac distance.

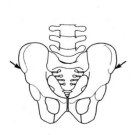
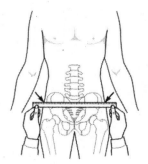

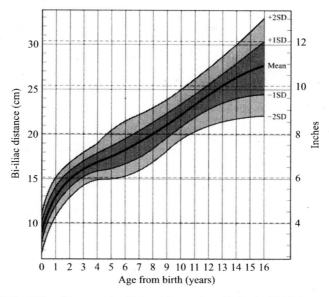

**Figure 9.20**   Bi-iliac distance, males, birth to 16 years. From Thelander (1966), by permission.

**Figure 9.21**   Bi-iliac distance, females, birth to 16 years. From Thelander (1966), by permission.

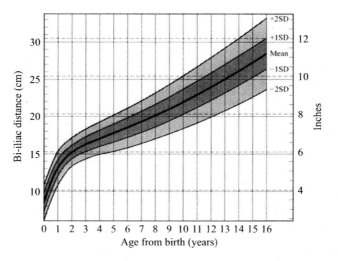

## Umbilical Cord Length

**Definition**   Length of the umbilical cord.

**Landmarks**   The umbilical cord should be measured from its attachment to the placenta to the trunk of the newborn infant.

**Instruments**   Tape-measure.

**Remarks**   The segments attached to the baby and placenta are measured and results added. Any part that has been cut out is also measured and added to give the total cord length.

The normal anatomy of the umbilicus is shown in Fig. 9.22. Normal values for umbilical cord length are shown in Fig. 9.23.

**Pitfalls**   In the presence of a supercoiled cord, once the cord is cut it should assume its true configuration, and stretching the cord will not be necessary.

**Figure 9.22**   Normal anatomy of umbilicus.

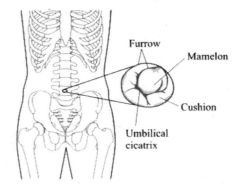

Furrow

Mamelon

Cushion

Umbilical cicatrix

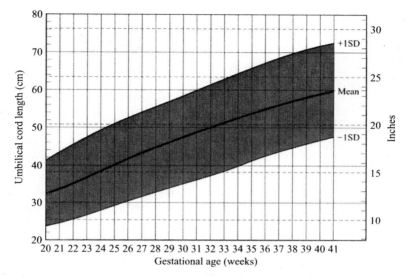

**Figure 9.23**   Umbilical cord length, both sexes, at birth. From Naeye (1985), by permission.

## Bibliography

Altshuler, G., Tsang, R.C., and Ermocilla, R. (1975). Single umbilical artery: correlation of clinical status and umbilical cord histology. *American Journal of Diseases in Children*, **129**, 697–700.

Demirjian and Jenickek (1983). In Roche and Malina. *Manual of physical status and performance in childhood. Vol. 1 B. Physical status*. Plenum Press, New York.

Feingold, M. and Bossert, W.H. (1974). Normal values for selected physical parameters: an aid to syndrome delineation. *Birth Defects: Original Articles Series*, **X(13)**, 1–15.

Maaser, R. (1977). In Bermann, R. Bergmann, K., Kollman, F., Maaser, R., and Hovels, D. *Wachstum atlas*. Papillon, Weisbaden, Germany.

Merlob, P., Sivan, Y., and Reisner, S.H. (1984). Anthropometric measurements of the newborn infant 27 to 41 gestational weeks. *Birth Defects: Original Article series*, **20**, 7.

Moore, K.L. (1982). *The developing human* (3rd ed). W.B. Saunders, Philadelphia.

Naeye, R.L. (1985). Umbilical cord length: clinical significance. *Journal of Pediatrics*, **107**, 278–281.

Pryor, H.B. (1966). Charts of normal body measurements and revised width weight tables in graphic form. *Journal of Pediatrics*, **68**, 615.

Roche, A.F. and Malina, R.M. (1983). *Manual of physical status and performance in childhood, Vol 1 B*, pp. 1008–1012. Plenum Press, New York.

Sivan, Y., Merlob, P., and Reisner, S.H. (1983). Sternum length, torso length, and internipple distance in newborn infants. *Pediatrics*, **72**, 523–525.

Thelander, H.E. (1966). Abnormal patterns of growth and development in mongolism. An anthropometric study. *Clinical pediatrics*, **5**, 493.

# Genitalia

10

## Introduction

### Prenatal Development

The first factor determining sexual differentiation during embryologic development is chromosomal sex. This is determined by which sex chromosome is present in the fertilizing sperm. The reproductive system develops from a common undifferentiated primordium. The primitive gonad has the potential to form either testis from its medullary portion or ovary from its cortical portion. The influence of a gene(s) on the Y chromosome (SRY), interacting with a gene(s) on the autosomes (SOX9, SF1, WT1, and others), determines that the medullary portion of the undifferentiated primordial gonad will develop into seminiferous tubules, which become recognizable between seven and eigth weeks of gestation. Absence of the testicular differentiating genes or a disturbance in the timing of various interactions will result in differentiation of the primordial gonad into an ovary. Recognition of ovarian tissue occurs by the 10th week of gestation. Even though early ovarian differentiation can take place when only one X chromosome is present, a second X chromosome is necessary for the complete development and maintenance of ovarian tissue. In Turner syndrome, where all or part of one X chromosome is missing, degeneration of some of the ovarian structures usually occurs before birth.

The second factor in sex differentiation is the gonadal sex. At about seven weeks of gestation, the testes in the male begin to secrete androgens which induce the development of the male internal ductal and genital structures, the epididymis, ductus deferens, and seminal vesicles from the Wolffian ducts. In the male, the structures of the Müllerian ducts degenerate under the influence of the nonsteroidal Müllerian inhibitory factor, which is secreted by the embryonic testes starting at about eight weeks of gestation. Inadequate production of androgens in a male fetus results in degeneration of the Wolffian ducts and Wolffian duct structures. Absence of Müllerian inhibitory factor results in Müllerian structures being present in the male. In the female fetus, the Müllerian duct differentiates autonomously into the fallopian tube, uterus, and proximal vagina. In the female, the Wolffian duct structures degenerate because of the lower level of androgen present.

In the male, under the influence of circulating androgens, the urogenital folds fuse to form a urethra, and the penis is formed by the growth of the genital tubercle (Fig. 10.1). The labioscrotal swellings develop into the scrotum, and the testes descend into the inguinal canal at about six months of gestation. Shortly before birth the testes enter the scrotum under the influence of gonadotropin stimulation. Failure of the testes to descend into the scrotum is called cryptorchidism and may be unilateral or bilateral. The internal ductal structures develop from the same primordia as the urinary tract. In the presence of androgens, the prostate gland develops from the vesicourethral canal.

In the female fetus, the clitoris (Fig. 10.1) develops from the genital tubercle; the urogenital groove remains open; the urogenital folds develop

**Figure 10.1**    Differentiation of external genitalia in the human fetus.

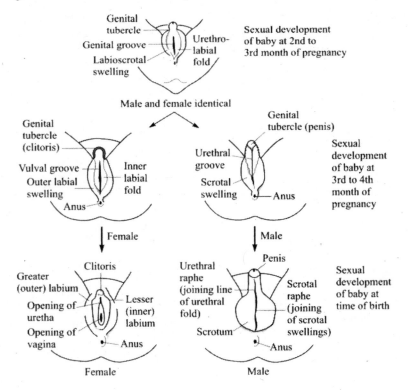

into the labia minora and the distal part of the vagina under the influence of estrogen; and the labioscrotal swellings form the labia majora.

There are many causes of aberrant sexual development, including prenatal hormonal disturbance or imbalance, absent cellular response to androgen or estrogen, chromosomal anomalies, and gene mutations.

## Puberty

In the early stages of male puberty, the testicles and adrenal glands synthesize increasing amounts of androgens, which stimulate the growth of the penis and scrotum; intiate the appearance of pubic, axillary, facial, and body hair; lead to the development of apocrine sweat glands; accelerate growth and maturation of the skeleton; and increase the muscle mass. Testicular growth antedates penile growth by 6 to 12 months. Enlarging testicular volume and the subsequent testicular sensitivity to pressure are the first signs of puberty in males.

In female puberty, estrogens produced by the ovary stimulate growth of the breast, uterus, fallopian tubes, and vagina. Androgens produced by the adrenal gland stimulate the growth of pubic and axillary hair, linear growth, and skeletal maturation. Apocrine sweating is usually the first sign of puberty in females.

## Stages of Puberty (Tanner Stages)

To assess how far an individual has progressed through puberty, a rating scale that describes the successive stages of growth of the genitalia and pubic hair in boys and breast development and pubic hair development in girls was introduced by Tanner (Fig. 10.2). The stage of development in the individual is compared with visual standards which are referred to as G-1 to G-5 for male genitalia development, B-1 to B-5 for breast development, and PH-1 to PH-5 for pubic hair development. The sequence and timing of stages is illustrated in Fig. 10.3.

(a)

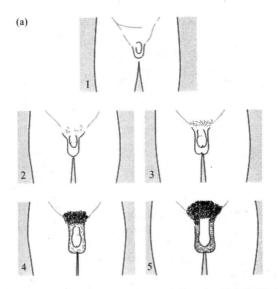

**Figure 10.2(a)** Male genital development (G-1 to G-5) and pubic hair (PH-1 to PH-5). Tanner stages. From Tanner (1975), by permission.

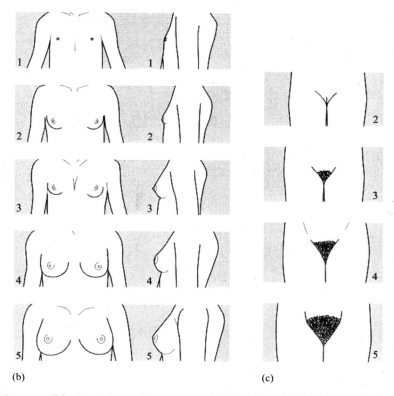

**Figure 10.2(b)**   Female breast development (B-1–B-5) and (c) pubic hair (PH-2 to PH-5). Tanner stages. From Tanner (1975), by permission.

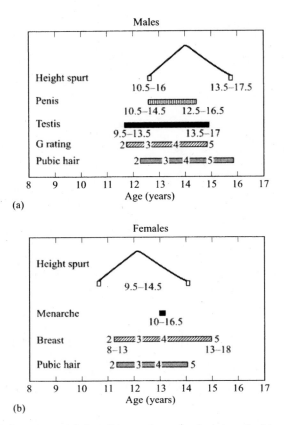

**Figure 10.3** Sequence and timing of Tanner stages of puberty in males (a), and females (b). From Tanner (1975), by permission.

**Fig. 10.3(c)**   Means and standard deviations in the timing of stages of puberty

| Stage | Mean age of onset ± 2 SD (yr) | Stage | Time between stages (yr) Mean | Percentile 5th | 95th |
|---|---|---|---|---|---|
| **Males** | | | | | |
| G-2 | 11.6 ± 2.1 | G2–G3 | 1.1 | 0.4 | 2.2 |
| G-3 | 12.9 ± 2.1 | PH2–PH3 | 0.5 | 0.1 | 1.0 |
| PH-2 | 13.4 ± 2.2 | G3–G4 | 0.8 | 0.2 | 1.6 |
| G-4 | 13.8 ± 2.0 | PH3–PH4 | 0.4 | 0.3 | 0.5 |
| PH-3 | 13.9 ± 2.1 | G4–G5 | 1.0 | 0.4 | 1.9 |
| PH-4 | .14.4 ± 2.2 | PH4–PH5 | 0.7 | 0.2 | 1.5 |
| G-5 | 14.9 ± 2.2 | G2–G5 | 3.0 | 1.9 | 4.7 |
| PH-5 | 15.2 ± 2.1 | PH2–PH5 | 1.6 | 0.8 | 2.7 |
| **Females** | | | | | |
| B-2 | 11.2 ± 2.2 | B2–B3 | 0.9 | 0.2 | 1.0 |
| PH-2 | 11.7 ± 2.4 | PH2–PH3 | 0.6 | 0.2 | 1.3 |
| B-3 | 12.2 ± 2.1 | B3–B4 | 0.9 | 0.1 | 2.2 |
| PH-3 | 12.4 ± 2.2 | PH3–PH4 | 0.5 | 0.2 | 0.9 |
| PH-4 | 12.9 ± 2.1 | B4–B5 | 2.0 | 0.1 | 6.8 |
| B-4 | 13.1 ± 2.3 | PH4–PH5 | 1.3 | 0.6 | 2.4 |
| PH-5 | 14.4 ± 2.2 | B2–B5 | 4.0 | 1.5 | 9.0 |
| B-5 | 15.3 ± 3.5 | PH2–PH5 | 2.5 | 1.4 | 3.1 |

*From Barnes (1975) by permission.*

**Figure 10.3(d)**   Racial differences in female pubertal development. Prevalence of breast development at Tanner stage 2 or greater by age and race; prevalence of pubic hair development at Tanner stage 2 or greater by age and race; and prevalence of menses by age and race. Adapted from Hermann-Giddens et al. (1997).

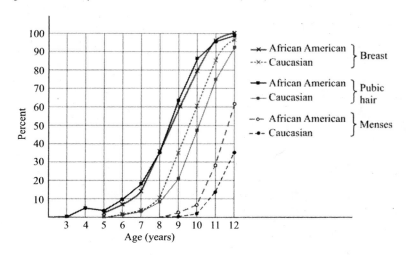

## Penile Length

**Definition**   The length of the gently stretched penis from the base of the tip.

**Landmarks**   Measure from the base of the penis (pubic ramus) to the tip of the glans with the penis gently stretched. The glans of the penis may need to be palpated through the foreskin in individuals who are not circumcised. Alternatively, the foreskin can be retracted (Fig. 10.4).

**Instruments**   A straight-edged clear plastic ruler, a tape-measure, or blunt calipers.

**Position**   Any comfortable position.

**Remarks**   The penis may appear small if there is a ventral insertion of the scrotum (shawl scrotum or webbing of the penis). This anomaly is believed to be due to failure of the scrotal swelling to shift caudally in fetal life. This penis is buried within the scrotal fold but can be palpated and is usually of normal size.

**Pitfalls**   If the fat pad at the base of the penis is not depressed so that the ruler touches the pubic ramus, a falsely short penile length will be perceived. If the penis is not gently stretched as a measurement is taken, the length of the penis may be as much as 2 cm shorter.

**Figure 10.4**   Measurement of penile length.

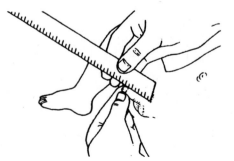

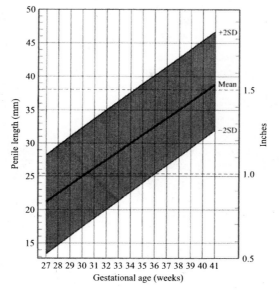

**Figure 10.5**  Penile length, 28–41 gestational weeks. From Feldmann and Smith (1975), by permission.

**Figure 10.6**  Penile length, 1 to 16 years. From Schonfeld (1943), by permission.

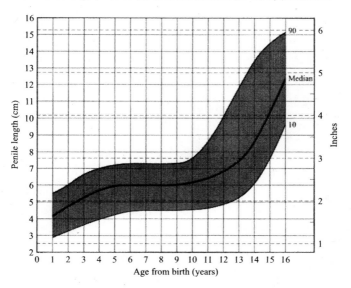

## Hypospadias

Usually the urethra leaves the penis shaft at the tip of the glans of the penis. Hypospadias is an abnormal placement of the outlet of the urethra on the penis shaft. The location of the urethral outlet can be best seen by pulling the ventral skin of the penis outward. Classification of hypospadias is shown in Fig. 10.7 and includes glandular, penile (along the shaft), penoscrotal (at the junction of the penis and scrotum), and perineal (the urethra opening on the perineum) outlet of the urethra. If the urethra opens on the dorsal side of the penis, this is called epispadias and again may have different degrees of severity.

**Figure 10.7** Types of hypospadias. From Alken and Soekeland (1976), by permission.

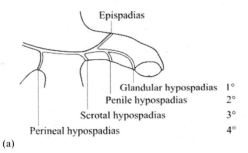

Epispadias

Glandular hypospadias 1°
Penile hypospadias 2°
Scrotal hypospadias 3°
Perineal hypospadias 4°

(a)

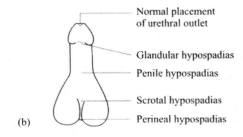

Normal placement of urethral outlet

Glandular hypospadias

Penile hypospadias

Scrotal hypospadias

Perineal hypospadias

(b)

## Testicular Volume

**Definition**   The volume of the testes.

**Landmarks**   The length and width of the testis can be measured along a vertical axis between the upper and lower pole of the testis and at the broadest width.

**Position**   The individual should be standing upright or lying supine.

**Instruments**   The size of the elliptical shaped testis is most easily estimated by palpation and comparison with standardized graded ellipsoid models of different volume sizes (Fig. 10.8). Since Prader developed and standardized these volume models, they are often referred to as "Prader beads." Several alternative methods for testis measurement are available, including blunt calipers, a tape-measure, or straight ruler, or the measurement may be made using ultrasonography.

**Remarks**   Comparative palpation with the orchidometer of Prader is a quick and fairly accurate way to estimate testicular size (Fig. 10.9). The volume in milliliters is clearly printed on each of the elliptical models. At young ages, intermediate volume size models can be obtained (0.5, 1.5, and 2.5 mL size), and very large volume size models have also been developed for macro-orchidism.

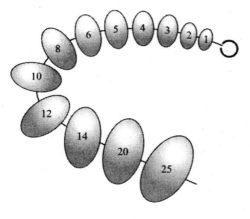

**Figure 10.8**   Prader orchidometer.

The use of a tape-measure or a straight ruler to determine the longest and widest diameters is less accurate. When these linear measurements are used the testicular volume must be calculated from comparison with age-matched normals. The calculation is made using the formula for ellipsoid volume:

$$\text{Testicular volume} = 0.71 \times \text{length}^2 \times \text{width}$$

If volumes are calculated or estimated, they should not be compared with the curves based on the measurements obtained from the orchidometer of Prader, because the calculation usually gives larger estimates of testicular volume. Only one method should be used to follow any individual patient over time and for comparison with other normal standards such as bone age (Fig. 10.10).

Testicular volumes for Japanese and Swiss males are compared Fig. 10.11.

Ultrasound measurements of testicular length and width have been utilized and seem to give the greatest accuracy and consistency of testicular volume.

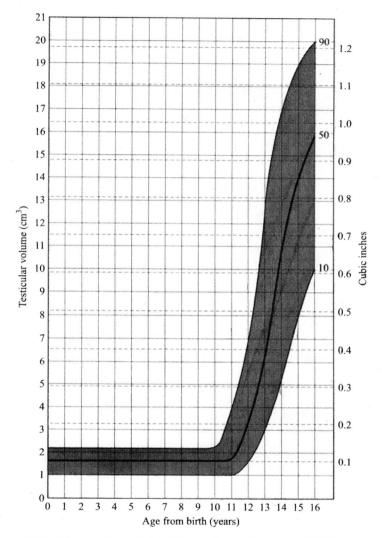

**Figure 10.9** Testicular volume, birth to 16 years. From Zachmann et al. (1974) and Goodman and Gorlin (1983), by permission.

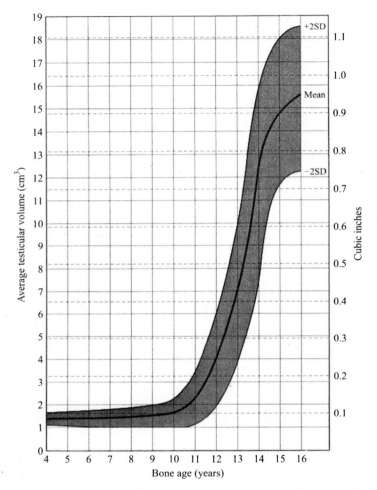

**Figure 10.10** Testicular volume from bone age, 4 to 16 years. From Waaler et al. (1974), by permission.

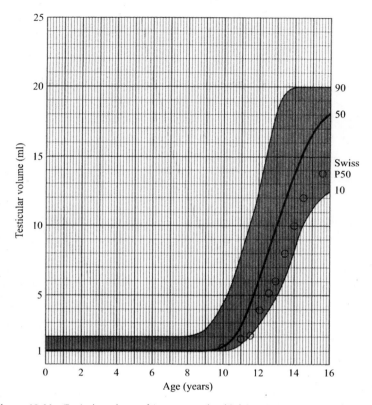

**Figure 10.11** Testicular volume of Japanese males, birth to 16 years, compared to Swiss 50th percentile. From Zachmann et al. (1974); adapted from Matsuo et al. (2000).

## Testicular Descent

**Definition**   Position of the testicle in its descent from the inguinal canal into the scrotum.

**Landmarks**   The base of the penis and the superior margin of the testicle are identified. The testicle is gently retracted away from the body. The distance from the base of the penis to the superior margin of the testicle is measured.

**Position**   This measurement is best taken when the patient is resting in the supine position.

**Instrument**   A plastic ruler or a tape-measure may be used.

**Remarks** Values for testicular descent are shown in relation to age in Fig. 10.12a and by Tanner stage in Fig. 10.12b.

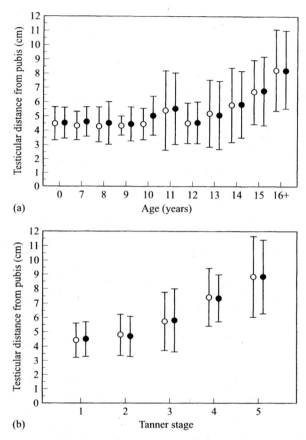

**Figure 10.12**   Testicular descent measurement by age (a) and by Tanner stage (b); symbol indicates mean measurement, and vertical line indicates two standard deviations from the mean. Open circles, right testicle; filled circles, left testicle. Adapted from Sack et al. (1993).

## Anal Placement

**Definition**   The position of the anus in relation to the vaginal introitus or beginning of scrotal tissue.

**Landmarks**   The distance between the posterior aspect of the introitus of the vagina (fourchette) in the female, or the end of scrotalized skin in the male, and the anterior border of the anal opening is measured.

**Position**   The small infant should be in a supine position with the hips and knees held flexed, allowing the gluteal folds to open. A child or older individual can bend forward at the hips or be prone with the legs drawn up toward the abdomen, opening the perineal area for measurement.

**Remarks**   Normal measurements are presented in Fig. 10.13 and 10.14. In the male an abnormality in anal placement usually presents as an anus that is anteriorly placed on the perineum, or as a skin-covered anus; in the female it is generally as a persistent fistula between the rectum and vagina or as an aberrant placement of the anus, with no space or too little space between the anus and the vaginal introitus.

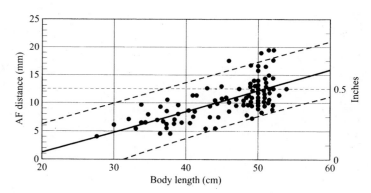

**Figure 10.13**   Anus-to-fourchette (AF) distance, related to body length in newborns, both sexes. From Callegari et al. (1987), by permission.

**Fig. 10.14** Clinical measurements

| | Anus–fourchette (AF)(mm) | Fourchette–clitoris (FC)(mm) | Anus–clitoris (AC)(mm) | AF/AC | FC/AC |
|---|---|---|---|---|---|
| Infants (*n* = 115) | 10.9 ± 3.5 | 19.4 ± 4.3 | 29.6 ± 6.3 | 0.37 ± 0.07 | 0.67 ± 0.07 |
| Adults (*n* = 10) | 30.1 ± 7.5 | 54.2 ± 11.1 | 84.0 ± 13.9 | 0.36 ± 0.07 | 0.64 ± 0.05 |

*Values represent mean ± SD.*
*From Callegari et al. (1987) by permission*

## Anal Diameter

A serious anal stenosis can be excluded by determining the anal diameter. This is done either by placing a gloved little finger into the anal opening or by the use of graduated sounding instruments (Hegar sounds). In the newborn, there is a correlation between anal diameter and weight (Fig. 10.15).

Incomplete development and separation of the cloaca into the urogenital sinus and the rectum will result in various anorectal anomalies. An international classification of anorectal anomalies is available (Fig. 10.16) that helps to relate the embryologic aberration with the clinical appearance and presentation of the anomaly.

**Figure 10.15** Mean anal diameter. From Haddad and Corkery (1985), by permission.

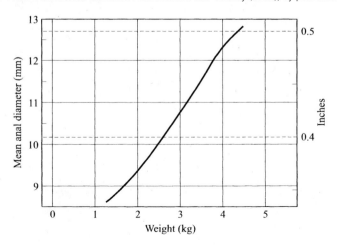

Male

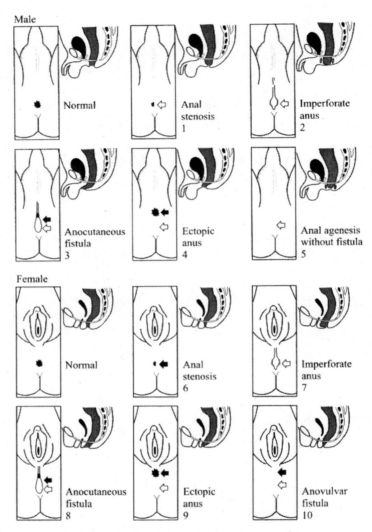

**Figure 10.16**  Anal anomalies. From Santulli et al. (1970), by permission.

## Breast and Nipple Size and Shape

### Introduction

The mammary gland develops from the mammary crest, which is of ecto-dermal origin. The mammary crest (milk line) extends from the axilla to the inguinal area on the developing trunk (see Fig. 9.1 in Chapter 9) but disappears in humans except in the pectoral area. During prenatal life the primary mammary bud is formed. From the deeper surface layers of the bud, 15–20 solid cellular cords, the secondary epithelial buds, proliferate into the mesenchyme. These subdivide and develop into a system of lact-iferous ducts. Parallel with the development of the cellular cords, the surface cells in the primary bud desquamate and form a central depression which, by the end of prenatal life, is everted through proliferation of the underlying dermis and forms the nipple.

The female breast undergoes physiological changes with age, starting with an infantile form, in which the areola and papilla of the nipple are visi-ble but flat. In the next stage, during early adolescence, a slight prominence of the nipple area ("pouting") can be observed, which is followed by primary development of breast tissue with continued prominence of the areola. During puberty the epithelial and fibrous tissues of the mammary gland proliferate under the influence of estrogens, and the stroma, fat, and connec-tive tissues develop, while the ducts grow. In the sexually developed female breast the nipple is integrated into the rounded shape of the adult breast.

The mammary gland consists of 15–20 lobes that radiate from the nipple. The ducts of the lobes unite and form a single excretory duct, which ends in the nipple. The size of the breast varies with age, nutritional state, and the number of pregnancies, as well as with ethnic and genetic background. It is difficult to establish a normal size. An average adult female breast size of 400 mL (range 120–600 mL) has been calculated for nonpregnant northern European women of normal weight using a Plexiglas cylinder to measure breast volume.

**Landmarks**   The female breast can be measured in a vertical diameter (length), measuring lateral to the breast along the trunk wall from the lower insertion along the base of the breast to the point of upper insertion, where a slight curve away from the thorax wall can be found (Fig. 10.17).

The prominence or protrusion of the breast is measured from the middle of the base of the breast on the chest wall to the point of elevation of the areola insertion (Fig. 10.17). Since the size of the nipple varies, it is not included in the measurement.

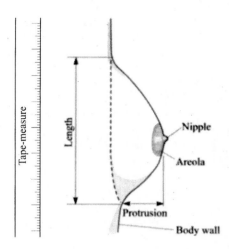

**Figure 10.17** Measurement of breast size.

## Measurement of Breast Volume

A variety of methods may be used to define the breast volume:

1. weighing the breast on a scale, which can be done with pendulous breasts;
2. using a water-filled container placed over the breast and into which the breast is placed. Since the volume of water in the container is known, the breast size can be calculated from the amount of water displaced;
3. making a cast of the breast, and the volume of the breast is measured from the cast;
4. measuring the breast size with a special breast-measuring cylinder of Plexiglas with a fitted domed piston and a scale, from which the breast size can be read.

**Instruments**   Calipers, tape-measure, solid ruler, or, for breast volume, a Plexiglas cylinder with a domed piston.

**Position**   The individual should stand or sit with the arms hanging loosely. The measurements with a tape-measure or calipers are taken from along the side of the breast.

If a cylinder is used to assess breast volume, the breast is placed in the cylinder, and the position of the piston is read off the scale.

**Remarks**   There are a variety of normal shapes of the female breast (Fig. 10.18). Usually the left breast is slightly larger than the right.

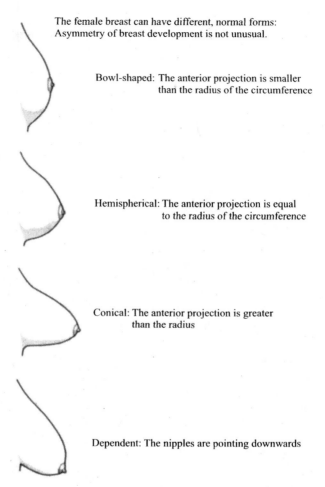

The female breast can have different, normal forms:
Asymmetry of breast development is not unusual.

Bowl-shaped: The anterior projection is smaller
than the radius of the circumference

Hemispherical: The anterior projection is equal
to the radius of the circumference

Conical: The anterior projection is greater
than the radius

Dependent: The nipples are pointing downwards

**Figure 10.18**   Breast shapes. From Martin and Saller (1962), by permission.

Asymmetric development (anisomastia) and overgrowth of breast tissue (macromastia) can be part of specific syndromes.

A small amount of breast development is often present in the newborn due to maternal hormones. It is usually not pathological. Mild breast development in males frequently occurs around puberty.

## Ptosis of the Breast

Ptosis of the breast means drooping of the breast, so that in an upright position the lower surface of the breast is below the lower insertion on the thorax (submammary fold) and the skin of the breast is in direct contact with the skin of the thorax. Ptosis of the breast occurs with aging and after nursing and multiple pregnancies. To measure ptosis of the breast, the woman is seated and a tape-measure is placed from the middle of the clavicle down to the nipple. Alternatively, an imaginary horizontal line can be drawn between the nipples and the distance from the top of the manubrium to the nipple line measured. The normal position of the nipple is 21–23 cm from the top of the manubrium.

## Areola Measurements

Areola measurements include diameter and prominence from the breast tissue. The diameter of the nipple is very variable, as is the diameter of the areola. On average, the adult female areola measures 3–4 cm in diameter.

**Instruments**   The nipple diameter can be measured with a plastic template circular cut-outs, calipers, or a transparent ruler.

**Remarks**   Significant differences in nipple diameter can be noted between stages B1 to B5 of breast development during puberty. Nipple size can be a useful measurement in girls with primary amenorrhoea. Girls with a large nipple diameter (greater than 0.7 cm) can be considered to have undergone hormonal stimulation.

Abnormalities of the nipple include extra or accessory nipples along the "milk line," absent or hypoplastic nipples (as in Poland anomaly, where part of the pectoral muscle and limb may also be missing), polythelia (more than one nipple on a breast), and inverted nipples (the tip of the nipple is directed inward and does not protrude from the areola). Hypoplasia or absence of the nipple and/or the mammary gland may be seen in ectodermal dysplasia.

# Bibliography

Alken, C.E. and Soekeland, J. (1976). *Urologie* (7th ed). Georg Thieme Veriag. Stuttgart, Germany.

Barnes, H.V.V. (1975). Physical growth and development during puberty. *Medical Clinics of North America*, **59**, 1305–1316.

Callegari, C., Everett, S., Ross, M., and Brasel, J.A. (1987). Anogenital ratio: measure of fetal virilization in premature and full-term newborn infants. *Journal of Pediatrics*, **11**, 240–243.

Feldmann, K.W. and Smith, D.W. (1975). Fetal phallic growth and penile standards for newborn male infants. *Journal of Pediatrics*, **86**, 395–398.

Goodman, R.M. and Gorlin, R.J. (1983). *The malformed infant and child*. Oxford University Press, Oxford.

Haddad, M.E. and Corkery, J.J. (1985). The anus in the newborn. *Pediatrics*, **76**, 927–928.

Herman-Giddens, M.E., Slora, E.J., Wasserman, R.C., Bourdon, C.J., Bhapkar, M.V., Koch, G.G., Hasen (1996) Secondary sexual characteristics and menses in young girls seen in office practice: a study from the Pediatric Research in Office Settings Network. *Pediatrics*, **99**, 505–512.

Laron, Z. and Zilka, E. (1969). Compensatory hypertrophy of testicle in unilateral cryptorchidism. *Journal of Clinical Endocrinology and Metabolism*, **29**, 1409–1413.

Martin, R. and Saller, K. (1962). *Lehrbuch der Anthropologie*, Gustav Fischer Verlag, Stuttgart, Germany.

Matsuo, N., Anzo, M., Sato, S., Ogata, T., and Kamimaki, T. (2000). Testicular volume in Japanese boys up to the age of 15 years. *European Journal of Pediatrics*, **159**, 843–845.

Prader, A. (1966). Die Hodengroesse. Beurteilung and klinische Bedeutung. *Triangel*, **7**, 240–243.

Sack, J., Reichman, B., and Fix, A.(1993). Normative values for testicular descent from infancy to adulthood. *Hormone Research*, **39**, 118–121.

Santulli, T.V., Kiesewetter, W.B., and Bill, A.H. (1970). Anorectal anomalies: a suggested international classification. *Journal of Pediatric Surgery*, **5**, 281–287.

Schonfeld, W.A. (1943). Primary and secondary sexual characteristics. *American Journal of Disease in Children*, **65**, 535–542.

Stroembeck, J.D. (1964). Macromastia in woman and its surgical treatment. *Acta chirurgica Scandinavica*, Supplement 341.

Tanner, J.M. (1975). Growth and endocrinology of the adolescent. In *Endocrine and genetic disease in childhood* (2nd ed), (ed. A. Gardner). W.B. Saunders, Philadelphia.

Waaler, E., Thorsen, T., Stoa, K.F., and Aarskog, D.(1974). Studies in male puberty. *Acta paediatrica Scandinavica*, supplement 249.

Zachmann, M., Prader, A., Kind, H.P., Haeflinger, H., and Budliger, H. (1974). Testicular volume during adolescence. *Helvetia paediatrica acta*, **29**, 61–72.

# Skin and Hair

## Introduction

The skin consists of two main layers: the superficial epidermis and the underlying dermis. They derive from two different germ line layers. The epidermis comes from the surface ectoderm. At about three weeks of gestation the epidermis consists of a single layer, while in the 4- to 6-week-old fetus two layers can be distinguished: the superficial periderm and the basal proliferative stratum germinativum. The periderm keratinizes and desquamates, giving rise to cells in the amniotic fluid and the vernix caseosa (the white cheese-like substance which covers the fetal skin until near term). By 8 to 11 weeks of gestation, proliferation of the stratum germinativum has produced several intermediate layers of epidermis, and at birth all the layers normally seen in adult epidermis, including a keratinized layer and the pigmentary cells (melanocytes), are present.

Most of the dermis derives from mesoderm. At about 11 weeks of gestation, mesenchymal cells in the dermis begin to produce collagen and elastin fibers. When the epidermal ridges grow down into the dermis at 11 to 12 weeks and begin to form the ridges and grooves that will produce dermatoglyphics, the dermis projects up into the epidermis, resulting in dermal papillae in which capillary loops and sensory nerve endings will form. A network of blood vessels forms in the fetal skin; some of these vessels are transitory and normally disappear.

The completely developed skin can be considered to have three layers: the epidermis, the dermis, and the subcutis, which is loose subcutaneous tissue. The surface of the epidermis is keratinized and covers an area of approximately 1.5 to 2 m², weighing 0.5 kg in an adult. There is variation in epidermal thickness, depending on the body area. The skin is thinner, for example, around the eyes and lips, and is thicker in the palmar and plantar areas. On average, the skin is 0.1 cm thick. The dermis is separated from the epidermis by a basal membrane. The dermis consists of collagen, elastin, and reticular fibers, as well as a variety of cell types and a matrix with many complex carbohydrates. The subcutis or subcutaneous tissue connects the skin with underlying tissue and structurally consists of a loose organization of fibers and septa. It contains a variable amount of fat, known as the panniculus adiposus. Skin turgor relates to the amount of subcutaneous fat. Thinning of the panniculus adiposus will result in an increased number of skin creases.

The surface of the skin is complex and varies in different body areas. Small lines can be found in the skin surface; they criss-cross the body surface. These lines are thought to be the result of the configuration of the dermal papillae, which reach up to the epidermis, the underlying collagen bundles, and the pull of muscles underneath the skin. Some regions of the skin are oilier than other, reflecting the presence of a variable number of sebaceous glands. Other areas are covered with numerous vellus hairs, like the superior helices of the ears, or the upper lip in females. Skin texture also depends on the number, function, and size of the sweat glands. Skin can be firm, soft, rough, moist, dry, or oily. The texture of skin changes with age, resulting in uneven atrophy and hyperplasia, development of yellowish thickened plaques and subcutaneous nodules, areas of erythema, telangiectasia, and brown macular irregular pigmented lesions. With aging, progressive degenerative changes in collagen can be seen on histology, and collagen is replaced by elastic fibers. Thinning of the overlying epidermis also occurs with aging.

## Extensibility of Skin

The extensibility of the skin varies with age and is greatest in older people. There are also differences between the sexes, apparently dependent on hormonal variations. Female skin is more extensible at all ages. There is variable extensibility in different parts of the body—the neck and elbow skin is looser than the skin on the forearms and hips. Extensibility depends on the collagen content of the skin. There are ways to measure precisely the extensibility of skin, which involve attaching a weight onto a piece of skin and measuring how far it stretches.

For clinical purpose, a subjective estimate of skin extensibility is usually sufficient. An easy way to estimate extensibility of skin is to pinch the outer side of the upper arm, holding the skin between the thumb and index finger, then lightly pulling it upward. If the skin stretches more than 1 cm, hyperextensibility should be suspected.

## Patterns Reflected by the Skin

Because the human embryo is originally segmental, various structures reflect a segmental pattern that can be appreciated on the surface of the body.

The melanin-producing cells are of neural crest origin and apparently migrate embryologically in a predictable pattern. The pattern was first described by Blaschko. When pigmented streaks reflecting that migration are seen, they are called "Blaschko lines" (Fig. 11.1). Disorders of pigmentation and mosaicism for two or more genetically different cell lines can be associated with the presence of these lines.

The sensory innervation of the skin is structured segmentally, according to the dermatomes (Fig. 11.2a,b). Some skin disorders, such as herpes zoster, may reflect this dermatome distribution. It is extremely useful to know the sensory nerve distribution of specific nerves when trying to pinpoint a neurological disorder. The distribution of motor nerves is also segmented but follows a different distribution than the sensory distribution.

**Figure 11.1** Blaschko lines.

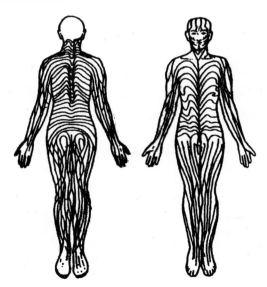

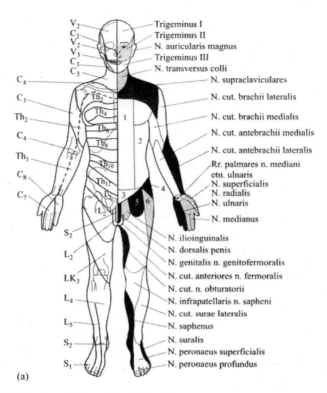

**Figure 11.2(a)**  Sensory innervation of the skin.

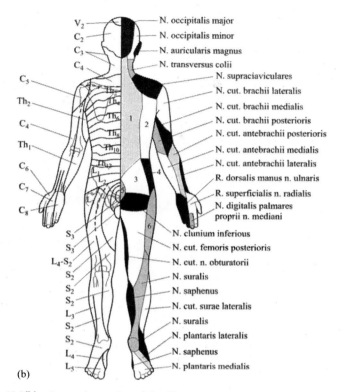

**Figure 11.2(b)**   Sensory innervation of the skin.

## Skin Color

**Origin and distribution**   Melanin is the black or brown pigment that is responsible for the color of the skin, hair, and local variation in pigmentation. It is produced only by the melanocytes. Melanocytes derive embryologically from melanoblasts. They migrate from the inner neural crest to the dermoepidermal junction. Mature melanocytes are essentially confined to the basal layers of the epidermis. In dark-skinned ethnic groups, pigment activity can be observed from the fourth fetal month.

The color of the skin depends on both the amount and distribution of the melanin in the epidermis (and occasionally in the dermis) and the vascularization of the skin. Additional factors that influence the skin color include hormones, such as melanocyte-stimulating hormone and the sex steroids, and exogenous factors, such as heat, injury, and exposure to ultraviolet light. Skin color can range from pale-yellow to gray-black. There are characteristic regional variations in skin color common to all ethnic groups, (e. g., palms are lighter than the rest of the hands, while around the eyes skin color is usually darker) as well as specific ethnic differences, such as pigment-free mucous membranes in Europeans.

**Describing Skin Color**   In describing skin color, it is essential to name the body area of observation (ventral, dorsal, chest, palms, etc.). Usually the skin is lighter on the ventral part of the body compared to the dorsum. In addition, the appearance of areas exposed to the sun versus protected areas should be described, as well as the differences between them. A skin color table may be helpful for special situations (see Bibliography).

**Remarks**   For documentation of skin color, a color photograph is useful. The color of tooth enamel, nails, iris, body, and scalp hair, as well as skin, should be recorded. The skin around the nipple, especially after pregnancy, may be darker due to hormonal influences. Genital skin and areas of apocrine sweating are usually darker. Pigment changes can occur in specific diseases, such as Addison disease (a bronze skin color) or albinism (where the skin and hair pigment may be reduced or absent).

**Pitfalls**   Skin color can be artificially altered and pigmented by make-up, dirt, and different forms of tattooing. Artificial light may give unusual tones or hues to the natural colors.

## Birthmarks

**Definition**   Various regionally limited congenital alterations of skin pigmentation or skin color are referred to as birthmarks. They may not be observed at birth, but usually they are obvious by several months of age. They can be due to the presence of an increased number of superficial lymph or blood vessels, increased pigment in the epidermis, aberrant tissue present in the skin, or pigment variation in the dermis.

### Local Variations in Pigmentation

**Café au Lait Spot**   Macular are of increased pigment:

- *Size*, a few millimeters to many centimeters
- *Frequency*, 5 percent of the population
- *Localization*, all body areas
- *Origin*, local melanocyte activity

- *Remarks*, may be a sign of neurofibromatosis if more than five café au lait spots greater than 0.5 cm before puberty or 1.5 cm after puberty are present

**Blue Nevus**   Bluish macular area:

- *Size*, usually larger than 5 cm
- *Synonym*, blue nevus; the blue color is an optical effect of deep-seated melanin
- *Frequency*, 9.6 percent in Caucasians, 95.5 percent in African Americans, 81 percent in Asians
- *Localization*, primarily over the sacrum and the gluteal region
- *Origin*, ectopic melanocytes in the dermis
- *Remarks*, no pathological significance; can be present from the fifth gestational month and usually disappears during childhood because of the loss of dermal pigment

**Depigmentation**   Macular area of reduced pigment:

- *Frequency*, 1 percent of the population
- *Localization*, can occur limited to circumscribed body areas or with a patchy distribution
- *Origin*, lack of functional melanocytes in this area
- *Remarks*, multiple small, leaf-shaped depigmented areas may be a sign of tuberous sclerosis

**Mole**   Circumscribed area of dark pigment:

- *Synonym*, lentigo, compound nevus
- *Frequency*, very common
- *Localization*, all body parts, usually present at birth but may occur later
- *Color*, varies from dark brown to black
- *Shape*, may be flat, elevated, verrucoid, domeshaped
- *Origin*, proliferation of melanocytes

**Capillary Hemangioma**

**Local Variation of Vasculature**   Pink macular area, commonly on the nape of the neck, eyelids, glabella, and midforehead in newborns:

- *Synonyms*, Unna's mark, nevus simplex, erythema nuchae, angel's kiss, salmon patch

- *Size*, very small fleck to several centimeters
- *Frequency*, very common; may be obvious at birth or appear within the first few days; persists throughout life but becomes less obvious with age
- *Origin*, dermal capillaries or telangiectases, representing fetal circulatory patterns in the skin

**Elevated Vascular Nevus**  Elevated irregular lesion of solid red color:

- *Synonym*, strawberry nevus, cavernous hemangioma, capillary hemangioma
- *Frequency*, 10 percent of the population
- *Localization*, single or multiple, all body areas
- *Origin*, enlarged or dilated vessels of the skin (nevus vascularis). Thrombosis may occur inside the nevus, which may resolve spontaneously, but rarely it may require therapeutic intervention, especially if a vital function or vision is disturbed.
- *Remarks*, usually not present at birth, but appears in the first few months of life, enlarging during the first year and then most often resolving spontaneously.

**Port Wine Nevus**  Large dark angioma; may start as pink-colored macula that later becomes purple and may be raised; at first it may be smooth but can become irregular later.

- *Synonym*, nevus flammeus
- *Frequency*, 0.3 percent of the population
- *Localization*, any area of the body, but usually anterior or lateral, not posterior; most frequently unilateral and rarely crosses the midline
- *Origin*, dilated mature capillaries of the dermis
- *Remarks*, can be a sign of Sturge–Weber syndrome if in the distribution of the first branch of the trigeminal nerve; does not resolve spontaneously.

**Telangiectasia**  Prominent blood vessel on the surface of the skin.

- *Origin*, results from a widening of the capillaries
- *Localization*, the main location is on the nose, the upper lip, conjunctiva, and the cheeks
- *Remarks*, the number increases with age; it can be seen in the ataxia–teleangiectasia syndrome and in hereditary hemorrhagic teleangiectasia

**Lymphangioma**  Overgrowth of lymphatic vessels.

- *Synonym*, cystic hygroma
- *Localization*, mostly found in the neck and tongue area
- *Origin*, results from lymphatic vessel anomalies
- *Remarks*, can lead to an excess of skin in the neck area when it occurs prenatally and subsequently resolves

## Other Anomalies of the Skin

**Nevus Sebaceous**  Raised waxy patch, often linear.

- *Synonym*, Jadassohn nevus
- *Origin*, organoid nevus of the epidermis with a preponderance of sebaceous glands
- *Frequency*, 0.2 percent of the population
- *Localization*, frequently on scalp or head
- *Remarks*, may be associated with mental retardation and seizures; may be seen in *Proteus* syndrome

**Cutis Aplasia**  Area of absence of skin:

- *Frequency*, rare, less than 0.1 percent
- *Localization*, usually in the midline at the vertex of the scalp
- *Origin*, possibly due to a vascular accident during development *in utero*. The area of the scalp in which it occurs most frequently is the spot from which the skin stretches when it grows and may be the first point to break down during abnormal development
- *Remarks*, frequent in trisomy 13, and Adams-Oliver syndrome

**Dimple**  Area in which the skin is attached to underlying structures:

- *Localization*, frequently over knuckles and on cheeks; occasionally at ankles, knees and elbows; rarely over buttocks or sacrum
- *Origin*, occurs in areas where there is unusually close proximity between bone, joints, or muscle and the skin during fetal life

**Congenital Alopecia**  Patch of skin without hair growth:

- *Localization*, may occur anywhere on the scalp or body
- *Origin*, absence or loss of hair follicles that may result from failure of hair follicles to develop or from follicles that produce a decreased amount of hair.

## Glands of the Skin

### Introduction

There are two kinds of glands in the skin: the sebaceous glands and the sweat glands (Fig. 11.3). Most sebaceous glands develop along the side of a developing epithelial root sheath of a hair follicle. A glandular bud grows

**Figure 11.3**  Development of sweat glands and sebaceous glands and the hair shaft. From Moore (1982), by permission.

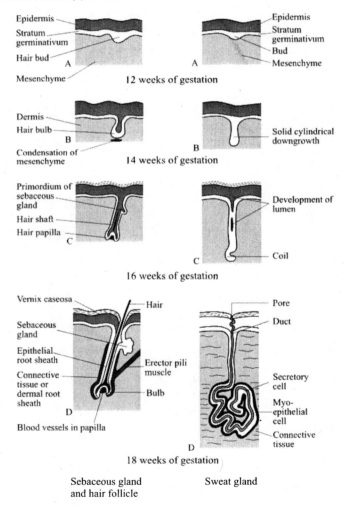

12 weeks of gestation

14 weeks of gestation

16 weeks of gestation

18 weeks of gestation

Sebaceous gland and hair follicle

Sweat gland

into the secondary connective tissue and forms alveoli. The central cells of the branched alveoli break down to form an oily secretion, the sebum. It is extruded into the hair follicle and then to the surface of the skin. In the fetus, sebum mixes with desquamated peridermal cells and forms the vernix caseosa. In the child and adult, it produces oil for the skin.

Two kinds of sweat glands occur: eccrine and apocrine sweat glands. The eccrine sweat glands develop first as solid epidermal downgrowths into the underlying dermis. The lower ends coil up and form the secretory portion of the gland. The central cells then degenerate, forming a lumen. The peripheral cells of the gland differentiate into secretory and myoepithelial cells. The myoepithelial cells are thought to form smooth muscles which help to expel the secreted sweat. The apocrine sweat glands are situated primarily in the axillary area, the pubic area, and around the nipple, but they also occur around the nose, in the outer ear canal, and on the eyelids. These glands form from the epidermis that gives rise to hair follicles. The ducts open, in contrast to the eccrine glands, not onto the skin surface but into the hair follicles just above the opening of the sebaceous glands. Developmental abnormalities in all three kinds of glands can occur.

## Quantitation of the Number of Sweat Glands

There are normally about 2 million sweat glands on the surface of the skin. To assess the number of sweat glands on the skin surface, several different techniques exist. Most ignore the apocrine sweat glands.

**Chemical Method**  A solution of *o*-phthaldialdehyde in xylene can be put on the skin. The chemical produces a black color if sweat is excreted, designating the sweat pores.

**Stereomicroscopy**  Using a 7× objective of a stereomicroscope, the sweat pores on the epidermal ridges of the fingertips can be quantitated by recording the number of pores along 0.5 cm of a dermal ridge. A transparent plastic template with an open square of 0.5 cm per side is used. The count should be performed on 10 ridges from 10 different fingers (Fig. 11.4).

**Electron Microscopy**  A more accurate way to quantitate sweat glands is to determine the number of glands seen on electron microscopic examination of a skin biopsy.

**Alternative**  A further method is to use a dermatoglyphic fingerprint and count the sweat pores on the fingerprint using a microscope or other high magnification device (Fig. 11.4).

**Fig. 11.4**  Average number of sweat pores in skin body area (per cm$^2$)

| Skin area | No. |
|---|---|
| Forehead | 113 (>60 years, 83) |
| Dorsum of hand | 130 (>60 years, 89) |
| Shoulder | 35 (>60 years, 27) |
| Upper arm | 36 (>60 years, 36) |
| Elbow, flexion side | 751 |
| Palmar | 373 |
| Breast | 155–250 |
| Backside | 57 |
| Fingertips | 32 (2–3 weeks) |
|  | 23 (18–30 years) |
|  | <20 (60–84 years) |

*From Fiedler (1969) and Frias and Smith (1968), by permission.*

**Remarks**  Different numbers of sweat glands occur in various parts of the body and decrease with age (Fig. 11.4). On average, before 20 years of age, there are 177 sweat pores/cm$^2$, whereas at 80 years of age there are only 101 sweat pores/cm$^2$.

In many forms of ectodermal dysplasia the glands of the skin do not form or do not function in a normal way. Normally, a single sweat gland secretes 0.003–0.01 ng/mm per day. In the course of a day, the skin may secret 800 ml of sweat. Sweating is important for thermal regulation, and without normal numbers of sweat glands an individual may become hyperpyrexic in hot weather.

## Hair

### Introduction

The total amount of body hair is difficult to estimate. The head alone has approximately 100,000 hairs. There are three phases in the life cycle of the hair that need to be distinguished:

1. the growing stage, called anagen;
2. the involution stage, called catagen;
3. the resting stage, called telogen.

Many factors, including general health, climate, drugs, hormones, and genetic programming, affect the growth of the hair. The rate of hair growth varies in different body regions (Fig. 11.5). On average, human hair grows 0.37 mm daily. In males, the scalp hair grows slower and the body hair grows faster than in females. Androgen increases the hair growth on the trunk and plays a role in male-pattern balding, however the exact mechanism is not fully understood. Seventy to 100 scalp hairs are shed daily in the normal telogen phase. In the ageing process, the hair also loses color because melanin fails to be synthesized in the hair matrix.

**Fig. 11.5**   Daily hair growth in different body areas

| Age (years) | Hair growth (mm) | | | |
| --- | --- | --- | --- | --- |
| | Frontal | Whorl | Occipital | Temporal |
| 5 | 0.25 | 0.27 | 0.40 | 0.31 |
| 25 | 0.44 | 0.35 | 0.39 | 0.39 |
| 30 | 0.35 | 0.39 | 0.41 | 0.37 |
| 60 | 0.27 | 0.28 | 0.28 | 0.23 |

*From Martin and Saller (1962), by permission.*

**Embryology and Hair Types**

The hair follicles develop from ectoderm and mesoderm (Fig. 11.3). They first appear in the third month of gestation, and continue to appear through the sixth month. The developing hair follicle grows downward from the epidermis and into the dermis. The deepest part of this hair bud will form the hair bulb. The hair bulb is invaginated by a hair papilla from the mesoderm. The peripheral cells of the hair follicle form the epithelial root sheath, and the surrounding mesenchymal cells differentiate into the dermal root sheath. The epithelial cells of the hair bulb produce the germinal matrix, which proliferates and pushes upward to become keratinized and form the hair shaft. Melanoblasts migrate into the hair bulb, and after differentiating into melanocytes they produce melanin. Hair is first recognizable at the eyebrow, upper lip, and chin areas at about the 20th week of gestation.

The first hair, called lanugo, is fine and colorless, and is usually lost during the perinatal period. It will be replaced by coarser hair, the vellus. This persists over most body areas except the axillary and pubic region, where it is replaced at puberty by coarse terminal hair. In males similar terminal hair appears on the chest and the face. From the mesenchyme around the hair bulb small bundles of smooth muscle form the erector pili muscle, which can make the hair rise off the surface of the skin.

All the hair follicles are present in the fetus. The distribution of hair in later life is mainly due to the difference in growth at the skin surface. Hair color, texture, and distribution need to be examined and recorded, particularly when an ectodermal dyplasia is suspected. The pattern of hair follicle distribution is discussed in Chapter 12.

**Hair Color**

Hair color depends on the degree of pigmentation. It can vary in different body areas; thus it is useful to record the color of eyebrow and eyelash hair as well as that of scalp and beard.

The hair color can be recorded by describing the shades of color. Examples are black, black-brown, dark-brown, red-brown, light-brown, dark-blond, fair, light, red, and albino. It can also be compared with hair color tables, as used by anthropologists (see Bibliography). Hair color can, of course, be altered by dyeing. The hair color charts for various hair dyes are also useful for recording the color. A sample of hair can also be taken and kept in an envelope in the patient's chart. The accurate color is preserved in such samples if they are not exposed to light.

## Hair Texture

Texture of the hair can vary greatly between individuals, even of the same ethnic group (Fig. 11.6). The twisting of a single hair shows great variance along its shaft. Physiologically significant differences in hair structure of various body areas also exist. Body hair is usually curlier than scalp hair. Curly hair is flatter in cross-section compared with straight hair, which is round. The major designations for hair texture also straight, wavy, curly, or narrow curls, but it can be further described as fine, coarse, wiry, stiff, flexible, and so on. Pathological structural anomalies of the hair can best be seen with the microscope (see Bibliography).

**Figure 11.6** Normal hair texture forms. From Martin and Saller (1962), by permission.

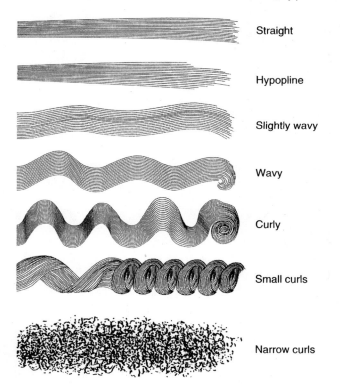

Straight

Hypopline

Slightly wavy

Wavy

Curly

Small curls

Narrow curls

## Balding

Balding occurs as part of the physiological process of aging. Timing of male baldness depends on the influence of androgens, age, and genetic predisposition. It usually occurs first in the frontoparietal area. This distribution is called "male-pattern" balding.

Female baldness usually occurs later, and the loss of hair is diffuse rather than starting with frontoparietal recession. Female balding is due to random atrophy of follicles and is associated with a decrease in circulating estrogen.

## Alopecia

There are various pathological forms of hair loss, the most common is alopecia, which is a premature loss of hair. It can be diffuse or circumscribed, and can involve areas of the scalp or the whole body. It can also be transient or permanent.

## Nails

### Embryology and Normal Structure

The nails begin to develop at the distal end of the digits at about 10 weeks of gestation. They appear as thickened areas of the epidermis (Fig. 11.7). These nail fields are surrounded by a fold of the epidermis, the nail fold. Cells from the proximal part (the nail bed) of the nail fold grow over the nail field and become keratinized, forming the nail or nail plate. New nail growth is produced by the nail bed in the proximal part of the nail field. The nail bed can be seen in some individuals as a white crescent at the base of the nail. The developing nail is covered by an epidermal layer, the eponychium, which later degenerates, except at the base of the nail, where it is called the cuticle. The fingernail plate grows to reach the fingertip at about 32 weeks of gestation. The toenail plate reaches the tip of the toe at 36 weeks. The size of the nail field is influenced by the size of the underlying distal phalanx.

In the newborn, the mean width of the index fingernail is $5.0 \pm 0$ and the length is $3.5 \pm 0.3$ mm.

With aging, the convexity of the nail plate increases, and the nail plate thickens and may develop ridges. These changes can sometimes be confused with a nail infection. The rate of nail growth is more rapid in warm climate, while nail growth slows down with infections and age.

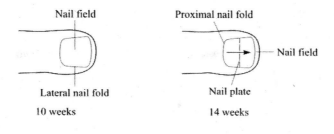

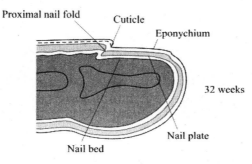

**Figure 11.7** Development of nails. From Moore (1982), by permission.

## Nail Size, Shape, Quality, and Color

The size of the nail in relation to the nail bed, the shape (e.g., round, oval, long, clubbed, broad [Fig. 11.8]), the quality (e.g., thick, thin, brittle, splitting, ridged, pitted), and any discoloration should be recorded. As with other body structures, photographs are often useful.

Specific changes can be seen in certain syndromes:

Longitudinal ridging occurs in cranio-fronto-nasal syndrome.

Longitudinal ridging and nail dystrophy with the thumbnails most severely affected, including absence of the lateral half of the thumbnail, may be seen in nail-patella syndrome.

Thickened, friable, and darkened fingernails and toenails are seen in pachyonychia congenita.

Ungual fibromata are seen in tuberous sclerosis.

**Figure 11.8**   Normal variation of fingernail configuration. From Martin and Saller (1962), by permission.

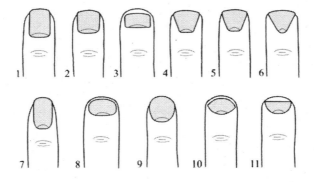

## Finger Clubbing

Clubbing of the finger and fingernail is an abnormal axial convex curved shape with enlargement of the distal finger and nail and loss of the angle at the nail fold. Clubbing of the fingers may be associated with an underlying pulmonary disease, as in cyanotic congenital heart disease, cystic fibrosis, and bronchial carcinoma. However, it can also be seen in Crohn disease, cirrhosis, and thyrotoxicosis. Finger clubbing can be an important clinical sign in the progress of a disease. Inherited differences in finger shape can also resemble pathological clubbing, but the angle at the proximal nail fold is intact. The degree of clubbing can be recorded in photographs taken from the side of the finger. A lateral photograph of the index finger will document the proximal nail fold, cuticle, and nail, as well as the curve of the nail itself (Fig. 11.9).

**Figure 11.9**  Schematic diagram of finger clubbing.

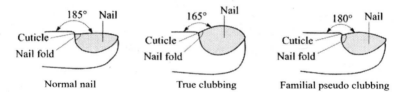

## Method to Estimate Nail Growth

Growth of a nail can be followed by marking an area of the nail with silver nitrate or by punching or cutting a hole or mark into the nail (nail plate) itself and measuring the distance from the cuticle over a period of time (see Bibliography).

The average thumbnail takes 150 days to grow from its cuticle to the free edge of the nail. The average rate of nail growth is between 0.10 and 0.123 mm/day. The nails of children grow faster than those of adults, and the rate varies with the season being slightly more rapid in the summer.

## Bibliography

Bean, W.B. (1974). Nail growth: 30 years of observation. *Archives of Internal Medicine*, **134**, 497–502.

Bentley, D., Moore, A., Shwachman, H. (1976). Finger clubbing: a quantitative survey by analysis of the shadowgraph. *Lancet*, **2**, 164–167.

Fiedler, H.P. (1969). *Der Schweiss*. Aulendorf Editio Cantor.

Frias, J.L. and Smith, D.W. (1968). Diminished sweat pores in hypohidrotic ectodermal dysplasia: a new method for assessment. *Journal of Pediatrics*, **72**, 606–610.

Gertler, W. (1970). Systematische Dermatologie und Grenzgebiete (Bd. I). Thieme Verlag, Leipzig.

Hamilton, J.B., Terada, H., and Mestler, G.E. (1955). Studies of growth throughout the lifespan in Japanese: growth and size of nails and their relationship to age, sex, heredity and other factors. *Journal of Geronotology*, **10**, 400.

Happle, R. (1985). Lyonization and the lines of Blaschko. *Human Genetics*, **70**, 200–206.

Hudson, V.K. (1988). Newborn nail size. *Dysmorphology and Clinical Genetics*, **1**, 145.

Jacobs, A.H. and Walton, R.G. (1976). The incidence of birthmarks in the neonate. *Pediatrics*, **58**, 218–222.

Jacobs, A.H. (1979). Birthmarks: I. Vascular nevi. *Pediatrics in Review*, **1**, 21–24.

Juhlin, L. and Shelley, W.B. (1967). A stain for sweat pores. *Nature*, **213**, 408.

Lau, J.T.K. and Ching, R.M.L. (1982). Mongolian spots in Chinese children. *American Journal of Diseases in Children*, **136**, 863–864.

Martin, R. and Saller, K. (1962). *Lehrbuch der Anthropologie*. Gustav Fischer Verlag, Stuttgart.

Moore, K.L. (1982). *The developing human,* pp. 432–446. W.B. Saunders, Philadelphia.

Smith, D.W. (1982). *Recognizable patterns of human malformation* (3rd ed), p. 576. W.B. Saunders, Philadelphia.

Tan, K.L. (1972). Nevus flammeus of the nape, glabella and eyelids. *Clinical Pediatrics,* **11**, 112–118.

# Dermatoglyphics and Trichoglyphics

**12**

## Dermatoglyphics: Introduction

In the sixth and seventh week of gestation, pads begin to develop on the palmar aspect of the fingertips, on the palm, in the inter-digital spaces, as well as on the radial (thenar) and ulnar (hypothenar) areas of the proximal palm (Fig. 12.1). These pads derive from mesenchymal cells and contain mucopolysaccharide–protein complexes that can bind water. The pads show great variation in size and symmetry. They influence the pattern of the developing dermal ridges. On the tips of the fingers, large fetal pads develop a whorl pattern, intermediate sized pads a loop pattern, while a smaller flat pad will usually give rise to an arch pattern (Fig. 12.2). During this gestational period, cells proliferating in the stratum germinativum of the epidermis grow down into the dermis and form epidermal ridges, which are established by the 17th gestational week. About that time the mesenchymal pads start to regress. The ridges and grooves form the dermatoglyphics on the surface of the palm, fingers, sole of the feet and toes. The permanent dermatoglyphic pattern is set by the 19th week of gestation.

The flexion creases in the skin of the body begin to develop in the second to third gestational month. Those of the limbs are usually present

**Figure 12.1** Distribution of pads at 10 weeks gestation. From Martin and Saller (1962), by permission.

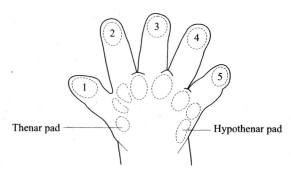

Thenar pad ———— Hypothenar pad

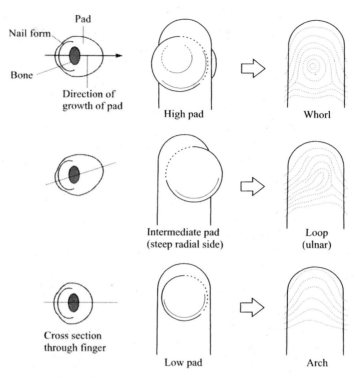

**Figure 12.2** Relation of pad height and dermatoglyphic pattern. From Mulvihill and Smith (1969), by permission.

by the sixth month of gestation. In the palms, the pattern of flexion creases appears to be influenced by the size of the pads in the thenar and hypothenar areas, the length of the bones, and intrauterine movement. The flexion creases of the palm do not all develop at the same time but from between the 8th and 13th weeks and are well defined by 13 weeks. They may consist of separate segments that later join (Fig. 12.3).

Strictly speaking, dermatoglyphics is the study of the epidermal ridge pattern of the skin but, in general use, both the epidermal ridge patterns and flexion creases are discussed together. They reflect structures and relationships that were present at the time they were forming. The epidermal ridge dermatoglyphic pattern consists of ridges (cristae superficiales) and grooves (sulci cutanei). A wide range of normal variation can be seen among dermal ridge patterns. The main patterns on the fingertips are

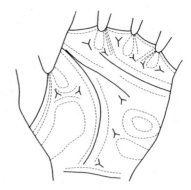

**Figure 12.3** Flexion creases in the hand of a 10-week old embryo. From Martin and Saller (1962), by permission.

described as arch, loop, and whorl (Fig. 12.2). Pattern variation is also seen in the thenar and hypothenar area.

## Methods to Record and Analyze Dermatoglyphics

There are several ways to record the dermal ridge patterns of the hands and feet. The first way is to evaluate the patterns with a magnifying glass, preferably one that has an integrated lamp like an otoscope, or a device used by stamp collectors. For recording the dermal ridge patterns, prints can be made in several ways.

**Ink staining**    Ink can be used to stain the patient's hands and feet, applied with a roller on a pre-inked pad, and distributed as evenly as possible (Fig. 12.4). The print is made by pressing a piece of paper against the

**Figure 12.4**    Recording dermatoglyphics by the ink staining method.

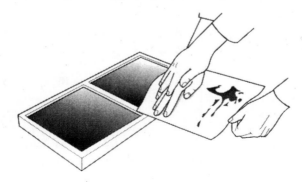

palm, or letting the patient stand on a piece of paper (it might be easier to have the patient roll the hand over a roller covered with a piece of paper large enough to obtain a print of the whole hand). Backing the paper with a soft material allows the fingers to "sink into" the paper and results in better prints. Usually each fingertip pattern is also recorded by rolling it separately from side to side.

**Photographic emulsion**   Instead of ink, a clear resensitizing fluid and photographic paper can be used. The technique for recording is the same. This method does not work as well for infants or on smooth lower ridges.

**Graphite**   Another alternative is to rub the patient's hands and feet with a soft graphite pencil. A print is taken by placing a broad piece of clear adhesive tape with the sticky side against the palm or sole. The adhesive tape is removed and can then be glued onto a white paper for better contrast and analysis. This method is particularly applicable for infants.

**Photocopying**   The hands and feet of an individual may be placed on a photocopying machine. The paper photocopies allow analysis of dermatoglyphics, but this is not a very precise method of obtaining dermatoglyphic data.

## Analysis of Ridge Patterns

**Dermal ridge count**   To count the dermal ridges of a particular pattern, a line is drawn from the middle or center of the pattern to a triradius (a point at which three converging patterns meet) (Fig. 12.5). The number of ridges which are crossed by this line or touch the line is counted. The total dermal ridge count for the individual is the sum of the ridge count of

**Figure 12.5**   Measuring dermal ridge count.

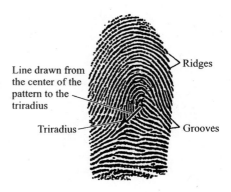

Line drawn from the center of the pattern to the triradius

Ridges

Triradius

Grooves

the 10 digits. If there are two triradii, as in a whorl, the line is drawn to the most distal triradius. Arch patterns have no ridge counts.

The average dermal ridge count in males is 144; in females 127.

**Triradii**   Triradii (or deltas) are the points at which three sets of converging ridge patterns meet. They are seen between the bases of the fingers, on the fingertips in loop and whorl patterns, and on the palm. Usually there is a triradius in the proximal part of the palm to the ulnar side of the center, just above the wrist flexion-crease: the proximal axial triradius ($t$). An angle can be established between the triradius at the base of the index finger ($a$), the proximal axial triradius ($t$), and the triradius at the base of the fifth finger ($d$). This is called the $atd$ angle. A distal palmar triradius ($t'$ or $t''$) may also be present. When the $at''d$ angle is calculated, it is usually much larger than the $atd$ angle. About 4 percent of Caucasians have a distal palmar triradius. Distal palmar triradii can be found in a number of syndromes, and their presence should alert the clinician to examine the dermatoglyphics more carefully.

**Thenar, hypothenar, and hallucal patterns**   Patterns may be present in the thenar and hypothenar areas of the palm. Unusual patterns may be helpful in making a specific diagnosis. A lack of ridges in the hypothenar region of the palm can be seen in Cornelia de Lange syndrome. On the soles of the feet, in the hallucal area, a pattern (loop or whorl) is usually seen. If no pattern is present (i.e., there is an arch), the hallucal area is said to have an "open field." Open hallucal fields are very rarely found in normal individuals, but are present in about 50 percent of patients with Down syndrome.

**Normal distribution of fingerprint patterns**   Evaluation of the fingertips generally reveals a variety of patterns on different fingertips (Fig. 12.6). The patterns tend to be familial. The most frequent patterns are whorls on the thumb and the fourth finger, and ulnar loops on fingers three and five. Among normal individuals, 0.9 percent have a predominance of arches on the fingertips, (i.e., 6 of 10 fingers show arches). However, this pattern is very frequently seen in patients with trisomy 18.

Three percent of normal individuals show 9–10 fingertips with a whorl pattern. Excessive whorl patterns derive from high fetal pads. They are seen frequently in patients with Turner syndrome or Noonan syndrome.

Radial loops on the fourth and fifth finger are unusual in normal individuals (1.5 percent) but are common in individuals with Down syndrome (12.4 percent).

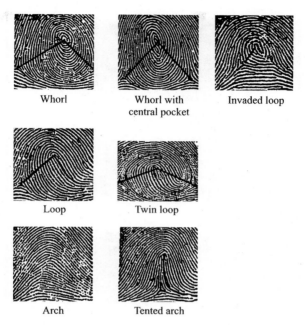

Whorl     Whorl with central pocket     Invaded loop

Loop     Twin loop

Arch     Tented arch

**Figure 12.6(a)**   Normal fingerprint patterns. From Martin and Saller (1962), by permission.

Racial differences exist: Asians and Native Americans have an increased number of whorls.

**Remarks** Alterations in the dermal ridge patterns or in the patterns of creases are recognizable in various syndromes (Fig. 12.7, and Bibliography). They are rarely pathognomonic but may provide an additional clue to the

**Fig. 12.6(b)**   Normal distribution of fingerprint pattern

|         | I(%)  | II(%) | III(%) | IV(%) | V(%)  | I–V(%)       |
|---------|-------|-------|--------|-------|-------|--------------|
| Figures |       |       |        |       |       |              |
| Arches  | 2.5   | 11.2  | 5.0    | 0.5   | 1.7   | 4.2 ± 2.1    |
| Loops   | 60.7  | 48.5  | 73.0   | 50.7  | 83.2  | 63.2 ± 1.3   |
| Whorls  | 36.7  | 40.2  | 22.0   | 48.7  | 15.0  | 32.5 ± 1.8   |
| Toes    |       |       |        |       |       |              |
| Arches  | 7.0   | 9.0   | 4.2    | 16.5  | 58.2  | 19.0 ± 2.0   |
| Loops   | 80.7  | 68.2  | 36.2   | 70.2  | 41.0  | 59.3 ± 1.4   |
| Whorls  | 12.2  | 22.7  | 59.5   | 13.2  | 0.7   | 21.7 ± 1.9   |

*From Martin and Saller (1962), by permission.*

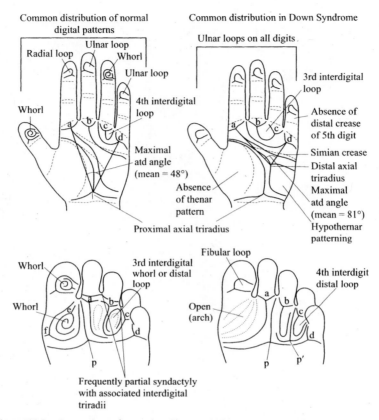

**Figure 12.7** Comparison of normal and Down syndrome patterns on hand and foot. From Smith (1982), by permission.

overall pattern of a malformation syndrome and may indicate the timing of a developmental anomaly. Any analysis of dermal ridges should include comparison with parental and/or family patterns.

## Analysis of Flexion Creases

The flexion creases of fingers reflect flexion at the interphalangeal joint; those of the palm reflect movement of the hand and the digits against the palm during early *in utero* development.

The flexion creases usually evaluated include those of the fingers and the major flexion creases of the palm. Each finger usually has three transverse

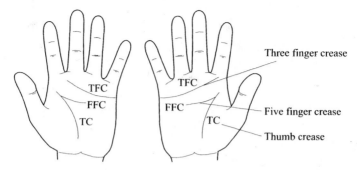

**Figure 12.8**   Normal flexion crease patterns. From Martin and Saller (1962), by permission.

creases of similar depth. If a crease is missing, or diminished, *in utero* movement of the underlying joint may have been absent or abnormal. There are usually three major creases in the palm (Fig. 12.8).

**The five finger crease (FFC)** This crease starts on the radial side of the hand near the insertion of the index finger and runs across the palm toward the ulnar side. If the FFC is long, it extends below the insertion of fingers 4 and 5. If it is of medium length, it extends below the insertion of the fourth finger, and if short it extends only to the third finger insertion.

**The three finger crease (TFC)** This crease starts on the ulnar side below the insertion of the fifth finger and runs across the palm distally, usually ending below the index and middle finger. The three finger crease is long if it reaches to the index finger insertion, of medium length if it reaches the interdigital area between the index and middle finger, and short if it only reaches the middle finger.

**The thumb crease (TC)** This crease starts together with the FFC from the radial side of the palm but runs proximally toward the mid-wrist. It is the consequence of oppositional flexion of the thumb. The thumb crease is long if it reaches down to the wrist crease.

Incomplete development of the FFC and the TFC may give rise to a single crease or simian crease (which may have different forms, being bridged or split). It may reflect alterations in the slope of the metacarpophalangeal plane of flexion or a short palm.

A single palmar crease (fusion of FFC and TFC) can be found unilaterally in 4 percent of the normal population and bilaterally in 1 percent of normal individuals. It is twice as common in males as in females. Single palmar creases are seen with increased frequency in Down syndrome.

A Sidney line is said to be present when the FFC extends all the way to the ulnar border.

## Trichoglyphics: Introduction and Embryology

The patterning of hair follicles is called trichoglyphics. The hair shaft directional slope is secondary to the plane of the stretch exerted on the skin when the hair follicles are forming. During the first two months of gestation, the embryo is completely hairless. Then the primary hair, called lanugo, starts to grow. The origin of the hair directional patterning is the original sloping angulation of the hair follicle. The hair follicles start to push downward into the underlying mesenchyme at 10–12 weeks of gestation (Fig. 12.9). On the scalp, the angle of the hair shaft reflects the prior plane of growth of the skin (e.g., the plane of growth present at the time when the follicle was forming). The plane of growth of the scalp skin is usually determined by the growth of the underlying brain.

The posterior parietal hair whorl is considered to be the focal point from which the growth stretch is exerted by the dome-like outgrowth of the brain during the time of hair follicle development. Central nervous system malformations that antedate hair follicle development, such as

**Figure 12.9** Time of hair patterning. From Smith and Gong (1974), by permission.

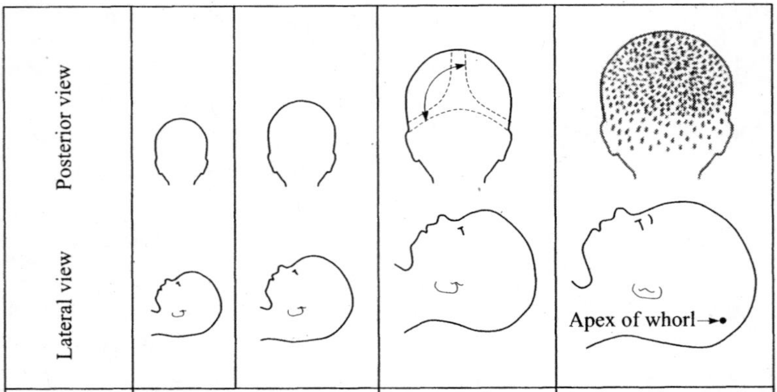

| | Early hair follicles with sloping downgrowth | | Hair being produced | Surface hair patterning evident |
|---|---|---|---|---|
| Hair | | | | |
| Gestational age | 11 weeks | 12½ weeks | 16½ weeks | 18 weeks |
| C–R length | 71 mm | 83 mm | 122 mm | 145 mm |

encephalocoele or microcephaly, would be expected to produce aberrations in scalp hair patterning, and these are indeed found. Eighty-five percent of patients with primary microcephaly have altered scalp hair patterning, indicating an early onset of the problem in brain development. Aberrant scalp patterning is also found frequently in association with established syndromes including Down syndrome. Thus, aberrant scalp hair patterning may be used as an indicator of altered size and/or shape of the brain before 12 weeks gestation.

On the forehead, two normal patterns of hair growth can be distinguished: the forehead stream (growing from the area of inner canthus upwards), and the parietal stream (growing from the parietal whorl to the supraorbital area). As the two steams meet, they give rise to the shape of the eyebrows. Eyebrow shape also reflects the underlying supraorbital ridge shape present in early fetal life. At 18 weeks of gestation, hair grows over the entire scalp and face. Later the hair growth in the eyebrow area and over the scalp will predominate, while hair growth over the remainder of the face suppressed.

Early anomalies in development of the eye and face can secondarily affect hair patterning over the eyebrow and frontal area, presumably related to altered growth tension of the skin during the period of hair follicle formation. Gross anomalies in development of the ear can also secondarily affect hair patterning, especially in the sideburn area.

## Normal and Abnormal Hair Patterns

The normal location of the parietal hair whorl is several centimeters anterior to the posterior fontanelle, the majority (56 percent) being located slightly to the left of the midline. Thirty percent of hair whorls in normal individuals are right sided, and 14 percent have a midline location. Five percent of individuals have bilateral hair whorls posteriorly. Ninety-four percent of hair whorls are clockwise and 5 percent are counter-clockwise.

From the posterior hair whorl, the hair sweeps anteriorly toward the forehead. The growth of the forebrain and the upper face influences the bilateral frontal hairstreams, which emerge from the ocular puncta and arch outward in a lateral direction. Usually the anterior and posterior hairstreams meet on the forehead. If they meet above the forehead, an anterior upsweep of hair will result (cowlick). A mild to moderate anterior upsweep is found in 5 percent of normal individuals.

Frontal upsweeps to the anterior hairline, as well as unruly hair patterns, have been linked to abnormalities of frontal lobe development.

A widow's peak along the frontal scalp line is probably the result of the bilateral periorbital fields of hair growth suppression intersecting lower than usual on the forehead. This can occur when the periorbital fields of hair growth suppression are smaller than usual, or when they are widely spaced. Wide spacing also explains the association between ocular hypertelorism and widow's peak. The only common anomaly of the posterior hairline is low placement with a squared distribution, which may be seen in Turner syndrome, in Noonan syndrome, and with abnormalities of cervical spine fusion or segmentation.

## Lanugo Hair Pattern

Persistence of lanugo hair whorls can be found over the entire back, particularly over the upper spine and in the coccygeal area. A hair whorl over the lower spine can be a sign of a defect of neural tube closure, a congenital tumor, or a neurofibroma. In the coccygeal area there may be a dimple at the point of the whorl (fovea coccygea). The coccygeal whorl may be related to the stretch point of an embryologically existing tail rudiment.

## Bibliography

Aase, J.M. and Lyons, R.B. (1971). Technique for recording dermatoglyphics. *Lancet*, 1, 432–433.

Martin, R. and Saller, K. (1962). *Lehrbuch der Anthropologie*. Gustav Fischer Verlag, Stuttgart, Germany

Moore, K.L. (1982). *The developing human*, pp. 432–446. W.B. Saunders, Philadelphia.

Mulvihill, J.J. and Smith, D.W. (1969). The genesis of dermatoglyphics. *Journal of Pediatrics*, 75, 579–589.

Rodewald, A. and Zankl, H. (1981). *Hautleistenfibel*. Gustav Fischer Verlag, Stuttgart, Germany

Smith, D.W. (1982), *Recognizable patterns of human malformation* (3rd ed), p. 576. W.B. Saunders, Philadelphia.

Smith, D.W. and Cohen, M.M. (1973). Widow's peak scalp-hair anomaly and its relation to ocular hypertelorism. *Lancet*, 2, 1127–1128.

Smith, D.W. and Gong, B.T. (1973). Scalp hair patterning as a clue to early fetal brain development. *Journal of Pediatrics*, 83, 374–400.

Smith, D.W. and Gong, B.T. (1974). Scalp-hair patterning: its origin and significance relative to early brain and upper facial development. *Teratology*, 9, 17–34.

Smith, D.W. and Greely, M.J. (1978). Unruly scalp hair in infancy: its nature and relevance to problems of brain morphogenesis. *Pediatrics,* **61**, 783–785.

Uchida, I. and Soltan, H./C. (1963). Evaluation of dermatoglyphics in medical genetics. *Pediatric Clinics of North America,* **10**, 409.

# Use of Radiographs for Measurement

13

## Introduction

Two techniques, bone age and pattern profiles, are time honored in describing growth and its variation in children. For other measurements and detailed discussions, the reader is referred to the Bibliography. Limb lengths, specific bone lengths, and asymmetry are often most accurately measured on radiographs. However, positioning of the limb or body part is critical to accuracy.

## Bone Age

Bone age is an attempt to quantify developmental age as seen in bone maturation on X-ray. In some ways it is a reflection of physiological growth and should be compared with height age and chronological age to assess the child's growth status. In normal children, bone age is an accurate reflection of physiological growth; however, in syndromes, growth disturbances, and osteochondrodysplasias (either undergrowth or overgrowth) it may be quite inaccurate. Assessment of bone age is further complicated by differences in the techniques used. Each technique is more or less useful under various circumstances. In spite of these problems, bone age assessment is an important and useful technique in describing the growth and physiological state of a child. It can also be used to predict ultimate height with some accuracy.

Assessment of bone age is dependent on the evolving appearance and growth of epiphyseal growth centers particularly in long bones. In the normal child, there is a predictable pattern of ossification and growth. Two main methods of determining bone age are used:

1. evaluation of the appearance of ossification centers throughout the body;
2. observation of growth and changes in a specific epiphysis or epiphyses and comparison with standards, such as for the hand (Greulich and Pyle) or the knee (Pyle and Hoerr).

In general, appearance of the ossification centers of the feet and knees is thought to be most useful in the young child. After two years of age, changes in specific epiphyses (such as in the hands) are most accurate.

## Ossification Centers

When taking X-rays to establish bone age, one should estimate approximate age to determine which will be the most useful films. Figure 13.1 will help to predict which areas should be studied. The observed areas of ossification are identified and compared to the expected age of ossification (Figs 13.2–13.6). The closest match is determined to be the present bone age.

**Figure 13.1** Region to sample for bone age related to chronological age. From Graham (1972), by permission.

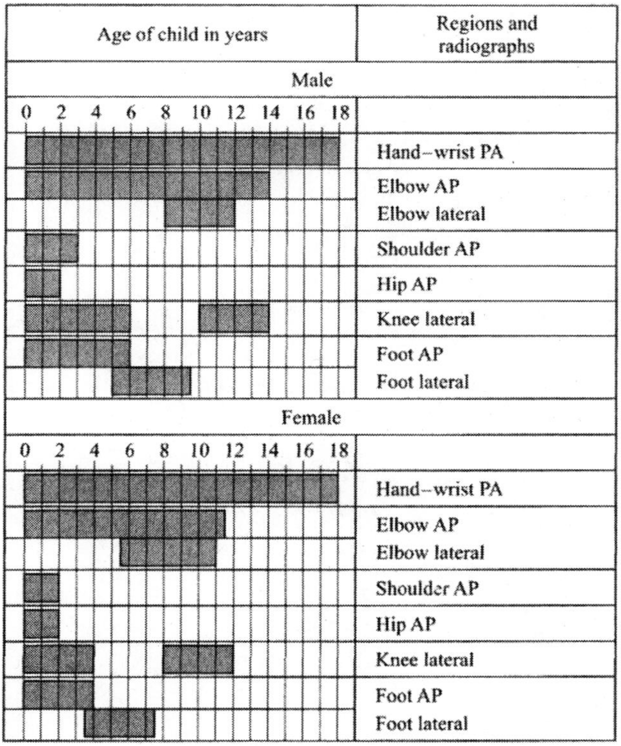

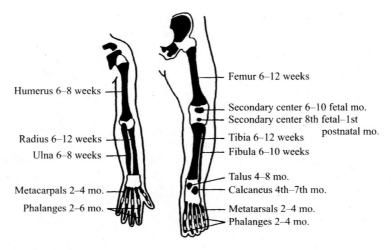

**Figure 13.2**    Fetal ossification centers. From Lowrey (1986), by permission.

**Comparison with established standards**    It is necessary to have the standard illustration present in the books by Greulich and Pyle (1959) and by Pyle and Hoerr (1969) to evaluate the shape and growth of phalangeal and knee epiphyses. By comparison with these standards, one arrives at a "best match" and establishes the bone age for the child.

**Fig. 13.3a**    Appearance time of ossification centers in the newborn (both sexes) in weeks of gestation

| Center | First seen | 5% | 50% | 95% |
|---|---|---|---|---|
| Humeral head epiphyses | 36 | 37 | — | 16 postnatal wk |
| Distal femoral epiphysis | 31 | 31 | 34 | 39 wk (male, 40 wk) |
| | 27 | — | — | |
| Proximal tibial epiphysis | 34 | 34 | 38–39 | 2 postnatal wk for female and 5 postnatal wk for male |
| Calcaneus | 22 | 22 | — | 25 after 26 wk, always present |
| Talus | 25 | 25 | — | 31 wk |
| | 26 | — | — | Talus may be absent until 34 wk |
| Cuboid | 31 | 37 | — | 8 postnatal wk in female and 16 postnatal wk in male |
| | — | 34 | — | |

**Fig. 13.3b**  Presence of six ossification centers in roentgenograms of newborns

| Ossification center | Birth weight (g) | | | | | |
|---|---|---|---|---|---|---|
| | Under 2000 | 2000–2499 | 2500–2999 | 3000–3499 | 3500–3999 | 4000 or more |
| **Calcaneus** | | | | | | |
| White boys | 100.0 | | | | | |
| girls | 100.0 | | | | | |
| African American boys | 100.0 | | | | | |
| girls | 100.0 | | | | | |
| **Talus** | | | | | | |
| White boys | 72.7 | 100.0 | | | | |
| girls | 83.3 | 100.0 | | | | |
| African American boys | 90.9 | 100.0 | | | | |
| girls | 100.0 | 100.0 | | | | |
| **Distal femoral epiphysis** | | | | | | |
| White boys | 9.1 | 75.0 | 85.3 | 100.0 | 100.0 | |
| girls | 50.0 | 91.7 | 98.0 | 100.0 | 100.0 | |
| African American boys | 18.2 | 88.5 | 90.7 | 94.0 | 100.0 | |
| girls | 50.2 | 93.8 | 99.0 | 100.0 | 100.0 | |
| **Proximal femoral epiphysis** | | | | | | |
| White boys | 0.0 | 18.8 | 52.9 | 78.8 | 84.1 | 97.1 |
| girls | 0.0 | 54.2 | 75.5 | 85.7 | 90.7 | 90.5 |
| African American boys | 0.0 | 38.5 | 62.7 | 76.0 | 80.0 | 92.9 |
| girls | 14.3 | 40.6 | 76.7 | 88.1 | 86.4 | 100.0 |
| **Cuboid** | | | | | | |
| White boys | 0.0 | 6.2 | 14.7 | 39.8 | 44.3 | 60.0 |
| girls | 0.0 | 37.5 | 57.1 | 65.2 | 70.4 | 76.2 |
| African American boys | 0.0 | 23.1 | 43.8 | 58.0 | 68.2 | 100.0 |
| girls | 21.4 | 37.5 | 68.0 | 78.2 | 81.8 | 75.0 |
| **Head of humerus** | | | | | | |
| White boys | 0.0 | 7.7 | 13.8 | 41.9 | 49.0 | 59.1 |
| girls | 0.0 | 5.6 | 25.8 | 41.9 | 69.0 | 86.7 |
| African American boys | 0.0 | 0.0 | 15.2 | 27.6 | 48.4 | 63.6 |
| girls | 0.0 | 10.7 | 22.7 | 52.6 | 38.9 | 100.0 |

*From Kuhns and Poznanski (1980) and Lowrey (1986), by permission.*

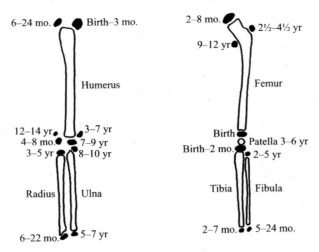

**Figure 13.4** Appearance of ossification centers in limbs, both sexes. From Lowrey (1986), by permission.

**Figure 13.5** Appearance of ossification centers in hands and feet, both sexes. Note: f.w. = fetal weeks; f.mo. = fetal months; b. = birth; mo. = postnatal months; y. = years. Phal. = phalange; Metac. = metacarpal; Hama. = hamate; Capit. = capitate; M. min. = multangular minor (trapezium); M. maj. = multangular major (trapezoid); Navic. = navicular; Trique. = triquetrum; Luna. = lunate; Pisif. = pisiform; Metat. = metatarsal; Cun. = cuneiform; Calca. = calcaneus. From Lowrey (1986), by permission.

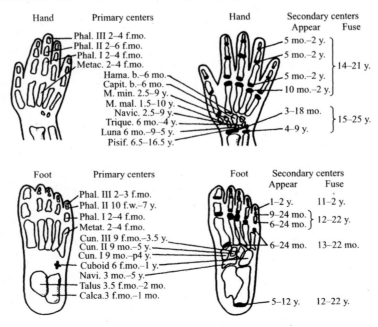

**Fig. 13.6** Age of appearance of perinatal ossification centers, both sexes

| | Boys (percentiles) | | | Girls (percentiles) | | |
|---|---|---|---|---|---|---|
| | 5th | 50th | 95th | 5th | 50th | 95th |
| **Wrist** | | | | | | |
| Capitate | Birth | 3m | 7m | Birth | 2m | 7m |
| Hamate | 2w | 4m | 10m | Birth | 2m | 7m |
| Distal radius | 6w | 1y1m | 2y4m | 5m | 10m | 1y8m |
| Triquetum | 6m | 2y5m | 5y6m | 3m | 1y8m | 3y9m |
| Lunate | 1y6m | 4y1m | 6y9m | 1y1m | 2y7m | 5y8m |
| Scaphoid | 3y7m | 5y8m | 7y10m | 2y4m | 4y1m | 6y |
| Trapezium | 3y6m | 5y10m | 9y | 1y11m | 4y1m | 6y4m |
| Trapezoid | 3y1m | 6y3m | 8y6m | 2y5m | 4y2m | 6y |
| Distal ulna | 5y3m | 7y1m | 9y1m | 3y3m | 5y4m | 7y8m |
| **Elbow** | | | | | | |
| Capitulum | 3w | 4m | 1y1m | 3w | 3m | 9m |
| Radial head | 3y | 5y3m | 8y | 2y3m | 3y10m | 6y3m |
| Medical epicondyle | 4y3m | 6y3m | 8y5m | 2y1m | 3y5m | 5y1m |
| Olecranon of ulna | 7y9m | 9y8m | 11y11m | 5y7m | 8y | 9y11m |
| Lateral epicondyle | 9y3m | 11y3m | 13y8m | 7y2m | 9y3m | 11y3m |
| **Shoulder** | | | | | | |
| Head of humerus | 37w* | | 16w | 37w* | | 16w |
| Coronoid | Birth | 2w | 4m | Birth | 2w | 5m |
| Tubercle of humerus | 3m | 10m | 2y4m | 2m | 6m | 1y2m |
| Acromion of scapula | 12y2n | 13y9m | 15y6m | 10y4m | 11y11m | 15y4m |
| Acromion of clavicle | 12y | 14y | 15y11m | 10y10m | 12y9m | 15y4m |
| **Hip** | | | | | | |
| Head of femur | 3w | 4m | 8m | 2w | 4m | 7m |
| Greater trochanter | 1y11m | 3y | 4y4m | 1y | 1y10m | 3y |
| Os acetabulum | 11y11m | 13y6m | 15y4m | 9y7m | 11y6m | 13y5m |
| Iliac crest | 12y | 14y | 15y11m | 10y10m | 12y9m | 15y4m |
| Ischial tuberosity | 13y7m | 15y3m | 17y1m | 11y9m | 13y11m | 16y |
| **Knee** | | | | | | |
| Distal femur | 31w* | | 40w* | 31w* | | 39w* |
| Proximal tibia | 34* | | 5w | 34w* | | 2w |
| Proximal fibula | 1y10m | 3y6m | 5y3m | 1y4m | 2y7m | 3y11m |
| Patella | 2y7m | 4y | 6y | 1y6m | 2y6m | 4y |
| Tibial tubercle | 9y11m | 11y10m | 13y5m | 7y11m | 10y3m | 11y10m |
| **Foot** | | | | | | |
| Calcaneus | 22w* | | 25w* | 22w* | | 25w* |
| Talus | 25w* | | 31w* | 25w* | | 31w* |
| Cuboid | 37w* | | 16w | 37w* | | 8w |
| Third cuneiform | 3w | 6m | 1y7m | Birth | 3m | 1y3m |
| Os calcis, apophysis | 5y2m | 7y7m | 9y7m | 3y6m | 5y4m | 7y4m |

\* *Prenatal age*
*From Poznanski et al. (1976) by permission.*

## Prediction of Adult Height

A number of methods have been developed to predict adult final height (see Chapter 4). Bone age is an important part of accurate predictions.

## Dental Age

Teeth can also be used to predict bone age (Fig. 13.7(a,b). They are sometimes called the 'poor man's bone age' because X-rays are not necessary. They can be used to predict bone age, however, they are not nearly as reliable as X-ray studies. Because tooth development starts *in utero* it also may reflect and date prenatal influences on shape, coloration, and enamel formation.

Ossification or molars in the jaw seen on X-ray can be used to predict bone maturation and gestational age as well. The first deciduous molar ossification can be seen at 32 weeks gestation. The second deciduous molar ossification occurs at 35 weeks gestation.

**Fig. 13.7(a)**  Dental development: Primary or deciduous teeth

|  | Initiation week *in utero* | Calcification begins, week *in utero* | Crown completed, month | Eruption |
|---|---|---|---|---|
|  |  |  |  | Maxillary |
| Central incisors | 7 | 14 (13–16) | 1–3 | 6–8 mo. |
| Lateral incisors | 7 | 16 (14$\frac{1}{2}$–16$\frac{1}{2}$) | 2–3 | 8–11 mo. |
| Cuspids (canine) | 7$\frac{1}{2}$ | 17 (15–18) | 9 | 16–20 mo. |
| First premolars | — | — | — | — |
| Second premolars | — | — | — | — |
| First molars | 8 | 15$\frac{1}{2}$(14$\frac{1}{2}$–17) | 6 | 10–16 mo. |
| Second molars | 10 | 18$\frac{1}{2}$ (16–23$\frac{1}{2}$) | 10–12 | 20–30 mo. |
| Third molars | — | — | — | — |

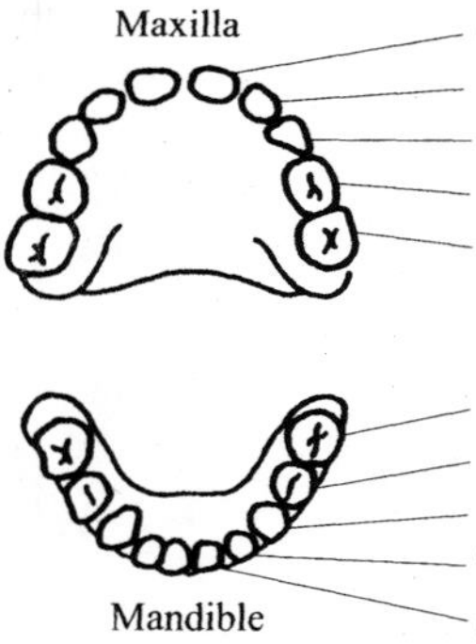

| | Age of eruption (mo.): | | | Average age of shedding (yr) |
|---|---|---|---|---|
| Maxilla | Early | Average | Late | |
| | 6 | 9.6 | 12 | 7.5 |
| | 7 | 12.4 | 18 | 8 |
| | 11 | 18.3 | 24 | 11.5 |
| | 10 | 15.7 | 20 | 10.5 |
| | 13 | 26.2 | 31 | 10.5 |
| | 13 | 26.0 | 31 | 11 |
| | 10 | 15.1 | 30 | 10 |
| | 11 | 18.2 | 24 | 9.5 |
| | 7 | 11.5 | 15 | 7 |
| Mandible | 5 | 7.8 | 11 | 6 |

**Figure 13.7(b)**  Sequence of primary tooth eruption and shedding. From Lowrey (1986), by permission.

**Fig. 13.7(c)**  Eruption and shedding of primary teeth

| Eruption Mandibular | Root completed, year | Root resorption begins, year | Shedding | |
|---|---|---|---|---|
| | | | Maxillary | Mandibular |
| 5–7 mo. | $1\frac{1}{2}$–2 | 5–6 | 7–8 yr | 6–7 |
| 7–10 mo. | $1\frac{1}{2}$–2 | 5–6 | 8–9 yr | 7–8 |
| 16–20 mo. | $2\frac{1}{2}$–$3\frac{1}{2}$ | 6–7 | 11–12 yr | 9–11 |
| — | — | — | — | — |
| — | — | — | — | — |
| 10–16 mo. | 2–$2\frac{1}{2}$ | 4–5 | 10–11 yr | 10–12 yr |
| 20–30 mo. | 3 | 4–5 | 10–12 yr | 11–13 yr |
| — | — | — | — | — |

*From Vaughn et al. (1979), by permission.*

**Fig. 13.7(d)** Secondary or permanent teeth

|  | Calcification | | Eruption | |
|---|---|---|---|---|
|  | Begins at | Complete at | Maxillary | Mandibular |
| Central incisors | 3–4 mo. | 9–10 yr | 7–8 yr | 6–7 yr |
| Lateral incisors |  |  |  |  |
|    Maxillary | 10–12 mo. | 10–11 yr | 8–9 yr | 7–8 yr |
|    Mandibular | 3–4 mo. |  |  |  |
| Canines | 4–5 mo. | 12–15 yr | 11–12 yr | 9–11 yr |
| First premolars | 18–21 mo. | 12–13 yr | 10–11 yr | 10–12 yr |
| Second premolars | 24–30 mos | 12–14 yr | 10–12 yr | 11–13 yr |
| First molars | Birth | 9–10 yr | 6–7 yr | 6–7 yr |
| Second molars | 30–36 mo. | 14–16 yr | 12–13 yr | 12–13 yr |
| Third molars |  |  |  |  |
|    Maxillary | 7–9 yr | 18–25 yr | 17–22 yr | 17–22 yr |
|    Mandibular | 8–10 yr |  |  |  |

*From Vaughan et al. (1979), by permission.*

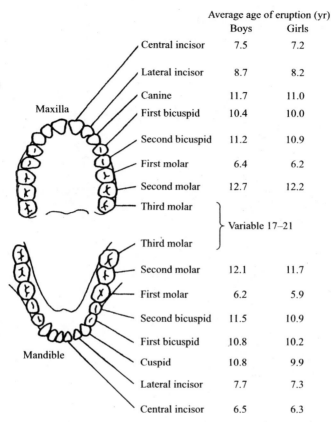

|  | Average age of eruption (yr) | |
|  | Boys | Girls |
|---|---|---|
| Central incisor | 7.5 | 7.2 |
| Lateral incisor | 8.7 | 8.2 |
| Canine | 11.7 | 11.0 |
| First bicuspid | 10.4 | 10.0 |
| Second bicuspid | 11.2 | 10.9 |
| First molar | 6.4 | 6.2 |
| Second molar | 12.7 | 12.2 |
| Third molar | Variable 17–21 | |
| Third molar | | |
| Second molar | 12.1 | 11.7 |
| First molar | 6.2 | 5.9 |
| Second bicuspid | 11.5 | 10.9 |
| First bicuspid | 10.8 | 10.2 |
| Cuspid | 10.8 | 9.9 |
| Lateral incisor | 7.7 | 7.3 |
| Central incisor | 6.5 | 6.3 |

**Figure 13.7(e)**  Average ages of eruption of secondary teeth, males and females. From Lowrey (1986), by permission.

## Pattern Profile of the Hand

Analysis of the pattern of hand bone lengths is a very useful technique for recognizing specific bone dysplasias, syndromes, and familial patterns that affect bone growth. By measuring the length of the 19 tubular bones of the hand from a standardized X-ray of the hand (Fig. 13.8a, b) one can construct a profile of the lengths of each bone in each digit (D1–D5). The lengths are then standardized by age. The measurement for each digit is then plotted by its deviation from normal for age (Fig. 13.8c–h) giving a profile of the hand.

The normal individual has a flat line with no deviations (Fig. 13.8d), but most syndromes have characteristic patterns. This method is a useful way to characterize and quantify dysmorphology of the hand in specific conditions. For specific examples, references at the end of this chapter should be consulted.

**Figure 13.8(a,b)**  Measuring finger bones. From Poznanski and Gartman (1983), by permission.

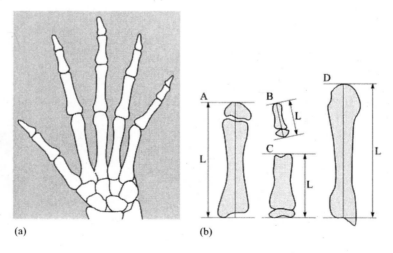

(a)                                        (b)

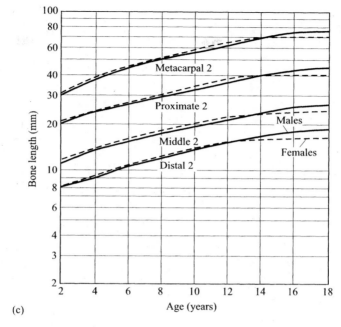

(c)

**Figure 13.8(c)**   Normal growth patterns of hand tubular bones.

**Figure 13.8(d)**   Normal family pattern profile of finger bones.

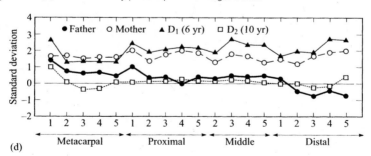

(d)

**Fig. 13.8e** Table of norms for finger bone lengths, age 2–10 years, males

Males

| Bones | | 2 Mean | 2 SD | 3 Mean | 3 SD | 4 Mean | 4 SD | 5 Mean | 5 SD | 6 Mean | 6 SD | 7 Mean | 7 SD | 8 Mean | 8 SD | 9 Mean | 9 SD | 10 Mean | 10 SD |
|---|---|---|---|---|---|---|---|---|---|---|---|---|---|---|---|---|---|---|---|
| Distal | 5 | 8.8 | — | 8.4 | 0.6 | 9.0 | 0.7 | 9.9 | 0.6 | 10.7 | 0.0 | 11.4 | 0.8 | 12.2 | 0.9 | 12.6 | 1.0 | 13.5 | 0.9 |
| | 4 | 9.2 | 0.7 | 9.9 | 0.8 | 10.5 | 0.8 | 11.5 | 0.9 | 12.3 | 0.9 | 13.1 | 1.0 | 13.9 | 1.0 | 14.4 | 1.0 | 15.3 | 1.2 |
| | 3 | 8.7 | 0.9 | 9.5 | 0.8 | 10.2 | 0.8 | 11.1 | 0.8 | 11.8 | 0.9 | 12.7 | 1.0 | 13.4 | 1.0 | 14.0 | 1.0 | 14.8 | 1.2 |
| | 2 | 8.2 | 0.5 | 8.8 | — | 9.4 | 1.0 | 10.1 | 0.9 | 10.8 | 0.9 | 11.6 | 1.0 | 12.4 | 1.0 | 13.0 | 1.0 | 13.7 | 1.1 |
| | 1 | — | — | 12.3 | — | 13.2 | 1.0 | 14.4 | 0.9 | 15.4 | 0.9 | 16.5 | 1.1 | 17.4 | 1.1 | 17.9 | 1.2 | 19.0 | 1.2 |
| Middle | 5 | — | — | — | — | 10.7 | 1.0 | 11.2 | 1.0 | 12.0 | 1.0 | 12.7 | 1.1 | 13.5 | 1.1 | 14.3 | 1.3 | 15.0 | 1.3 |
| | 4 | — | — | — | — | 15.8 | 1.0 | 16.5 | 1.0 | 17.7 | 1.1 | 18.7 | 1.2 | 19.8 | 1.2 | 20.9 | 1.4 | 21.6 | 1.4 |
| | 3 | 14.1 | 0.8 | 15.1 | 1.0 | 16.5 | 1.0 | 17.6 | 1.0 | 18.7 | 1.1 | 19.8 | 1.2 | 20.9 | 1.2 | 22.0 | 1.2 | 22.9 | 1.4 |
| | 2 | 11.2 | 0.8 | 12.3 | 1.1 | 13.5 | 1.0 | 14.4 | 0.9 | 15.3 | 1.0 | 16.1 | 1.1 | 17.1 | 1.1 | 18.1 | 1.2 | 18.8 | 1.2 |
| Proximal | 5 | 16.1 | 0.7 | 17.8 | 0.9 | 19.2 | 1.0 | 20.6 | 1.0 | 21.8 | 1.0 | 23.0 | 1.1 | 24.2 | 1.3 | 25.2 | 1.5 | 26.4 | 1.5 |
| | 4 | 20.5 | 0.9 | 22.8 | 1.0 | 24.7 | 1.2 | 26.4 | 1.2 | 27.9 | 1.2 | 29.5 | 1.4 | 31.0 | 1.6 | 32.3 | 1.9 | 33.9 | 1.8 |
| | 3 | 21.8 | 1.0 | 24.2 | 1.1 | 26.3 | 1.4 | 28.1 | 1.4 | 29.8 | 1.4 | 31.5 | 1.6 | 33.2 | 1.8 | 34.7 | 2.2 | 36.1 | 1.9 |
| | 2 | 19.5 | 1.0 | 21.9 | 1.1 | 23.7 | 1.3 | 25.4 | 1.4 | 26.8 | 1.5 | 28.3 | 1.6 | 29.7 | 1.8 | 31.4 | 1.9 | 32.5 | 1.9 |
| | 1 | 15.2 | — | 15.9 | 1.1 | 17.2 | 1.1 | 18.3 | 1.2 | 19.6 | 1.2 | 20.8 | 1.3 | 21.8 | 1.3 | 23.1 | 1.5 | 24.2 | 1.4 |
| Metacarpal | 5 | 23.9 | 1.0 | 26.3 | 1.5 | 28.9 | 1.9 | 32.1 | 2.2 | 34.6 | 2.2 | 36.7 | 2.1 | 38.8 | 2.5 | 40.6 | 2.5 | 42.7 | 2.9 |
| | 4 | 25.5 | 1.1 | 28.9 | 1.5 | 31.7 | 2.1 | 35.0 | 2.5 | 37.9 | 2.7 | 40.1 | 2.5 | 42.2 | 3.1 | 44.1 | 2.8 | 46.5 | 3.5 |
| | 3 | 28.6 | 1.3 | 32.3 | 1.8 | 35.6 | 2.3 | 39.3 | 2.8 | 42.6 | 2.9 | 45.3 | 2.8 | 47.6 | 3.5 | 49.8 | 3.0 | 52.3 | 3.7 |
| | 2 | 30.6 | 1.5 | 34.5 | 1.7 | 37.9 | 2.3 | 41.6 | 2.7 | 44.9 | 2.9 | 47.7 | 2.8 | 50.2 | 3.4 | 52.6 | 3.0 | 55.0 | 3.9 |
| | 1 | 19.6 | 1.3 | 22.0 | 1.2 | 24.1 | 1.6 | 26.7 | 1.6 | 29.0 | 1.7 | 30.9 | 1.8 | 32.7 | 2.1 | 34.4 | 2.1 | 36.3 | 2.3 |

**Fig. 13.8f** Table of norms for finger bone lengths, age 2–10 years, females

| Years | | 2 | | 3 | | 4 | | 5 | | 6 | | 7 | | 8 | | 9 | | 10 | |
|---|---|---|---|---|---|---|---|---|---|---|---|---|---|---|---|---|---|---|---|
| Bones | | Mean | SD | Mean | SD | Mean | SD | Mean | SD | Mean | SD | Mean | SD | Mean | SD | Mean | SD | Mean | SD |
| **Females** | | | | | | | | | | | | | | | | | | | |
| Distal | 5 | 7.8 | 0.6 | 8.4 | 0.6 | 9.1 | 0.7 | 9.9 | 0.7 | 10.6 | 0.8 | 11.4 | 0.9 | 12.1 | 1.0 | 12.7 | 1.1 | 13.5 | 1.2 |
| | 4 | 9.1 | 0.7 | 9.9 | 0.7 | 10.6 | 0.8 | 11.5 | 0.9 | 12.4 | 1.0 | 13.2 | 1.1 | 14.0 | 1.0 | 14.4 | 1.2 | 15.5 | 1.4 |
| | 3 | 8.8 | 0.7 | 9.9 | 0.8 | 10.2 | 0.7 | 11.1 | 0.9 | 12.2 | 1.3 | 12.7 | 1.1 | 13.0 | 1.1 | 14.1 | 1.1 | 15.0 | 1.4 |
| | 2 | 8.0 | 0.8 | 8.6 | 0.7 | 9.4 | 0.7 | 10.1 | 0.8 | 10.9 | 0.9 | 11.7 | 1.0 | 12.3 | 1.1 | 13.1 | 1.1 | 13.8 | 1.4 |
| | 1 | 11.3 | 0.8 | 12.5 | 0.8 | 13.2 | 0.8 | 14.4 | 1.0 | 15.4 | 1.1 | 16.3 | 1.2 | 17.3 | 1.1 | 17.8 | 1.3 | 19.0 | 1.6 |
| Middle | 5 | 9.0 | 1.2 | 9.8 | 1.1 | 10.5 | 1.1 | 11.2 | 1.1 | 12.2 | 1.2 | 12.9 | 1.3 | 13.6 | 1.3 | 14.2 | 1.4 | 15.2 | 1.6 |
| | 4 | 13.5 | 0.9 | 14.9 | 1.0 | 15.8 | 1.1 | 16.9 | 1.2 | 18.1 | 1.3 | 19.1 | 1.4 | 20.1 | 1.4 | 20.9 | 1.5 | 22.2 | 1.7 |
| | 3 | 14.2 | 0.9 | 15.6 | 1.1 | 16.6 | 1.2 | 17.9 | 1.2 | 19.2 | 1.3 | 20.3 | 1.4 | 21.4 | 1.4 | 22.1 | 1.6 | 23.6 | 1.8 |
| | 2 | 11.6 | 0.9 | 12.8 | 1.0 | 13.6 | 1.1 | 14.8 | 1.1 | 16.0 | 1.2 | 16.8 | 1.3 | 17.8 | 1.4 | 18.1 | 1.5 | 19.6 | 1.7 |
| Proximal | 5 | 16.3 | 1.0 | 17.9 | 1.1 | 19.1 | 1.1 | 20.6 | 1.3 | 22.0 | 1.4 | 23.1 | 1.6 | 24.4 | 1.4 | 25.2 | 1.6 | 27.1 | 2.0 |
| | 4 | 20.7 | 1.1 | 22.9 | 1.3 | 24.6 | 1.3 | 26.3 | 1.5 | 28.2 | 1.7 | 29.7 | 1.9 | 31.2 | 1.6 | 32.4 | 2.0 | 34.5 | 2.4 |
| | 3 | 22.2 | 1.2 | 24.5 | 1.3 | 26.4 | 1.4 | 28.3 | 1.8 | 30.4 | 1.8 | 32.1 | 2.0 | 33.7 | 2.0 | 35.0 | 2.2 | 37.3 | 2.6 |
| | 2 | 20.1 | 1.2 | 22.3 | 1.3 | 24.0 | 1.8 | 25.8 | 1.7 | 27.7 | 1.7 | 29.2 | 1.9 | 30.7 | 2.2 | 31.5 | 2.4 | 34.0 | 2.4 |
| | 1 | 14.9 | 1.0 | 16.3 | 1.1 | 17.2 | 1.3 | 18.8 | 1.3 | 20.2 | 1.3 | 21.4 | 1.5 | 22.7 | 2.0 | 23.5 | 2.0 | 25.5 | 2.1 |
| Metacarpal | 5 | 23.7 | 1.5 | 26.9 | 2.1 | 29.4 | 1.8 | 32.6 | 2.0 | 35.1 | 2.1 | 37.2 | 2.4 | 39.4 | 1.6 | 40.8 | 2.5 | 43.8 | 2.8 |
| | 4 | 26.0 | 1.9 | 29.6 | 2.7 | 32.2 | 2.0 | 35.6 | 2.5 | 38.4 | 2.7 | 40.5 | 2.8 | 43.1 | 3.0 | 44.3 | 2.8 | 47.5 | 3.5 |
| | 3 | 29.4 | 2.1 | 33.4 | 2.9 | 36.3 | 2.2 | 40.3 | 2.7 | 43.3 | 3.1 | 45.8 | 3.1 | 48.7 | 3.2 | 49.9 | 3.2 | 53.6 | 3.8 |
| | 2 | 31.3 | 1.9 | 35.2 | 2.7 | 38.2 | 2.3 | 42.3 | 2.7 | 45.6 | 3.2 | 48.1 | 3.3 | 51.2 | 3.3 | 52.6 | 3.4 | 56.6 | 4.1 |
| | 1 | 19.9 | 1.6 | 22.7 | 1.6 | 24.8 | 1.7 | 27.3 | 1.8 | 29.6 | 1.9 | 31.5 | 2.0 | 33.5 | 2.1 | 34.8 | 2.4 | 37.4 | 2.6 |

\* For each sex N = 150 at age 4, 124 at age 9, 78 in adulthood, and 30–85 at intermediate ages. All values are in millimeters.

**Fig. 13.8g** Table of norms for finger bone lengths, ages 11 years to adult, males

| Years | 11 | | 12 | | 13 | | 14 | | 15 | | 16 | | 17 | | 18 | | Adults | |
|---|---|---|---|---|---|---|---|---|---|---|---|---|---|---|---|---|---|---|
| Bones | Mean | SD | Mean | SD | Mean | SD | Mean | SD | Mean | SD | Mean | SD | Mean | SD | Mean | SD | Mean | SD |
| **Males** | | | | | | | | | | | | | | | | | | |
| Distal | | | | | | | | | | | | | | | | | | |
| 5 | 14.2 | 0.9 | 15.0 | 0.9 | 15.8 | 0.9 | 16.8 | 1.0 | 17.6 | 1.1 | 17.9 | 1.0 | 18.1 | 1.0 | 18.1 | 1.2 | 18.7 | 1.3 |
| 4 | 16.1 | 1.2 | 17.0 | 1.3 | 17.8 | 1.4 | 18.8 | 1.3 | 19.6 | 1.4 | 20.0 | 1.3 | 20.3 | 1.3 | 20.0 | 1.3 | 20.5 | 1.2 |
| 3 | 15.6 | 1.2 | 16.4 | 1.2 | 17.1 | 1.3 | 18.2 | 1.3 | 19.0 | 1.4 | 19.3 | 1.4 | 19.5 | 1.3 | 19.4 | 1.3 | 20.1 | 1.2 |
| 2 | 14.3 | 1.1 | 15.0 | 1.0 | 15.7 | 1.4 | 16.7 | 1.2 | 17.5 | 1.2 | 17.8 | 1.3 | 18.2 | 1.3 | 18.1 | 1.3 | 18.8 | 1.4 |
| 1 | 19.7 | 1.2 | 20.6 | 1.3 | 21.7 | 1.4 | 22.8 | 1.3 | 24.1 | 1.4 | 24.5 | 1.4 | 24.9 | 1.4 | 24.8 | 1.5 | 25.2 | 1.4 |
| Middle | | | | | | | | | | | | | | | | | | |
| 5 | 15.7 | 1.4 | 16.5 | 1.5 | 17.5 | 1.5 | 18.9 | 1.6 | 19.9 | 1.4 | 20.5 | 1.4 | 20.6 | 1.4 | 21.0 | 1.4 | 21.6 | 1.6 |
| 4 | 22.6 | 1.5 | 23.6 | 1.5 | 24.8 | 1.7 | 26.5 | 1.6 | 27.7 | 1.5 | 28.4 | 1.5 | 28.7 | 1.4 | 29.1 | 1.5 | 29.6 | 1.6 |
| 3 | 24.0 | 1.8 | 24.9 | 1.4 | 26.3 | 1.6 | 28.0 | 1.5 | 29.2 | 1.6 | 30.5 | 1.6 | 30.2 | 1.6 | 30.6 | 1.8 | 31.1 | 1.8 |
| 2 | 19.8 | 1.7 | 20.4 | 1.3 | 21.6 | 1.6 | 23.2 | 1.5 | 24.3 | 1.5 | 25.0 | 1.5 | 25.3 | 1.4 | 25.6 | 1.7 | 26.1 | 1.6 |
| Proximal | | | | | | | | | | | | | | | | | | |
| 5 | 27.6 | 2.0 | 28.9 | 2.0 | 30.5 | 2.4 | 32.9 | 2.4 | 34.9 | 2.0 | 35.6 | 1.8 | 36.1 | 1.8 | 35.9 | 2.0 | 36.3 | 2.0 |
| 4 | 35.3 | 2.3 | 37.0 | 2.4 | 38.8 | 2.8 | 41.6 | 2.8 | 43.7 | 2.6 | 44.9 | 2.3 | 45.4 | 2.2 | 45.2 | 2.5 | 45.5 | 2.3 |
| 3 | 37.8 | 2.1 | 39.5 | 2.6 | 41.5 | 2.9 | 44.4 | 2.8 | 46.6 | 2.5 | 47.8 | 2.4 | 48.3 | 2.3 | 48.2 | 2.7 | 48.5 | 2.6 |
| 2 | 33.9 | 1.6 | 35.5 | 2.4 | 37.2 | 2.6 | 39.8 | 2.6 | 41.8 | 2.2 | 42.8 | 2.0 | 43.3 | 2.1 | 43.4 | 2.4 | 43.7 | 2.2 |
| 1 | 25.4 | 2.8 | 26.7 | 2.0 | 28.5 | 2.2 | 30.9 | 2.2 | 32.9 | 1.8 | 33.8 | 1.5 | 34.6 | 2.6 | 34.7 | 1.8 | 35.0 | 1.9 |
| Metacarpal | | | | | | | | | | | | | | | | | | |
| 5 | 44.6 | 3.1 | 47.1 | 3.2 | 49.1 | 4.0 | 52.2 | 3.9 | 55.4 | 3.6 | 57.1 | 2.8 | 57.9 | 2.5 | 57.5 | 2.9 | 58.0 | 3.0 |
| 4 | 48.4 | 3.4 | 5.10 | 3.7 | 53.1 | 4.6 | 56.4 | 4.5 | 59.5 | 4.1 | 61.5 | 3.7 | 62.6 | 3.1 | 61.7 | 3.4 | 62.1 | 3.5 |
| 3 | 54.6 | 3.5 | 57.3 | 4.0 | 59.5 | 5.1 | 63.1 | 4.9 | 66.7 | 4.4 | 68.7 | 4.1 | 69.7 | 3.3 | 69.0 | 3.7 | 69.0 | 3.8 |
| 2 | 57.3 | 2.4 | 60.6 | 3.9 | 63.5 | 5.1 | 67.1 | 4.8 | 70.6 | 4.3 | 73.2 | 3.8 | 74.2 | 2.9 | 73.9 | 3.5 | 73.7 | 3.8 |
| 1 | 38.2 | | 40.2 | 2.7 | 42.5 | 3.0 | 45.1 | 2.8 | 47.6 | 2.6 | 48.8 | 2.3 | 49.5 | 2.1 | 49.4 | 2.7 | 49.6 | 2.9 |

**Fig. 13.8h** Table of norms for finger bone lengths, age 11 years to adult, females

| Bones | | 11 Mean | 11 SD | 12 Mean | 12 SD | 13 Mean | 13 SD | 14 Mean | 14 SD | 15 Mean | 15 SD | 16 Mean | 16 SD | 17 Mean | 17 SD | 18 Mean | 18 SD | Adults Mean | Adults SD |
|---|---|---|---|---|---|---|---|---|---|---|---|---|---|---|---|---|---|---|---|
| **Females** | | | | | | | | | | | | | | | | | | | |
| Distal | 5 | 14.2 | 1.3 | 15.0 | 1.3 | 15.4 | 1.3 | 15.6 | 1.3 | 15.9 | 1.4 | 15.9 | 1.4 | 16.2 | 1.3 | 16.0 | 1.2 | 16.2 | 1.2 |
| | 4 | 16.2 | 1.4 | 17.1 | 1.4 | 17.6 | 1.2 | 17.9 | 1.3 | 18.0 | 1.4 | 18.0 | 1.3 | 18.1 | 1.4 | 17.9 | 1.3 | 18.0 | 1.3 |
| | 3 | 15.8 | 1.3 | 16.6 | 1.4 | 17.1 | 1.4 | 17.3 | 1.3 | 17.6 | 1.5 | 17.5 | 1.4 | 17.6 | 1.4 | 17.4 | 1.3 | 17.7 | 1.3 |
| | 2 | 14.4 | 1.3 | 15.2 | 1.5 | 15.7 | 1.5 | 15.8 | 1.5 | 16.1 | 1.6 | 16.0 | 1.6 | 16.3 | 1.5 | 16.2 | 1.3 | 16.6 | 1.3 |
| | 1 | 20.0 | 1.7 | 20.9 | 1.7 | 21.4 | 1.6 | 21.7 | 1.6 | 22.0 | 1.7 | 22.0 | 1.7 | 22.1 | 1.8 | 22.0 | 1.6 | 22.1 | 1.6 |
| Middle | 5 | 16.2 | 1.8 | 17.2 | 1.7 | 17.9 | 1.8 | 18.1 | 1.6 | 18.4 | 1.7 | 18.5 | 1.7 | 18.5 | 1.9 | 18.6 | 1.7 | 18.7 | 1.7 |
| | 4 | 23.4 | 1.9 | 24.7 | 1.8 | 25.7 | 1.9 | 25.9 | 1.6 | 26.3 | 1.8 | 26.4 | 1.8 | 26.5 | 1.9 | 26.3 | 1.8 | 26.4 | 1.7 |
| | 3 | 24.9 | 1.8 | 26.2 | 1.9 | 27.2 | 2.0 | 27.5 | 1.7 | 28.1 | 1.8 | 28.0 | 1.9 | 28.0 | 1.8 | 27.8 | 1.8 | 27.9 | 1.7 |
| | 2 | 20.9 | 2.1 | 21.8 | 1.9 | 22.7 | 1.8 | 23.0 | 1.8 | 23.5 | 2.2 | 23.3 | 1.9 | 23.4 | 1.9 | 23.1 | 1.6 | 23.2 | 1.6 |
| Proximal | 5 | 28.7 | 2.5 | 30.5 | 2.2 | 31.9 | 2.2 | 32.3 | 2.1 | 32.9 | 2.5 | 32.8 | 2.3 | 32.8 | 2.3 | 32.5 | 2.0 | 32.5 | 1.9 |
| | 4 | 36.5 | 2.7 | 38.8 | 2.6 | 40.3 | 2.5 | 40.9 | 2.3 | 41.5 | 2.6 | 41.6 | 2.6 | 41.7 | 2.6 | 41.1 | 2.2 | 40.8 | 2.4 |
| | 3 | 39.5 | 2.6 | 41.7 | 2.8 | 43.5 | 2.8 | 44.1 | 2.4 | 44.8 | 2.6 | 44.8 | 2.7 | 44.8 | 2.6 | 44.2 | 2.4 | 44.0 | 2.3 |
| | 2 | 35.9 | 2.3 | 38.0 | 2.6 | 39.5 | 2.6 | 39.9 | 2.4 | 40.6 | 2.0 | 40.6 | 2.6 | 40.7 | 2.7 | 39.9 | 2.3 | 40.0 | 2.3 |
| | 1 | 27.2 | 2.9 | 29.2 | 2.4 | 30.6 | 2.2 | 31.1 | 1.9 | 31.8 | 2.0 | 31.7 | 2.1 | 31.9 | | 31.3 | 1.9 | 31.4 | 2.0 |
| Metacarpal | 5 | 46.3 | 3.8 | 48.7 | 2.9 | 50.8 | 2.8 | 52.1 | 2.8 | 52.6 | 3.0 | 52.8 | 3.0 | 53.0 | 3.5 | 52.0 | 2.7 | 51.9 | 3.6 |
| | 4 | 50.2 | 4.0 | 52.8 | 3.7 | 55.1 | 3.6 | 56.2 | 3.6 | 56.9 | 3.6 | 57.2 | 3.9 | 57.2 | 4.0 | 56.1 | 2.9 | 56.0 | 3.5 |
| | 3 | 56.5 | 4.3 | 59.5 | 4.2 | 62.1 | 4.0 | 63.4 | 3.9 | 63.9 | 3.9 | 64.3 | 4.0 | 64.5 | 4.1 | 63.2 | 3.4 | 62.6 | 4.0 |
| | 2 | 59.9 | 3.0 | 63.2 | 4.4 | 66.2 | 4.2 | 67.4 | 3.9 | 68.1 | 4.2 | 68.6 | 4.3 | 68.9 | 2.6 | 67.5 | 3.4 | 66.9 | 4.3 |
| | 1 | 39.7 | | 42.0 | 3.0 | 43.8 | 2.7 | 44.4 | 2.5 | 45.3 | 2.4 | 45.0 | 2.8 | 45.0 | | 44.6 | 2.2 | 44.2 | 2.6 |

*For each sex N= 150 qt age 4, 124 at age 9, 78 in adulthood, and 30–85 at intermediate ages. All values are in mm.
From Garn et al. (1972) by permission.

## Carpal Angle

The angle that the carpal bones make at the wrist is useful in alerting the clinician to disproportionate growth elsewhere. Norms have been established for age, sex, and racial group.

The carpal angle is defined as the angle resulting from the intersection of two lines, one tangent to the proximal edge of the lunate and scaphoid and one tangent to the proximal edge of the lunate and triquetrum.

Imaginary lines are drawn on the X-ray, and the angles are measured (Fig. 13.9a). The angle should be compared with normal standards (Fig. 13.9b).

**Figure 13.9(a)**    Measurement of carpal angle using X-rays.

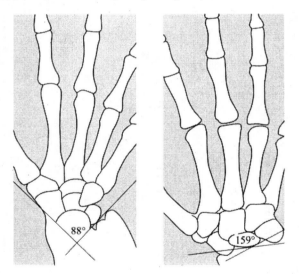

**Fig. 13.9b**   Carpal angle—norms

| Age groups (years) | Sample size | Percentiles 5th | 50th | 95th | Sample size | Percentiles 5th | 50th | 95th |
|---|---|---|---|---|---|---|---|---|
| | | | | **Carpal angle in degrees** | | | | |
| | | | White males | | | | White females | |
| 4–6 | 10 | 116.0 | 122.0 | 132.5 | | 120.0 | 126.5 | 143.0 |
| 6–8 | 36 | 111.0 | 124.0 | 153.5 | | 115.0 | 130.5 | 147.5 |
| 8–10 | 25 | 122.0 | 133.5 | 147.0 | | 115.5 | 129.5 | 139.5 |
| 10–12 | 24 | 155.5 | 133.0 | 143.0 | | 123.0 | 134.0 | 152.5 |
| 12–14 | 24 | 117.0 | 132.0 | 142.5 | | 116.0 | 130.0 | 143.0 |
| 14–24 | 49 | 119.0 | 134.0 | 149.0 | | 115.0 | 129.0 | 139.5 |
| 24–40 | 30 | 114.0 | 136.0 | 145.5 | | 112.0 | 130.5 | 142.5 |
| 40–83 | 33 | 113.5 | 134.0 | 146.5 | | 113.0 | 130.5 | 149.0 |
| | | | African American males | | | | African American females | |
| 4–6 | 9 | 124.0 | 131.0 | 143.0 | 16 | 116.5 | 130.5 | 140.5 |
| 6–8 | 32 | 119.0 | 128.5 | 147.5 | 22 | 121.0 | 133.0 | 146.5 |
| 8–10 | 31 | 128.0 | 139.0 | 142.0 | 16 | 125.0 | 139.0 | 155.0 |
| 10–12 | 28 | 121.0 | 138.0 | 152.5 | 23 | 125.5 | 138.5 | 151.0 |
| 12–14 | 32 | 125.5 | 141.0 | 143.0 | 28 | 123.0 | 141.0 | 153.5 |
| 14–24 | 52 | 128.0 | 146.0 | 139.5 | 67 | 123.0 | 139.0 | 150.0 |
| 24–40 | 14 | 128.0 | 136.0 | 142.5 | 18 | 127.0 | 136.5 | 151.0 |
| 40–83 | 32 | 125.5 | 140.0 | 149.0 | 46 | 126.5 | 140.5 | 153.5 |

*From Harper et al. (1974) by permission.*

## Bibliography

Garn, S.M., Hertzog, K.P., Poznanski, A.K. and Nagy, J.M. (1972). Metacarpophalangeal length in the evaluation of skeletal malformation. *Radiology*, **105**, 375–381.

Graham, C.B. (1972). Assessment of bone maturation—methods and pitfalls. *Radiologic Clinics of North America*. **10**, 185–202.

Greulich, W.W. and Pyle, S.I. (1959) *Radiographic atlas of skeletal development of the hand and wrist* (2nd ed). Standford University Press, Standford, Calif.

Harper, H.A.S., Poznanski, A.K., and Garn, S.M. (1974). The carpal angle in American populations. *Investigative Radiology*, **9**, 217–221.

Kuhns, L.R. and Poznanski, A.K. (1980). Radiological assessment of maturity and size of the newborn infant. *CRC Critical Reviews in Diagnostic Imaging, Vol. 0*, 245–308.

Lowrey, G.H. (1986). *Growth and development of children* (8th ed). Year Book Medical Publishers, Chicago.

Lunt, R.C. and Law, D.B. (1974). A review of the chronology of calcification of the deciduous teeth. *Journal of the American Dental Association*, **89**, 599–606.

Poznanski, A.K., Kuhns, L.R., and Garn, S.M. (1976). *Radiology evaluation of maturation. Practical approaches to pediatric radiology.* pp. 293–310. Year Book Medical Publishers, Chicago.

Poznanski, A.K., Garn, S.M. Nagy, J.M., and Gal, J.C., Jr. (1972). Metacarpophalangeal pattern profiles in the evaluation of skeletal malformations. *Radiology*, **104**, 1–11.

Poznanski, A.K. Garn, S.M., and Shaw, H.A. (1975). The carpal angle in the congenital malformation syndromes. *European Society of Pediatric Radiology*, **19**, 141–150.

Poznanski, A.K. and Gartman, S. (1983). Pattern profile comparisons: differences and similarities. *European Society of Pediatric Radiology*, 89–96.

Pyle, S.I. and Hoerr, N.L. (1969). *Radiographic standard reference for the growing knee.* Charles C. Thomas, Springfield, Il.

Vaughn, V.C., McKay, R.J., Behrman, R.E., (1979). *Nelson's textbook of pediatrics*, pp. 32. W.B. Saunders, Philadelphia.

# Developmental Data

14

## Introduction

Behavioral development depends on the growth and functional maturation of the central nervous system. In the evaluation of the infant or child, there is considerable overlap between the neurological and the behavioral aspects. The behavioral or developmental assessment is a measure of a person's achievements or accomplishments in functional areas. This involves a steady, largely predictable increase of abilities with increasing age as a result of the interaction between the central nervous system and environmental experiences. The neurological assessment measures the integrity of neural mechanisms appropriate to the age of the subject. Although these two different assessments will usually parallel or complement each other, exceptions can exist.

Evaluation of the individual actually begins *in utero* with documentation of appropriate growth and movement (see Chapter 15). The fetus exhibits reflex movements in a very crude way as early as 8 or 9 weeks. These consist of flexion of the trunk, retraction of the head, and retraction or backward movement of the arms. By 14 to 16 weeks, the fetus is quite active, showing elementary movements of short excursion involving the extremities, trunk, and neck. The motor and most of the reflex behavior in later fetal life is mainly under the control of the medulla and spinal cord. Many of the so-called primitive reflexes, especially those involving the limbs, depend on the tonic and myotactic reflexes—that is, recoil from stretch. These reflexes appear by or after 32 weeks of gestation. One of the earliest reflex patterns to crystallize is that of sucking. By 14 to 16 weeks gestation, the fetus will protrude the lips in unmistakable preparation for sucking. The tongue and pharynx can adequately adapt to swallowing by this time. Figure 14.1 provides detail of the evolution of neonatal reflexes.

After birth, the first neurodevelopmental assessment is the assignment of an Apgar score based on heart rate, respiratory effort, muscle tone, color, and reflex (Fig. 14.2). At birth tonicity and activity are equal bilaterally, and the resting position assumed is one in which there is a

**Fig. 14.1**   Evolution of neonatal reflexes

| Reflex | Appears (fetal week) | Disappears (postnatal mo.) |
| --- | --- | --- |
| Tonic-neck | 20 | 7–8 |
| Moro | 28 | 2–3 |
| Palmar grasp | 28 | 3–4 |
| Trunk in-curve | 28 | 4–5 |
| Doll's eyes* | 32 | 10 days |
| Babinski | 38 | 12–16 |

*Eyes open, head is rotated from side to side. Positive response is contraversive conjugate deviation of eyes.*
*From Lowrey (1986), by permission.*

tendency for all extremities to be flexed in an attitude of the fetal position. There is usually good tone throughout the body, and this is particularly exemplified by the resistance to extension of all extremities. Full details of the various neonatal reflexes will not be provided here.

Figure 14.3 outlines a clinical estimation of gestational age at birth.

**Fig. 14.2**   Apgar test

| Score | Heart rate | Respiratory effort | Muscle tone | Color | Reflex |
| --- | --- | --- | --- | --- | --- |
| 2 | Over 100 | Strong cry | Good, active movement | Completely pink | Irritability (response to stimulation of foot) Normal cry |
| 1 | Below 100 | Slow, irregular respirations | Fair, some flexion of limbs | Baby pink limbs blue | Moderately depressed grimace |
| 0 | No beat obtained | No respirations | Flaccid | Blue, pale | Absent |

**Weeks gestation**

| Physical findings | | 20–48 weeks descriptions |
|---|---|---|
| Vermix (Vernix) | | Appears (21) · Covers body, thick layer (23–37) · Scant, in creases (40–41) · On back, scalp, in creases (39) · No vermix (44–48) |
| Breast tissue and areola | | Areola & nipple barely visible no palpable breast tissue (24–29) · Areola raised (34) · 1–2 mm nodule (36–37) · 3–5 mm (38) · 5–6 mm (39) · 7–10 mm (42) · ?12 mm (46) |
| Ear | Form | Beginning incurving superior (34–35) · Incurving upper 2/3 Pinna (37–38) · Well-defined incurving to lobe (44–45) |
| | Cartilage | Pinna soft, stays folded (24–27) · Cartilage scant returns slowly from folding (33–34) · Thin cartilage springs back from folding (38) · Pinna firm, remains erect from head (43) |
| Sole creases | | Smooth soles & creases (24–28) · 1–2 anterior creases (33–34) · 2–3 anterior creases (35) · Creases anterior 2/3 sole (37) · Creases involving heel (41) · Deeper creases over entire sole (44) |
| Skin | Thickness & appearance | Thin translucent skin, plethoric, venules over abdomen edema (24–29) · Smooth thicker no edema (34–35) · Pink (37) · Few vessels (39) · Some desquamation pale pink (41) · Thick pale desquamation over entire body (44) |
| | Nail plates | Appear (20) · Appears on head (24) · Nails to finger tips (37) · Nails extend well beyond finger tips (45) |
| Hair | | Eye brows & lashes (25–28) · Fine, woolly, bunches out from head (30–34) · Silky, single strands lays flat (38) · ?Receding hairline or loss of baby hair short, fine underneath (43) |
| Lanugo | | Appears (20) · Covers entire body (26–28) · Vanishes from face (34) · Present on shoulders (38) · No lanugo (45) |
| Genitalia | Testes / Scrotum | Testes palpable in inguinal canal (30–31) · In upper scrotum (37) · In lower scrotum (43) |
| | | Few rugae (32) · Rugae, anterior position (37) · Rugae cover (41) · Pendulous (45) |
| | Labia & clitoris | Prominent clitoris labia majora small widely separated (32–34) · Labia majora larger nearly cover clitoris (37) · Labia minora & clitoris covered (43) |
| Skull firmness | | Bones are soft (24–28) · Soft to 1" from anterior fontanelle (30–31) · Spongy at edges of fontanelle center firm (36) · Bones hard sutures easily displaced (39) · Bones hard, cannot be displaced (44) |
| Posture | Resting | Hypotonic lateral decubitus (22–23) · Hypotonic (27) · Beginning flexion thigh (30–31) · Stronger hip flexion (32–33) · Frog-like (34) · Flexion all limbs (37) · Hypertonic (39) · Very hypertonic (44) |
| | Recoil-Leg | No recoil (25–26) · Partial recoil (34) · Prompt recoil (43) |
| | Arm | No recoil (27–28) · Begin flexion no recoil (34–35) · Partial recoil (35) · Prompt recoil may be inhibited (38) · Prompt recoil after 30 inhibition (46) |
| Horizontal positions | | Hypotonic arms & legs straight (29–30) · Arms & legs flexed (36) · Head & back even flexed extremities (38) · Head above back (44) |

| 20 | 21 | 22 | 23 | 24 | 25 | 26 | 27 | 28 | 29 | 30 | 31 | 32 | 33 | 34 | 35 | 36 | 37 | 38 | 39 | 40 | 41 | 42 | 43 | 44 | 45 | 46 | 47 | 48 |

**Figure 14.3** Clinical estimation of gestational age. From Lubchenko (1987), by permission.

Weeks gestation (20–48)

| | Physical findings | Progression across weeks gestation |
|---|---|---|
| **Tone** | Heel to ear | No resistance (≈27–28) → Some resistance (≈31) → Impossible (≈35) |
| | Scarf sign | No resistance (≈23–25) → Elbow passes midline (≈31–32) → Elbow at midline (≈37–38) → Elbow does not reach midline (≈43) |
| | Neck flexors (head lag) | Absent (≈27) → Hand in plane of body (≈40) → Holds head (≈44) |
| | Neck extensors | Head begins to right itself from flexed position (≈34–35) → Good righting cannot hold it (≈37) → Holds head few seconds (≈39) → Keeps head in line with trunk >40° (≈42–43) → Turns head from side to side (≈46) |
| | Body extensors | Straightening of legs (≈33) → Straightening of trunk (≈38) → Straightening of head & trunk together (≈45) |
| | Vertical positions | When held under arms, body slips through hands (≈30) → Arms hold baby legs extended? (≈34) → Legs flexed good support with arms (≈43) |
| **Flexion angles** | Popliteal | No resistance (≈24) → 150° (≈30) → 110° (≈33) → 100° (≈36) → 90° (≈39) → 80° (≈44) |
| | Ankle | 90° (≈30) → 60° (≈34) → 45° (≈36) → 20° (≈38) → 0 (≈41); A pre-term who has reached 40 weeks still has a 40° angle |
| | Wrist (square window) | 90° (≈31) → 45° (≈37) → 30° (≈39) → 0 (≈41) |
| **Reflexes** | Sucking | Weak not synchronized with swallowing (≈28) → Stronger synchronized (≈33) → Perfect (≈36) |
| | Rooting | Long latency period flow, imperfect (≈28) → Hand to mouth (≈32) → Brisk complete, durable (≈38) → Complete (≈45) |
| | Group | Finger grasp is poor strength is poor (≈30) → Stronger (≈35) → Can lift baby off bed involves arms (≈39) → Perfect hand to mouth (≈40) → Hands open (≈47) |
| | Mono | Barely apparant (≈23) → Weak not elicited every time (≈28) → Stronger (≈33) → Complete arm extension open fingers, cry (≈37) → Arm adduction added (≈40) → Begins lose mono (≈47) |
| | Crossed extension | Flexion & extension in a random, purposeless pattern (≈28) → Extension but no adduction (≈33) → Still incomplete (≈37) → Extension adduction fanning of toes (≈40) → Complete (≈45) |
| | Automatic walk | Minimal (≈31) → Begin tiptoeing good support on sole (≈34) → Fast tiptoeing (≈37) → Heal-toe progression whole sole of foot (≈39) → A pre-term who has reached 40 weeks walks on toes (≈44) → ? Begins to lose automatic walk (≈47) |
| | Pupillary reflex | Appears (≈30) → Present (≈39) |
| | Glabellar tap | Appears (≈30) → Present (≈40) |
| | Tonic neck reflex | Appears (≈33) → Present after 37 weeks (≈42) |
| | Neck-righting | Absent (≈24–28) → Appears (≈36) |

**Figure 14.3, cont'd**

## Intelligence

Most people would probably agree that individuals vary in "brightness" or "intelligence," in their capacity for adaptive thinking and action. There is considerable controversy about the extent to which these variations in intelligence are genetically determined, the extent to which they remain constant throughout the life cycle, and the point in development at which such variations become measurable and predictable entities. The reliability and validity of infant intelligence tests are questionable. During the first two years of life, there is rarely consistency between an infant's performances on the same test at different times, or between an individual's performance on different tests given at the same time. At any given point in development, it is not possible to predict from a child's score on one test what his or her score might be on another test. Infants test scores are poor indices of performance on intelligence tests for older children such as the Stanford Binet and the Wechsler Intelligence Scale for Children (WISC). This may be explained by the fact that infant tests measure primarily sensorimotor functions, while tests at later age levels are based on verbal and reasoning skills.

A general rule of thumb in interpreting infant intelligence test scores is that their predictive value increases directly as the age of the child increases and inversely with the amount of time between successive testings. Infant tests can also reveal children who are at the extremes, those who are exceedingly advanced or who are exceedingly slow. Where infant tests are less useful is in the middle range of intellectual ability, where finer discriminations are necessary. Unfortunately, it is in just this middle range where tests are most needed, since the experienced clinician does not usually need a mental test to recognize the exceptional child at either end of the ability scale.

General intellectual functioning is defined as an intelligence quotient (IQ) obtained by assessment with one or more of the individually administered general intelligence tests. Figure 14.4 outlines the suggested age at which many of these available tests are applicable. Each test measures specific areas and has particular strengths and weaknesses. The interested reader is referred to literature cited at the end of this chapter for more detailed information.

Significantly subaverage intellectual functioning is defined as an IQ of 70 or less on an individually administered IQ test. Since any measurement is fallible, an IQ score is generally thought to involve an error of measurement of approximately 5 points. Hence, an IQ of 70 is considered to represent a band or zone of 65 to 75. An IQ level of 70 was chosen because most people with IQs below 70 require special services and care, particularly

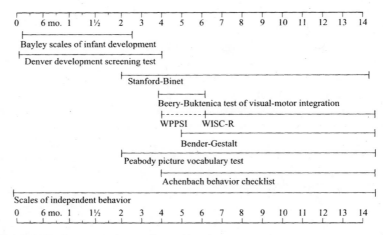

**Figure 14.4** Age-appropriate psychometric testing.

during the school age years. The arbitrary IQ ceiling values outlined in Figure 14.5 are based on data indicating a positive association between intelligence and adaptive behavior at lower IQ levels. This association declines at the mild and moderate levels of mental retardation.

Adaptive functioning refers to the person's effectiveness in areas such as social skills, communication, and daily living skills, and how well he or she meets the standards of personal independence and social responsibility expected of certain age level or cultural group. Adaptive functioning in people with mental retardation is influenced by personality characteristics,

**Fig. 14.5** Classification of mental retardation and intelligence

| Degree of severity | IQ |
| --- | --- |
| Mild | 50–55~70 |
| Moderate | 35–40 to 50–55 |
| Severe | 20–25 to 35–40 |
| Profound | Below 20 or 25 |
| Intelligence | |
| Borderline | 70–79 |
| Dull average/normal | 80–89 |
| Average | 90–109 |
| Upper average/bright | 110–119 |
| Superior | 120 or above |

*From American Psychiatric Association (1987) by permission.*

motivation, education, and social and vocational opportunities. Adaptive behavior is more likely to improve with remedial efforts than is IQ, which tends to remain more stable.

The Expanded Interview of the Vineland Adaptive Behavior Scales II assesses the personal and social skills of disabled and nondisabled individuals, ranging in age from birth to 90 (Sparrow et al., 2004).

## Developmental Screening

Developmental screening is viewed as a necessary strategy in the primary prevention of developmental disabilities and their sequelae. Screening is "the presumptive identification of unrecognized disease or defects by the application of tests, examinations, or other procedures which can be applied rapidly." Early detection can be adequately met only by the use of standardized, valid, reliable instruments to assess the developmental status of young children. If one relies on a developmental history and a child's performance in a clinical situation, mild developmental delay is frequently overlooked. This situation may be compounded by denial by the physicians or parents.

Because of a need for standardized screening for early detection of developmental delay, in order that the suspected child may then have further detailed investigation and increased opportunities for effective treatment, the Denver Developmental Screening Test (DDST) was devised in 1967. It was revised in 1981. The test is simple to administer, easy to score and interpret, and useful for repeated evaluations. A graphic format was designed so that the user could easily compare the individual with the standard for age. Each item was represented by a horizontal bar marked to indicate the 25th, 50th, 75th, and 90th percentiles. Four categories were designated: gross motor, fine motor–adaptive, language, and personal–social. The results were validated by good correlation with the Yale Developmental Schedule.

Failure to pass a particular item may represent inability to pass or unwillingness to pass secondary to illness, fatigue, or fear of separation from the parent. The separation of items into developmental domains has important prescriptive, diagnostic, and predictive value. The normally developing infant may demonstrate uniformity across all domains of growth, but the delayed or handicapped infant exhibits unique patterns and inconsistencies. A single global score will not provide enough information to indicate the direction of further assessment and intervention.

The revised DDST (R-DDST) is easy to use (Fig. 14.6). Through its agreement with diagnostic tests such as the Stanford Binet or the revised Bayley, the R-DDST attains predictive validity. More than 78 percent of the children who initially fail a DDST have educational retardation and low intelligence or learning problems in school. The R-DDST is a valid and reliable developmental screening instrument. It requires that the clinician be trained to proficiency in the administration and interpretation of the R-DDST. Improper administration or interpretation of test items invalidates the R-DDST norms. The DDST and its abbreviated modifications tap only a limited number of developmental aspects. For instance, it does not evaluate the young child's home environment, which is a major determinant of later development. Thus, nonsuspect DDST scores for a particular child who seems to be having a developmental problem should not lull the clinician into a false sense of assurance, since the test does not tap all aspects of development and the results may be in error. Furthermore, even if a child's development seems to be progressing appropriately, it is important to realize that development is an ongoing, dynamic process which requires periodic rescreening.

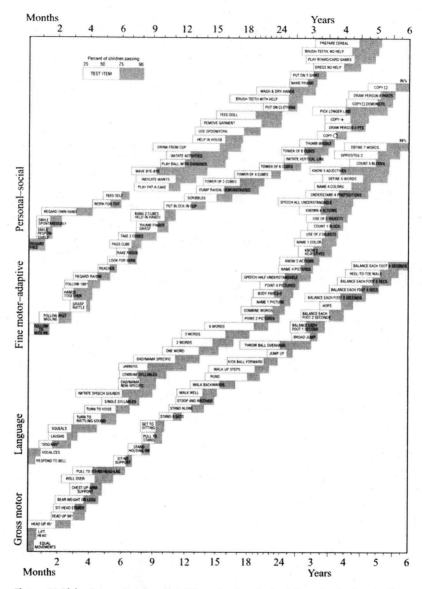

**Figure 14.6(a)** Denver Developmental Screening Test–Revised. From Frankenburg and Dodds (1990), by permission.

## DIRECTIONS FOR ADMINISTRATION

1. Try to get child to smile by smiling, talking or waving.  Do not touch him/her.
2. Child must stare at hand several seconds.
3. Parent may help guide toothbrush and put toothpaste on brush.
4. Child does not have to be able to tie shoes or button/zip in the back.
5. Move yarn slowly in an arc from one side to the other, about 8" above child's face.
6. Pass if child grasps rattle when it is touched to the backs or tips of fingers.
7. Pass if child tries to see where yarn went.  Yarn should be dropped quickly from sight from tester's hand without arm movement.
8. Child must transfer cube from hand to hand without help of body, mouth, or table.
9. Pass if child picks up raisin with any part of thumb and finger.
10. Line can vary only 30 degrees or less from tester's line.
11. Make a fist with thumb pointing upward and wiggle only the thumb.  Pass if child imitates and does not move any fingers other than the thumb.

| 12. Pass any enclosed form.  Fail continuous round motions. | 13. Which line is longer? (Not bigger.)  Turn paper upside down and repeat. (pass 3 of 3 or 5 of 6) | 14. Pass any lines crossing near midpoint. | 15. Have child copy first. If failed, demonstrate. |

When giving items 12, 14, and 15, do not name the forms.  Do not demonstrate 12 and 14.

16. When scoring, each pair (2 arms, 2 legs, etc.) counts as one part.
17. Place one cube in cup and shake gently near child's ear, but out of sight.  Repeat for other ear.
18. Point to picture and have child name it.  (No credit is given for sounds only.)
    If less than 4 pictures are named correctly, have child point to picture as each is named by tester.

19. Using doll, tell child:  Show me the nose, eyes, ears, mouth, hands, feet, tummy, hair.  Pass 6 of 8.
20. Using pictures, ask child: Which one flies?... says meow?... talks?... barks?... gallops? Pass 2 of 5, 4 of 5.
21. Ask child: What do you do when you are cold?... tired?... hungry?  Pass 2 of 3, 3 of 3.
22. Ask child:  What do you do with a cup?  What is a chair used for?  What is a pencil used for?
    Action words must be included in answers.
23. Pass if child correctly places and says how many blocks are on paper. (1, 5).
24. Tell child: Put block on table; under table; in front of me, behind me.  Pass 4 of 4.
    (Do not help child by pointing, moving head or eyes.)
25. Ask child: What is a ball?... lake?... desk?... house?... banana?... curtain?... fence?... ceiling?  Pass if defined in terms of use, shape, what it is made of, or general category (such as banana is fruit, not just yellow).  Pass 5 of 8, 7 of 8.
26. Ask child: If a horse is big, a mouse is __?  If fire is hot, ice is __?  If the sun shines during the day, the moon shines during the __? Pass 2 of 3.
27. Child may use wall or rail only, not person.  May not crawl.
28. Child must throw ball overhand 3 feet to within arm's reach of tester.
29. Child must perform standing broad jump over width of test sheet (8 1/2 inches).
30. Tell child to walk forward, ⟳⟳⟳→  heel within 1 inch of toe.  Tester may demonstrate.
    Child must walk 4 consecutive steps.
31. In the second year, half of normal children are non-compliant.

**OBSERVATIONS:**

**Figure 14.6(b)**   Denver Developmental Screening Test–Revised. From Frankenburg and Dodds (1990), by permission.

# Bibliography

American Psychiatric Association (1987). *Diagnostic and statistical manual of mental disorders* (3rd ed), pp. 28–33. American Psychiatric Association, Washington, DC.

Elkind, D. (1973). Infant intelligence. *American Journal of Diseases in Children*, **126**, 143–144.

Frankenburg, W.K., and Dodds, J.B. (1967). The Denver Developmental Screening Test. *Journal of Pediatrics*, **71**, 181–191.

Frankenburg, W.K., Dick, N.P., and Carland, J. (1975). Development of preschool-aged children of different social and ethnic groups: implications for developmental screening. *Journal of Pediatrics*, **87**, 125–132.

Frankenburg, W.K., Fandal, A.W., Sciarillo, W., and Burgess, D. (1981). The newly abbreviated and revised Denver Developmental Screening Test. *Journal of Pediatrics*, **99**, 995–999.

Katoff, L. and Reuter, J. (1980). Review of developmental screening tests for infants. *Journal of Clinical Child Psychology*, **9**, 30–34.

Lowrey, G.H. (1986). Behaviour and personality. In *Growth and development of children* (8th ed), pp. 143–219. Year Book Medical Publishers, Chicago.

Lubchenko, L. (1986). In Lowery, G.H. *Growth and development of children* (8th ed). Year Book Medical Publishers, Chicago.

Sattler, J.M. (1982). *Assessment of children's intellect and special abilities* (2nd ed). Allyn and Bacon, Boston.

Sparrow, S.S., Cicchetti, D.V., and Balla, D.A. (2004). Vineland Adaptive Behavior Scales. American Guidance Service, Circle Pines, Minn.

# Prenatal Ultrasound Measurements

**15**

## Introduction

With the advent of prenatal diagnosis, standards for intrauterine growth have become important. Ultrasound measurements of the fetus help not only to establish the gestational age but also to determine whether the fetus is growing in a normal way. Comparison of measurements in different areas of the body can establish normal proportions in the fetus, in the same manner as postnatal measurements. Comparisons over time can establish normal or abnormal growth patterns, which often allow specific diagnosis and improved pregnancy management.

Accurate norms for various body structures at different stages of gestation are available. However, the quality and accuracy of the measurements in a particular case are very much a function of the experience of the technician and the quality of the equipment used. Most ultrasound departments, with a large volume of prenatal diagnostic studies, establish their own age-related norms.

## Choice of Measurement in Relation to Gestational Age

At different gestational ages, different measurements are most accurate. Studies should be adapted to the gestational age and the particular circumstances of the case. Measurements can be made and compared with the appropriate standards, given in Figures 15.1–15.23.

*From 7 to 10 weeks:*
• Crown–rump length (Fig. 15.5)

*From 10 to 14 weeks:*
• Crown–rump length (Fig. 15.5)
• Biparietal diameter (Fig. 15.6)
• Femur Length (Fig. 15.8)
• Humerus length (Fig. 15.9)

*From 15 to 28 weeks:*
- Biparietal diameter (Fig. 15.6)
- Femur length (Fig. 15.8)
- Humerus length (Fig. 15.9)
- Binocular distance (Fig. 15.19)
- Other long bone lengths (Figs. 15.10–15.14)

*After 28 weeks*
- Biparietal diameter (Fig. 15.6)
- Femur length (Fig. 15.8)
- Humerus length (Fig. 15.19)
- Other long bone lengths (Figs. 15.10–15.14)
- Binocular distance (Fig. 15.19)

**Figure 15.1**   Positions of ultrasound measurements.

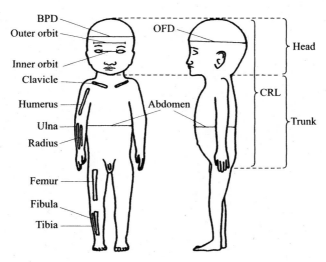

**Fig. 15.2**  Fetal biometric data from ultrasound measurements

| Week | BPD | OFD | HC | TTD | AC | Femur | CRL | Weight |
|------|------|------|------|------|------|-------|------|--------|
| 12 | 2.0cm | — | — | 1.7 | 5.3 | — | 4.7 | — |
| 13 | 2.4 | — | — | 2.0 | 6.3 | 1.0 | 6.0 | 14g |
| 14 | 2.8 | 3.1 | 10.6 | 2.4 | 7.5 | 1.2 | 7.3 | 25 |
| 15 | 3.2 | 3.8 | 11.5 | 2.7 | 8.5 | 1.6 | 8.6 | 50 |
| 16 | 3.5 | 4.1 | 12.7 | 3.1 | 9.7 | 1.8 | 9.7 | 80 |
| 17 | 3.8 | 4.6 | 14.0 | 3.4 | 10.7 | 2.2 | 11.0 | 100 |
| 18 | 4.2 | 5.0 | 15.2 | 3.7 | 11.6 | 2.5 | 12.0 | 150 |
| 19 | 4.6 | 5.4 | 16.4 | 4.0 | 12.6 | 2.8 | 13.0 | 200 |
| 20 | 4.9 | 5.8 | 17.6 | 4.4 | 13.5 | 3.1 | 14.0 | 250 |
| 21 | 5.2 | 6.3 | 19.0 | 4.7 | 14.5 | 3.4 | CHL | 300 |
| 22 | 5.6 | 6.7 | 20.3 | 5.0 | 15.5 | 3.6 | ▼ | 350 |
| 23 | 5.9 | 7.2 | 21.5 | 5.3 | 16.5 | 3.9 | 28 | 450 |
| 24 | 6.2 | 7.6 | 22.6 | 5.6 | 17.3 | 4.1 | | 530 |
| 25 | 6.5 | 8.0 | 24.0 | 5.9 | 18.3 | 4.4 | ⌐31 | 700 |
| 26 | 6.8 | 8.4 | 25.1 | 6.2 | 19.1 | 4.7 | | 850 |
| 27 | 7.1 | 8.8 | 26.3 | 6.5 | 20.2 | 4.9 | 34 | 1000 |
| 28 | 7.4 | 9.1 | 27.4 | 6.9 | 21.1 | 5.1 | | 1100 |
| 29 | 7.7 | 9.5 | 28.4 | 7.2 | 22.2 | 5.4 | 37 | 1250 |
| 30 | 8.0 | 9.8 | 29.3 | 7.4 | 23.0 | 5.6 | | 1400 |
| 31 | 8.2 | 10.0 | 30.3 | 7.8 | 24.0 | 5.9 | 40 | 1600 |
| 32 | 8.5 | 10.3 | 31.1 | 8.1 | 24.9 | 6.1 | | 1800 |
| 33 | 8.7 | 10.5 | 31.8 | 8.3 | 25.8 | 6.3 | 43 | 2000 |
| 34 | 8.9 | 10.7 | 32.5 | 8.6 | 26.8 | 6.5 | | 2250 |
| 35 | 9.1 | 10.9 | 33.2 | 8.9 | 27.7 | 6.7 | 45 | 2550 |
| 36 | 9.3 | 11.1 | 33.7 | 9.2 | 28.7 | 6.9 | | 2750 |
| 37 | 9.5 | 11.2 | 34.0 | 9.4 | 29.6 | 7.1 | 47 | 2950 |
| 38 | 9.6 | 11.3 | 34.4 | 9.7 | 30.6 | 7.3 | | 3100 |
| 39 | 9.8 | 11.4 | 34.7 | 9.9 | 31.5 | 7.4 | 50 | 3250 |
| 40 | 9.9 | 11.5 | 34.9 | 10.1 | 32.0 | 7.5 | | 3400 |

*From Hansmann (1985), by permission.*
*BPD, biparietal diameter; OFD, occipilsfrontal diameter; HC, head circumference; TTD, transthoracic diameter; AC, abdominal circumference; CRL, crown–rump length; CHL, hand–heel length.*

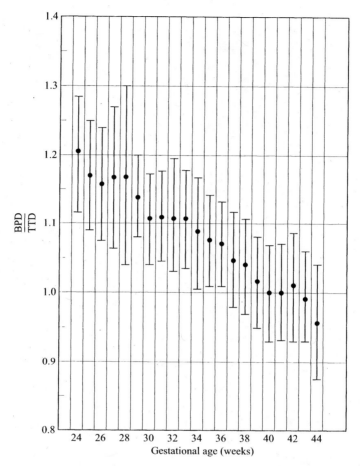

**Figure 15.3** Head-to-trunk ratio as a function of gestational age. Note: BPD = biparietal diameter; TTD = transthoracic diameter. From Hansmann (1985), by permission.

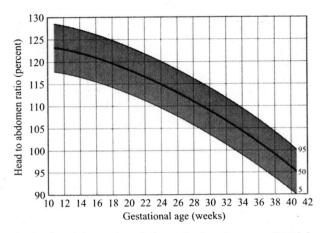

**Figure 15.4**  Head-to-abdomen circumference ratio. From Hansmann (1985), by permission.

**Figure 15.5**  Crown–rump length as a function of gestational age. From Hansmann (1985), by permission.

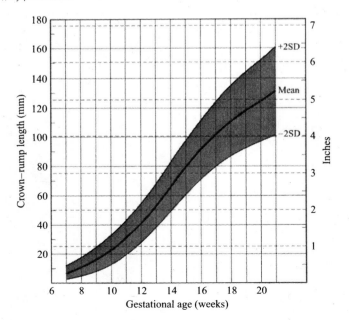

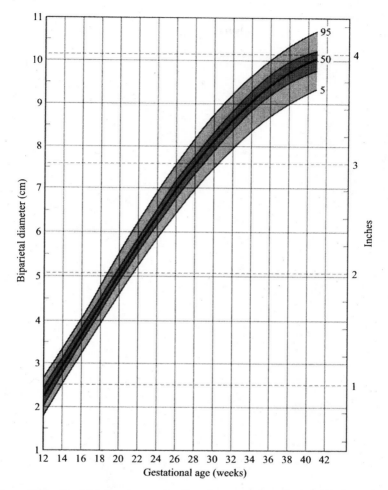

**Figure 15.6** Biparietal diameter as a function of gestational age. From Sabbagha et al. (1978), by permission.

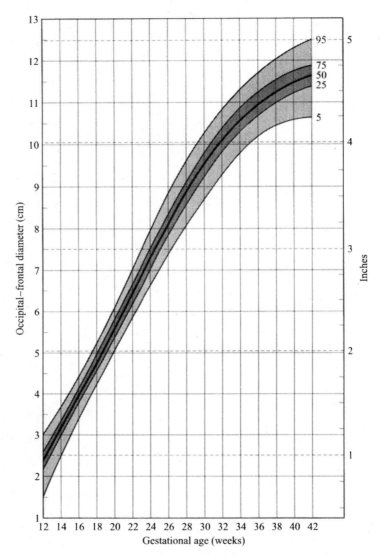

**Figure 15.7**  Occipital–frontal diameter—percentile growth curves. From Hansmann (1985), by permission.

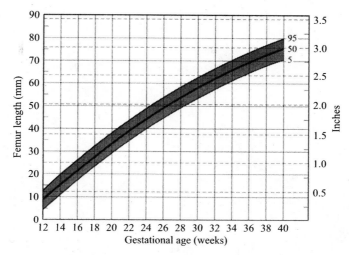

**Figure 15.8**   Growth of femur as a function of gestational age. From Hansmann (1985), by permission.

**Figure 15.9**   Growth of humerus length as a function of gestational age. From Jeanty and Romero (1984), by permission.

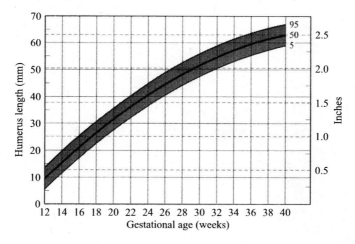

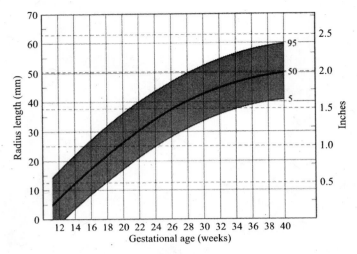

**Figure 15.10**  Growth of radius length as a function of gestational age. From Jeanty and Romero (1984), by permission.

**Figure 15.11**  Growth of ulna length as a function of gestational age. From Jeanty and Romero (1984), by permission.

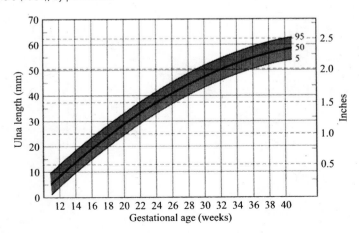

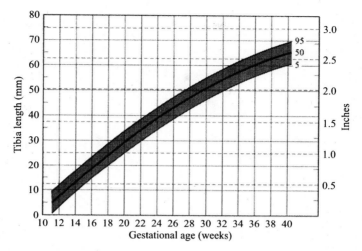

**Figure 15.12**   Growth of tibia length as a function of gestational age. From Jeanty and Romero (1984), by permission.

**Figure 15.13**   Growth of fibula length as a function of gestational age. From Jeanty and Romero (1984), by permission.

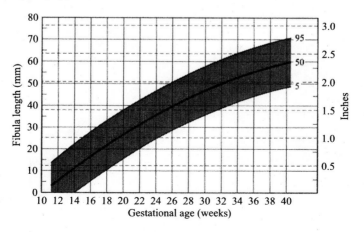

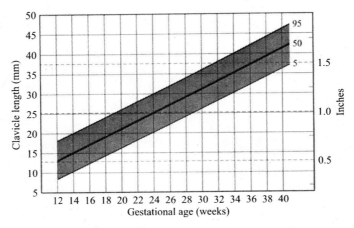

**Figure 15.14**   Growth of clavicle length as a function of gestational age. From Hansmann (1985), by permission.

**Figure 15.15**   Growth of kidney length as a function of gestational age. From Hansmann (1985), by permission.

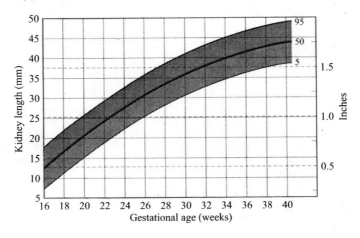

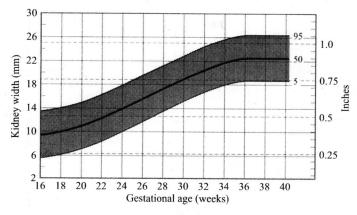

**Figure 15.16** Growth of kidney width as a function of gestational age. From Hansmann (1985), by permission.

**Figure 15.17** Growth of splenic length as a function of gestational age. From Hansmann (1985), by permission.

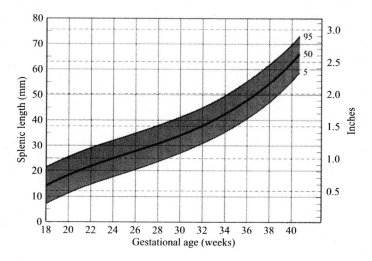

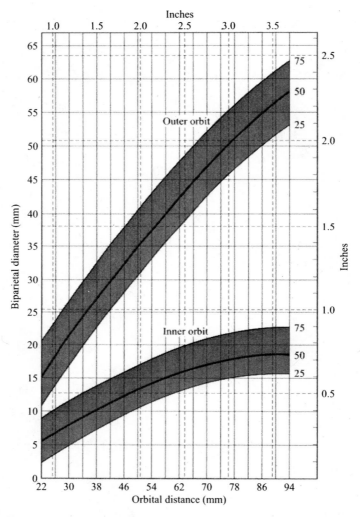

**Figure 15.18** Growth of orbit size in relation to biparietal diameter. From Mayden et al. (1982), by permission.

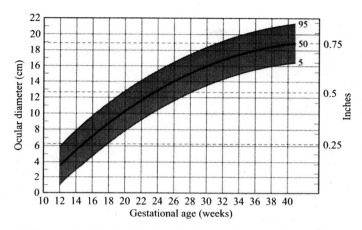

**Figure 15.19**  Growth of ocular diameter as a function of gestational age. From Mayden et al. (1982), by permission.

**Figure 15.20**  Growth of abdominal circumference as a function of gestational age. From Hadlock et al. (1982), by permission.

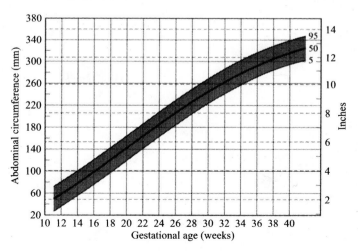

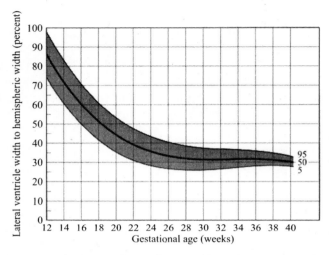

**Figure 15.21**   Lateral ventricle width as a function of hemispheric width. From Hansmann (1985), by permission.

**Figure 15.22**   Growth of transverse cardiac diameter as a function of gestational age. From Hansmann (1985), by permission.

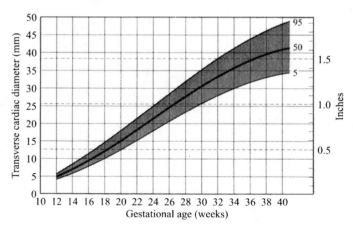

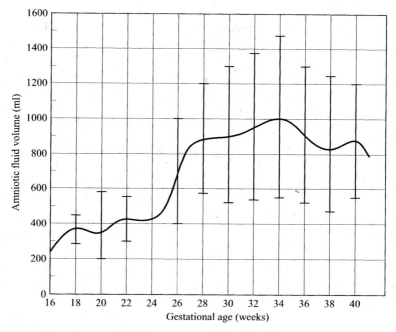

**Figure 15.23** Amniotic fluid volume in relation to gestational age. At 20 weeks, the fetus swallows about 12 ml of amniotic fluid every 24 hours and urinates 15–17 ml of urine into the amniotic fluid every 24 hours. From Hansmann (1985), by permission.

## Prenatal Measurements

In general, ultrasound measurements use the longest dimension of a particular structure, whether it is a bone such as the femur or an organ such as the kidney. Ratios help to determine whether there is disproportionate growth, undergrowth, or overgrowth of a structure. When assessing brain growth, ventricular size must be evaluated (Fig. 15.21), and when assessing renal size and function, the amount of amniotic fluid must be evaluated (Fig. 15.23).

## Normal Fetal Activity During Gestation

Patterns of fetal activity indicate fetal well-being and help to determine maturation.

**Fig. 15.24**   Fetal movement during gestation.

| Type of movement | Normal activity | Movement observed |
|---|---|---|
| Embryo movement | From 7 wk | |
| Limb movement | From 10 wk, increases up to 20 wk | Mean movement 120/hr |
| | Decreases from 20–40 wk | Mean movement 60–80/hr |
| Breathing | 12–24 wk | Seen 5–17% of time |
| | 28–40 wk | Present 30% of time; episodic and irregular; may go up to 2 hr without breathing movements |
| | 30 wk onwards | 20–60 breaths/min |
| | | Coordinated and synchronized breathing movements |
| Hiccoughing | From 12 wk | Abrupt thoracic and abdominal movement |
| Sucking | From 12 wk | Hands are held around the face; regular thumb sucking in third trimester |
| Swallowing | From 12 wk | Amniotic fluid increases if no swallowing occurs |
| Bladder emptying | From 12 wk | Fills over 45 min period, then empties |

# Bibliography

Abramovich, D.R. (1970). The volume of amniotic fluid in early pregnancy. *British Journal of Obstetrics and Gynaecology*, **77**, 865.

Campbell, S., Waldimiroff, J.W., and Dewhyrst, C.J. (1973). The antenatal mesurements of fetal urine production. *British Journal of Obstetrics and Gynaecology*, **80**, 680.

Campbell, S., and Newman, G.B. (1973). Growth of the fetal biparietal diameter during normal pregnancy. *British Journal of Obstetrics and Gynaecology*, **78**, 513.

de Vries, J.I.P., Visser, G.H.A., and van Prechtl, H.F.R., (1982). *Behavioural states in the human fetus during labour.* Proceedings, 1st Conference, The Society for the Study of Fetal Physiology, Oxford.

Hadlock, F.P., Deter, R.L., Harrist, R.B., and Park, S.K. (1982). Fetal abdominal circumference as a predictor of menstrual age. *AJR, American Journal of Roentgenology*, **139(2)**, 367–370.

Hansmann, M. (1985). *Ultrasonic diagnosis in obstetrics and gynecology.* Springer, Berlin.

Jeanty, P. and Romero, R. (1984). *Obstetrical ultrasound.* McGraw-Hill, New York.

Levi, S. (1973). Intra-uterine fetal growth studied by ultrasonic biparietal measurement. The percentiles of biparietal distribution. *Acta obstetrica Gynecologica Scandinavica*, **52**, 193.

Mayden, K.L., Tortora, M., Berkowitz, R.L., Braken, M., and Hobbins, J.C. (1982). Orbital diameters. *American Journal of Obstetrics and Gynecology*, **144**, 289–297.

Meire, H.B. (1981). Ultrasound assessment of fetal growth patterns. *British Medical Bulletin*, **37**, 253–258.

Queenan, J.T., and Thompson, P. (1972). Amniotic fluid volumes in normal pregnancies. *American Journal of Obstetrics and Gynecology*, **114**, 34–48.

Sabbagha, R.E., and Hughey, M. (1978). Standardization of sonar cephalometry and gestational age. *Obstetrics & Gynecology*, **52(4)**: 402–406.

# Postmortem Organ Weights

16

## Embryo and Fetal Pathology

Intrauterine fetal death during the late second or third trimester of pregnancy is reported to occur once in every 100 births. Although the risk is less with improved fetal surveillance and testing, a stillbirth remains an alarming event to both the parents-to-be and the physician, requiring thorough investigation for proper patient counseling. After delivery, obvious abnormalities are uncommon on gross inspection of the fetus or placenta. The clinical history is often unremarkable, and any preexisting antepartum medical or obstetric complications may not relate directly to the cause of the stillbirth. Therefore, the cause is often subtle and frequently bewildering to the parents.

In 25 percent of stillbirths, there is a fetal abnormality. One half of these have a single-gene, chromosomal, or polygenic cause with a risk for recurrence. In approximately twothirds, the recurrence risk is greater than 1 percent. In 25 %, the recurrence risk is greater than 10 percent. Prenatal diagnosis is possible in 50 percent of those cases where there is a risk of recurrence.

Current recommendations for evaluation of all stillbirths and infants dying within 24 hours after birth (neonatal deaths) include gross and microscopic autopsy of the fetus and the placenta, postmortem photography and radiography, analysis of bacterial cultures, karyotyping of the fetal tissues, and saving tissue for DNA studies when indicated (Fig. 16.1).

Detailed clinical examination of the placenta will reveal abnormalities in more than 80 percent of cases, autopsy examination of the placenta will reveal abnormalities in 70 percent of cases and placental histological evaluation will reveal abnormalities in 98 percent of cases. The placental abnormalities are the sole findings in 10 percent of cases. The most frequent placental anomalies are haemorrhagic endovasculitis, severe acute chorioamnionitis, retroplacental hematomas, erythroblastosis/hydrops, and villus changes indicative of uteroplacental vascular insufficiency. Certain abnormalities of the umbilical cord may be best appreciated histologically.

A two-vessel cord, which may be associated with underlying congenital anomalies, may go undetected without microscopic examination.

Often the single most useful tool for establishing a specific diagnosis is the gross postmortem examination. Careful and complete histopathological evaluation may further understanding of the mechanisms of embryogenesis, pregnancy loss, and early neonatal mortality in addition to providing a specific diagnosis in an isolated case. Since full details of specific organ weights proportional to total fetal body weight at varying gestational ages are not widely available, the data are provided here (Figs. 16.2–16.9).

**Figure 16.1**   Protocol for selective evaluation of stillbirths and early neonatal deaths. From Mueller et al. (1983), by permission.

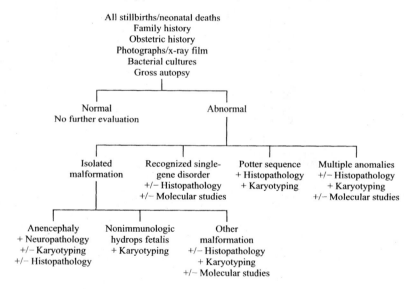

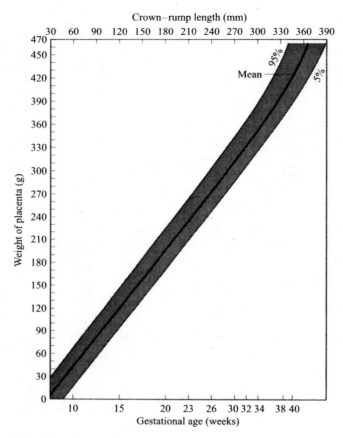

**Figure 16.2**   Placental weight at term; average weight is 500 g (range 350–600 g).

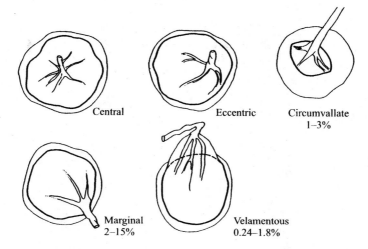

Central          Eccentric          Circumvallate
                                     1–3%

Marginal                   Velamentous
2–15%                      0.24–1.8%

| Menstrual age (week) | Umbilical cord length (cm ± 1 SD) |
|---|---|
| 20 to 21 | 32.4 ± 8.6 |
| 22 to 23 | 36.4 ± 9.0 |
| 24 to 25 | 40.1 ± 10.1 |
| 26 to 27 | 42.5 ± 11.3 |
| 28 to 29 | 45.0 ± 9.7 |
| 30 to 31 | 47.6 ± 11.3 |
| 32 to 33 | 50.2 ± 12.1 |
| 34 to 35 | 52.5 ± 11.2 |
| 36 to 37 | 55.6 ± 12.6 |
| 38 to 39 | 57.4 ± 12.6 |
| 40 to 41 | 59.6 ± 12.6 |
| 42 to 43 | 60.3 ± 12.7 |
| 44 to 45 | 60.4 ± 12.7 |
| 46 to 47 | 60.5 ± 13.0 |

**Figure 16.3**   Placenta cord insertion and umbilical cord length. From Naeye (1985), by permission.

(a) Monochorionic monoamniotic placenta indicative of fertilization of one ovum by one sperm and separation into two embryonic discs 8 days or more after ovulation. About 1% of all twin pregnancies. About 7% of monozygous twin pregancies.

(b) Monochorionic diamniotic placenta indicative of fertilization of one ovum by one sperm and separation into two embryonic discs between 3 and 8 days after ovulation. 20–30% of all twin pregnancies. 70–75% of all monozygous twin pregnancies.

(c) Fused dichorionic diamniotic placenta (35–40% of all twin pregnancies) indicative of: (i) fertilization of one ovum by one sperm and early separation of the blastomere (0–3 days post-ovulation) 10% of all monozygous twin pregnancies; (ii) fertilization of two ova by two sperm and implantation in juxtaposition. 35–40% of all dizygous twin pregnancies.

(d) Separate dichorionic diamniotic placentas (35–50% of all twin pregnancies) indicative of: (i) fertilization of one ovum by one sperm, early separation of blastomeres and separate implantation sites (0–3 days post-ovulation) 15% of all monozygous twin pregnancies; (ii) fertilization of two ova by two sperm which implant at separate sites 60–65% of all dizygous twin pregnancies.

(e)

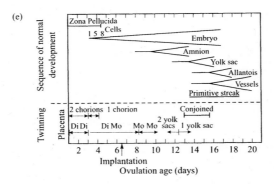

**Figure 16.4** Twinning, timing and membranes. From MacGillivay et al. (1975), by permission.

**Fig. 16.5a** Fetal organ weights by ovulation age

| Ovulation age (days) | Weight (g) | CR length (mm) | Brain (g) | Heart (g) | Lungs (g) | Liver (g) | Kidneys (g) | Adrenals (g) | Thymus (g) | Spleen (g) | Pancreas (g) |
|---|---|---|---|---|---|---|---|---|---|---|---|
| 49 | 0–4 | 3 | 0.8 | 0.1 | 0.1 | 0.2 | 0.1 | 0.1 | — | — | — |
| 66 | 5–9 | 5 | 1.2 | 0.1 | 0.1 | 0.2 | 0.1 | — | — | — | — |
| 67 | 10 | 6 | 1.5 | 0.2 | 0.3 | 0.7 | 0.1 | 0.1 | — | — | — |
| 71 | 15 | 6 | 2.6 | 0.2 | 0.4 | 0.8 | 0.1 | 0.1 | — | — | — |
| 73 | 20 | 7 | 4.3 | 0.3 | 0.4 | 1.1 | 0.2 | 0.1 | — | — | — |
| 76 | 25 | 7 | 4.8 | 0.4 | 0.7 | 1.1 | 0.2 | — | — | — | — |
| 79 | 30 | 8 | 5.4 | 0.4 | 1.0 | 1.3 | 0.2 | 0.2 | — | — | — |
| 84 | 35 | 9 | 6.2 | 0.5 | 1.4 | 2.0 | 0.3 | 0.2 | — | — | — |
| 88 | 40 | 9 | — | — | — | — | — | — | — | — | — |
| 89 | 45 | 9 | 7.4 | 0.5 | 1.9 | 2.5 | 0.4 | 0.4 | 0.1 | 0.1 | 0.1 |
| 90 | 50 | 10 | 8.5 | 0.5 | 1.9 | 3.0 | 0.5 | 0.5 | 0.2 | 0.1 | 0.1 |
| 91 | 60 | 10 | 10 | 0.5 | 2.5 | 3.4 | 0.6 | 0.6 | 0.2 | 0.1 | 0.2 |
| 92 | 70 | 11 | 11 | 0.6 | 3.0 | 3.6 | 0.8 | 0.6 | 0.2 | 0.2 | 0.2 |
| 96 | 80 | 11 | 12 | 0.7 | 3.0 | 4.3 | 0.8 | 0.6 | 0.2 | 0.2 | 0.2 |
| 100 | 90 | 12 | 14 | 0.9 | 3.0 | 4.7 | 0.9 | 0.7 | 0.2 | 0.2 | 0.2 |
| 105 | 100 | 12 | 17 | 1.1 | 3.9 | 5.6 | 1.4 | 0.7 | 0.3 | 0.2 | 0.2 |
| 109 | 125 | 13 | 23 | 1.3 | 4.1 | 7.4 | 1.4 | 0.7 | 0.3 | 0.2 | 0.2 |
| 115 | 150 | 14 | 23 | 1.4 | 5.3 | 9.2 | 1.4 | 0.8 | 0.3 | 0.3 | 0.2 |
| 117 | 175 | 14 | 23 | 1.4 | 5.6 | 11 | 1.8 | 0.8 | 0.3 | 0.4 | 0.4 |
| 118 | 200 | 15 | 33 | 1.7 | 7.2 | 12 | 2.2 | 1.1 | 0.4 | 0.4 | 0.4 |
| 124 | 250 | 16 | 39 | 2.2 | 9.1 | 15 | 2.7 | 1.2 | 0.4 | 0.5 | 0.4 |
| 130 | 300 | 17 | 46 | 2.4 | 10 | 17 | 3.1 | 1.5 | 0.7 | 0.6 | 0.5 |
| 133 | 350 | 18 | 54 | 2.9 | 11 | 21 | 3.8 | 2.0 | 0.8 | 0.7 | 0.5 |
| 143 | 400 | 18 | 61 | 3.4 | 11 | 23 | 4.2 | 2.2 | 1.0 | 0.8 | 0.6 |
| 149 | 450 + | 19 | 70 | 3.4 | 12 | 23 | 4.7 | 2.3 | 1.0 | 0.8 | 0.6 |

*After Potter and Craig (1975), by permission.*

**Fig. 16.5b**  Fetal organ weights, by body weight

| Body weight (g) | Organ weights (g) | | | | | | | | | |
|---|---|---|---|---|---|---|---|---|---|---|
| | Brain | Heart | Lungs | Liver | Kidneys | Adrenals | Thymus | Spleen | Pancreas | Thyroid |
| 500–999 | 109 ± 45 | 6 ± 2 | 18 ± 6 | 39 ± 11 | 7 ± 3 | 3 ± 1 | 2 ± 1 | 2 ± 3 | 1.0 ± 1.3 | 0.8 ± 0.7 |
| 1000–1499 | 180 ± 53 | 9 ± 5 | 27 ± 7 | 60 ± 16 | 12 ± 4 | 4 ± 1 | 4 ± 2 | 3 ± 3 | 1.4 ± 1.0 | 0.8 ± 0.8 |
| 1500–1999 | 250 ± 55 | 13 ± 5 | 38 ± 10 | 76 ± 17 | 16 ± 4 | 5 ± 2 | 7 ± 3 | 5 ± 3 | 2.0 ± 1.3 | 0.9 ± 0.6 |
| 2000–2499 | 308 ± 76 | 15 ± 5 | 44 ± 10 | 98 ± 25 | 20 ± 4 | 6 ± 2 | 8 ± 4 | 7 ± 5 | 2.3 ± 1.1 | 1.0 ± 0.7 |
| 2500–2999 | 359 ± 67 | 19 ± 5 | 49 ± 11 | 127 ± 31 | 23 ± 5 | 8 ± 3 | 9 ± 4 | 9 ± 4 | 3.0 ± 1.2 | 1.3 ± 0.9 |
| 3000–3499 | 403 ± 60 | 21 ± 4 | 55 ± 13 | 155 ± 33 | 25 ± 5 | 10 ± 3 | 11 ± 4 | 10 ± 4 | 3.5 ± 1.2 | 1.6 ± 0.9 |
| 3500–3999 | 421 ± 72 | 23 ± 5 | 58 ± 12 | 178 ± 38 | 28 ± 7 | 11 ± 3 | 13 ± 5 | 12 ± 5 | 4.0 ± 1.5 | 1.7 ± 0.8 |
| 4000–4499 | 424 ± 55 | 28 ± 5 | 66 ± 15 | 215 ± 36 | 31 ± 7 | 12 ± 4 | 14 ± 5 | 14 ± 5 | 4.6 ± 2.1 | 1.9 ± 0.9 |
| 4500 + | 406 ± 56 | 36 ± 10 | 74 ± 16 | 275 ± 54 | 33 ± 8 | 15 ± 4 | 17 ± 6 | 17 ± 7 | 6.0 ± 6.2 | 2.3 ± 1.1 |

*After Potter and Craig (1975), by permission.*

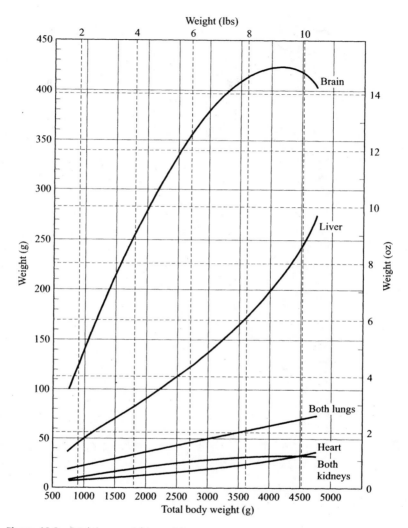

**Figure 16.6** Fetal tissue weights, part 1.

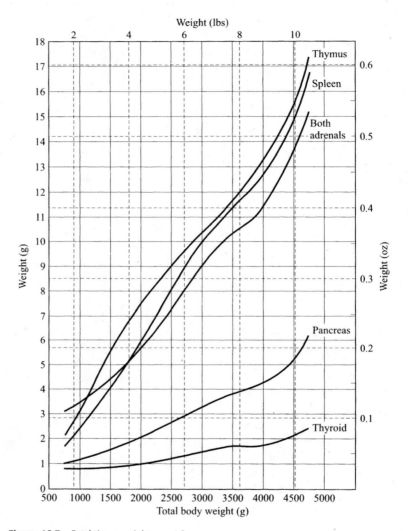

**Figure 16.7** Fetal tissue weights, part 2.

**Fig. 16.8** Normal mean organ weight by age

| Age | Sex | Weight (kg) | Length (cm) | Brain (g) | Heart (g) | Lungs Right (g) | Lungs Left (g) | Liver (g) | Kidneys Right (g) | Kidneys Left (g) | Adrenals (g) | Thymus (g) | Spleen (g) | Pancreas (g) |
|---|---|---|---|---|---|---|---|---|---|---|---|---|---|---|
| Birth-3 days | Both Sexes | 3.4 | 49 | 335 | 17 | 21 | 18 | 78 | 13 | 14 | | | 8 | |
| 3–7 days | | | 49 | 355 | 18 | 24 | 22 | 96 | 14 | 14 | | | 9 | |
| 1–3 weeks | | | 52 | 382 | 19 | 29 | 26 | 123 | 15 | 15 | 5.0 | 7.2 | 10 | 6.1 |
| 3–5 weeks | | | 52 | 413 | 20 | 31 | 27 | 127 | 16 | 16 | | | 12 | |
| 5–7 weeks | | | 53 | 422 | 21 | 32 | 28 | 133 | 19 | 18 | | | 13 | |
| 7–9 weeks | | | 55 | 489 | 23 | 32 | 29 | 136 | 19 | 18 | | | 13 | |
| 3 months | | 6.5 | 56 | 516 | 23 | 35 | 30 | 140 | 20 | 19 | 4.9 | 8.0 | 14 | 7.2 |
| 4 months | | | 59 | 540 | 27 | 37 | 33 | 160 | 22 | 21 | 4.9 | | 16 | 8.0 |
| 5 months | | | 61 | 614 | 29 | 38 | 35 | 188 | 25 | 25 | | 9.8 | 16 | 10.0 |
| 6 months | | 8.5 | 62 | 660 | 31 | 42 | 39 | 200 | 26 | 25 | 4.9 | 13.0 | 17 | 11.0 |
| 7 months | | | 63 | 691 | 34 | 49 | 41 | 227 | 30 | 30 | 5.3 | 10.0 | 99 | 11.0 |
| 8 months | | | 65 | 714 | 37 | 52 | 45 | 254 | 31 | 30 | 5.3 | | 20 | |
| 9 months | | 9.8 | 67 | 750 | 37 | 53 | 47 | 260 | 31 | 30 | 5.4 | | 20 | 11.0 |
| 10 months | | | 69 | 809 | 39 | 54 | 51 | 274 | 32 | 31 | 5.7 | | 22 | 14 |
| 11 months | | 10.8 | 70 | 852 | 40 | 59 | 53 | 277 | 34 | 33 | 6.1 | | 25 | 15 |
| 12 months | | | 73 | 925 | 44 | 64 | 57 | 288 | 36 | 35 | 6.2 | | 26 | 14 |
| 14 months | | | 74 | 944 | 45 | 66 | 60 | 304 | 36 | 35 | | | 26 | |
| 16 months | | | 77 | 1010 | 48 | 72 | 64 | 331 | 39 | 39 | | | 28 | |
| 18 months | | | 78 | 1042 | 52 | 72 | 65 | 345 | 40 | 43 | | 26.6 | 30 | |
| 20 months | | | 79 | 1050 | 56 | 80 | 74 | 370 | 43 | 44 | | | 30 | |
| 22 months | | | 82 | 1059 | 56 | 83 | 75 | 380 | 44 | 44 | | | 33 | |
| 3 years | | 15.2 | 88 | 1141 | 59 | 89 | 77 | 418 | 48 | 49 | | | 39 | |
| 4 years | | 17.3 | 99 | 1191 | 73 | 90 | 85 | 516 | 55 | 56 | | | 47 | |
| 5 years | | 19.4 | 108 | 1237 | 85 | 107 | 104 | 596 | 65 | 64 | | | 58 | |
| 6 years | | 21.9 | 109 | 1243 | 94 | 121 | 122 | 642 | 68 | 67 | | | 66 | |

Continued

**Fig. 16.8** Normal mean organ weight by age—cont'd

| Age | Sex | Weight (kg) | Length (cm) | Brain (g) | Heart (g) | Lungs Right (g) | Lungs Left (g) | Liver (g) | Kidneys Right (g) | Kidneys Left (g) | Adrenals (g) | Thymus (g) | Spleen (g) | Pancreas (g) |
|---|---|---|---|---|---|---|---|---|---|---|---|---|---|---|
| 7 years | | 24.6 | 113 | 1263 | 100 | 130 | 123 | 680 | 69 | 70 | | | 69 | |
| 8 years | | 27.7 | 119 | 1273 | 110 | 150 | 140 | 736 | 74 | 75 | | | 73 | |
| 9 years | | 31.0 | 125 | 1275 | 115 | 174 | 152 | 756 | 82 | 83 | | | 85 | |
| 10 years | | 34.8 | 130 | 1290 | 116 | 177 | 166 | 852 | 92 | 95 | | | 87 | |
| 11 years | | 38.8 | 135 | 1320 | 122 | 201 | 190 | 909 | 94 | 95 | | | 93 | |
| 12 years | | 43.2 | 139 | 1351 | 124 | — | — | 936 | 95 | 96 | | | — | |
| 17–19 | M | | | 1340 | 219 | | | | | | 25 | 190 | | |
| | F | | | 1242 | 210 | | | | | | | 120 | | |
| 20–29 | M | | | 1396 | | | | 1820 | | | | | | |
| | F | | | 1234 | | | | 1440 | | | | | | |
| 30–39 | M | | | 1365 | | | | 1830 | | | | 20 | 155 | |
| | F | | | 1233 | | | | 1460 | | | | | 120 | |
| 40–49 | M | | | 1366 | | | | 1840 | | | | | 145 | |
| | F | | | 1240 | | | | 1440 | | | | | 120 | |
| 50–59 | M | | | 1375 | | | | 1840 | | | | 16 | 145 | |
| | F | | | 1200 | | | | 1430 | | | | | 110 | |
| 60–69 | M | | | 1323 | | | | 1740 | | | | | | |
| | F | | | 1178 | | | | 1380 | | | | | | |
| 70–85 | M | | | 1279 | | | | 1380 | | | | 6 | | |
| | F | | | 1121 | | | | 1180 | | | | | | |
| All adult ages | Both sexes | | | | | 450 | 375 | | | | | | | |
| | M | | | | 300 (270–360) | | | 1840 (900–3000) | | 313 (230–440) | | 9.7 (7–20) | 145 (75–245) | 110 (60–135) |
| | F | | | | 250 (200–280) | | | 1700 (910–2130) | | 288 (240–350) | | 8.3 (7–18) | 115 (55–190) | |

From Sunderman and Boerner (1949), by permission.

**Fig. 16.9**  Miscellaneous organ sizes

| Organ | Age | Weight (g) | Length (cm) |
|---|---|---|---|
| Thyroid | adult | 40 (30–70) | |
| Parathyroids | adult | 0.12–0.18 | |
| Pituitary | 10–20 yrs | 0.56 | |
| | 20–70 yrs | 0.61 | |
| | pregnancy | 0.95 (0.84–1.06) | |
| Combined ovaries | birth–5 yrs | 0.4–2.1 | |
| | 6yrs–10yrs | 2.2–3.1 | |
| | 11yrs–16 yrs | 3.3–4.0 | |
| | adult | 14 | |
| Combined testes | Birth–5yrs | 0.4–1.8 | |
| | 6 yrs–10 yrs | 1.6–3.0 | |
| | 11 yrs–16yrs | 3.0–13.0 | |
| | adult | 25 (20–27) | |
| Uterus | birth– | 4.6 | |
| | 1 mth–5yrs | 1.9–2.9 | |
| | 6 yrs–10 yrs | 2.9–3.4 | |
| | 11 yrs–16 yrs | 5.3–25 | |
| | adult | 35 (33–41) | |
| | after pregnancy | 110 (102–117) | |
| Prostate | birth–5yrs | 0.9–1.2 | |
| | 6 yrs–10yrs | 1.2–1.4 | |
| | 11 yrs–16 yrs | 2.3–6.1 | |
| | 20 yrs–30 yrs | 15 | |
| | 31 yrs–50 yrs | 20 | |
| | 51 yrs–80 yrs | 40 | |
| Gastrointestinal tract (adults): | | | |
| Esophagus | | 25 | |
| Duodenum | | 30 | |
| Small intestine | | 550–650 | |
| Colon | | 150–170 | |
| Spinal cord | | Average weight 27 g | Average length 45 cm |
| | | **Frontal** | **Sagittal** |
| | Cervical | 1.3–1.4 cm | Average 0.9 |
| | Thoracic | Average 1.0 cm | Average 0.8 |
| | Lumbar | Average 1.2 cm | Average 0.9 |

*From Minckler and Boyd (1968) and Sunderman and Boerner (1949), by permission.*

## Bibliography

Kissane, J.M. (1975). *Pathology of infancy and childhood* (2nd ed). C.V. Mosby Company, St Louis.

Kronick, J.B., Scriver, C.R., Goodyer, P.R., and Kaplan, P.B. (1983). A perimortem protocol for suspected genetic disease. *Pediatrics*, **71**, 960–963.

MacGillivray, Nylander, and Corney (1975). *Human multiple reproduction.* W.B. Saunders Company, Philadelphia.

MacLeod, P.M., Dill, F., and Hardwick, D.F. (1979). Chromosomes, syndromes, and perinatal deaths: The genetic counseling value of making a diagnosis in a malformed abortus, stillborn and deceased newborn. *Birth Defects*, **15(5A)**, 105–111.

Minckler, T.M. and Boyd, E. (1968). Physical growth of the nervous system and its coverings. In *Pathology of the nervous system* (ed. J. Minckler) Vol. 1, pp. 120–137. McGraw-Hill Book Company, New York.

Moore, K.L. (1982). *The developing human* (3rd ed). W.B. Saunders Company, Philadelphia.

Mueller, R.F., Sybert, V.P., Johnson, J., Brown, Z.A., and Chen, W.-J. (1983). Evaluation of a protocol for post-mortem examination of stillbirths. *New England Journal of Medicine*, **309**, 586–590.

Naeye, R.L. (1985). Umbilical cord length: Clinical significance. *Journal of Pediatrics*, **107(2)**, 278–281.

Poland, B.J. and Lowry, R.B. (1974). The use of spontaneous abortuses and stillbirths in genetic counseling. *American Journal of Obstetrics and Gynecology*, **118**, 322–331.

Potter, E.L., and Craig, J.M. (1975). *Pathology of the fetus and the infant* (3rd ed). Year Book Medical Publishers.

Rayburn, W., Sander, C., Barr, M. Jr., and Rygiel, R. (1985). The stillborn fetus: Placental histologic examination in determining a cause. *Obstetrics and Gynecology*, **65**, 637–641.

Sunderman, F.W. and Boerner, F. (1949). *Normal values in clinical medicine.* W.B. Saunders Company, Philadelphia.

# Measurements for Specific Syndromes

## Introduction

As the natural history of various specific conditions begins to be defined, it is possible to generate growth curves for those conditions. Although inevitably there are many problems with such growth curves (e.g., heterogeneity, lack of longitudinal data, complicating factors as part of the natural history), they are still very useful because they allow comparison between the individual and what is considered "normal" for the specific condition.

We are including the available growth curves for some of the more common syndromes in the hope that they will be useful and will also encourage the collection of additional data to enlarge the number of cases and the number of disorders for which such information is available.

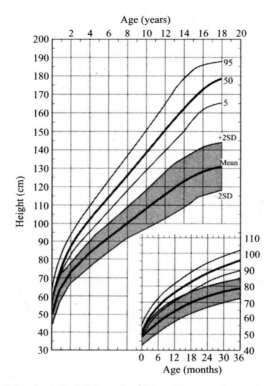

**Figure 17.1**  Achondroplasia, height, males, birth to 18 years. Mean and two standard deviations are depicted as indicated. For comparison, range of measurements in typical persons is included. Adapted from Horton et al. (1978).

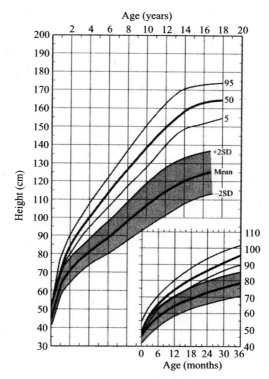

**Figure 17.2** Achondroplasia, height, females, birth to 18 years. Mean and two standard deviations are depicted as indicated. For comparison, range of measurements in typical persons is included. Adapted from Horton et al. (1978).

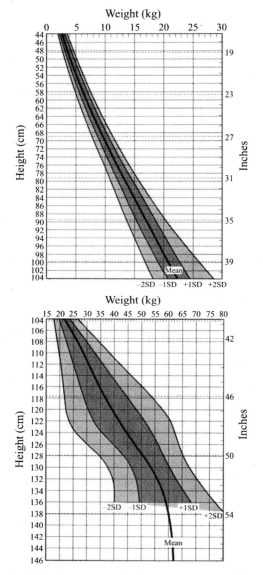

**Figure 17.3** Achondroplasia, weight for height, males. Mean, 1SD, and 2SD are shown. Adapted from Hunter et al. (1996a).

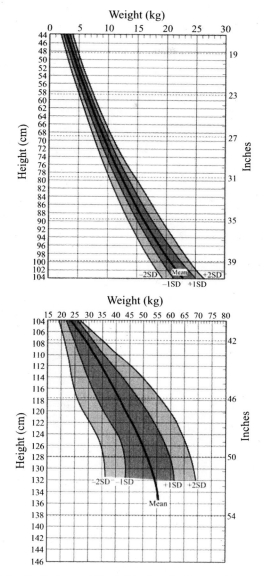

**Figure 17.4** Achondroplasia, weight for height, females. Mean, 1SD, and 2SD are shown. Adapted from Hunter et al. (1996a).

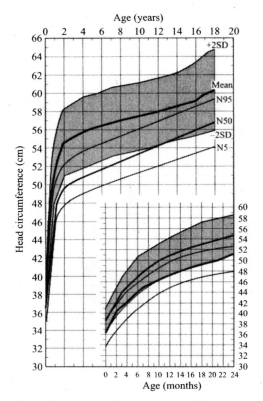

**Figure 17.5** Achondroplasia, head circumference, males, birth to 18 years. Mean and two standard deviations are depicted as indicated. For comparison, range of measurements in typical persons is included. Adapted from Horton et al. (1978).

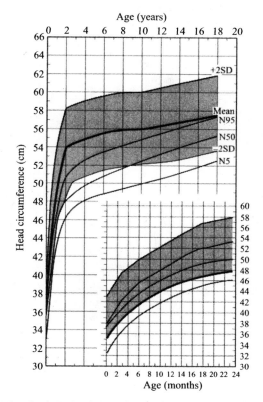

**Figure 17.6** Achondroplasia, head circumference, females, birth to 18 years. Mean and two standard deviations are depicted as indicated. For comparison, range of measurements in typical persons is included. Adapted from Horton et al. (1978).

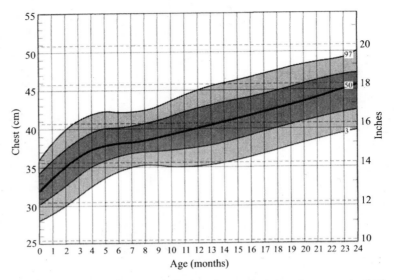

**Figure 17.7** Achondroplasia, smoothed curve of mean chest circumference, males, birth to 24 months. Adapted from Horton et al. (1978).

**Figure 17.8** Achondroplasia, smoothed curve of mean chest circumference, females, birth to 24 months. Adapted from Horton et al. (1978).

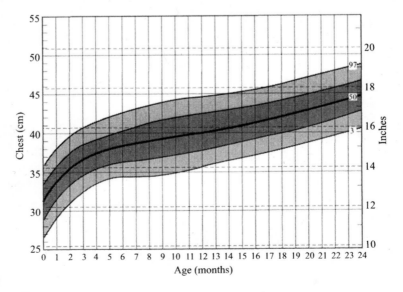

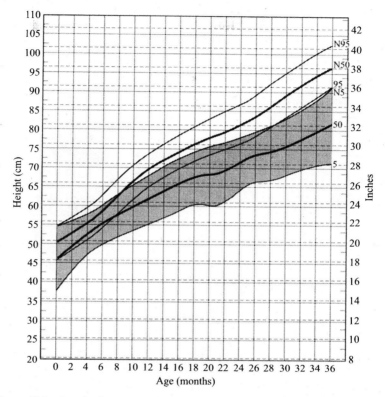

**Figure 17.9**    Cornelia de Lange syndrome, height, males, birth to 36 months. For comparison, range of measurements in typical persons (N) is included. Adapted from Kline et al. (1993).

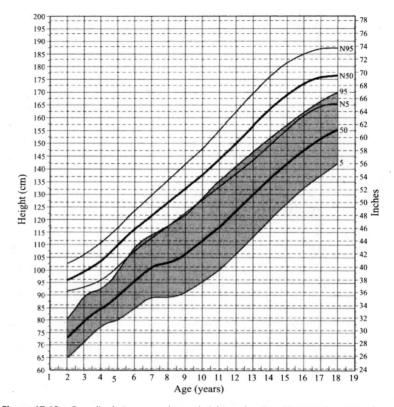

**Figure 17.10** Cornelia de Lange syndrome, height, males, 2 to 18 years. For comparison, range of measurements in typical persons (N) is included. Adapted from Kline et al. (1993).

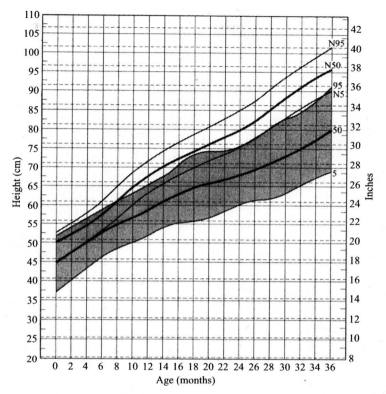

**Figure 17.11**   Cornelia de Lange syndrome, height, females, birth to 36 months. For comparison, range of measurements in typical persons (N) is included. Adapted from Kline et al. (1993).

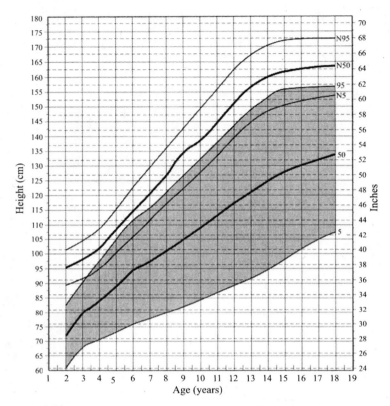

**Figure 17.12**   Cornelia de Lange syndrome, height, females, 2 to 18 years. For comparison, range of measurements in typical persons (N) is included. Adapted from Kline et al. (1993).

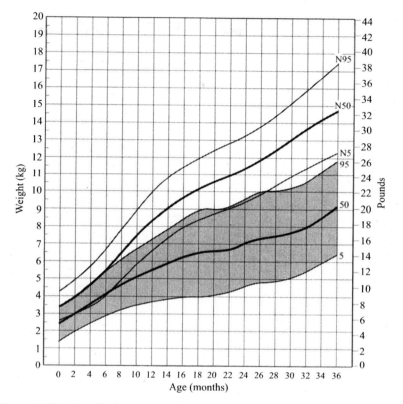

**Figure 17.13**   Cornelia de Lange syndrome, weight, males, birth to 36 months. For comparison, range of measurements in typical persons (N) is included. Adapted from Kline et al. (1993).

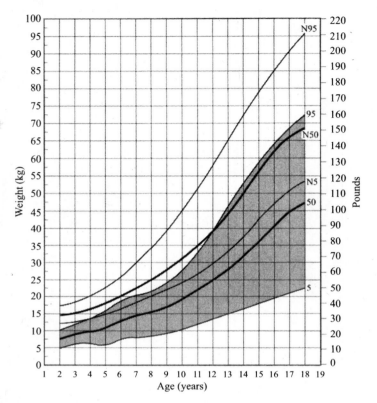

**Figure 17.14**    Cornelia de Lange syndrome, weight, males, 2 to 18 years. For comparison, range of measurements in typical persons (N) is included. Adapted from Kline et al. (1993).

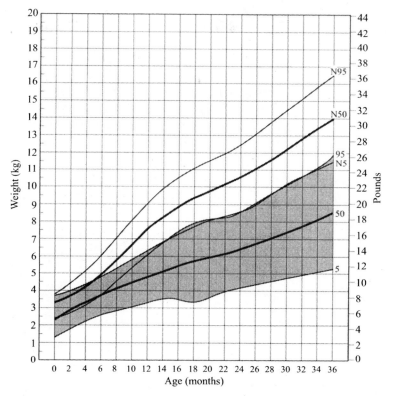

**Figure 17.15**   Cornelia de Lange syndrome, weight, females, birth to 36 months. For comparison, range of measurements in typical persons (N) is included. Adapted from Kline et al. (1993).

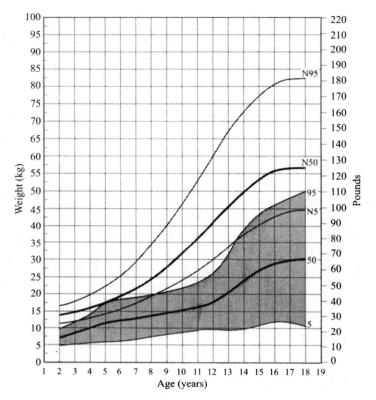

**Figure 17.16** Cornelia de Lange syndrome, weight, females, 2 to 18 years. For comparison, range of measurements in typical persons (N) is included. Adapted from Kline et al. (1993).

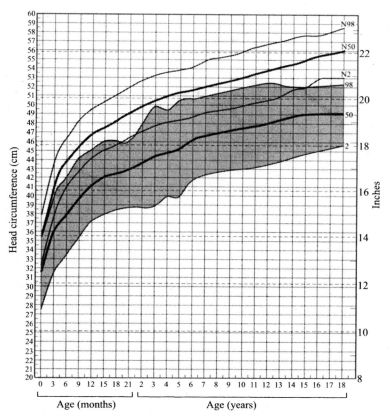

**Figure 17.17**   Cornelia de Lange syndrome, head circumference, males, birth to 18 years, compared with normal males (N). Adapted from Kline et al. (1993).

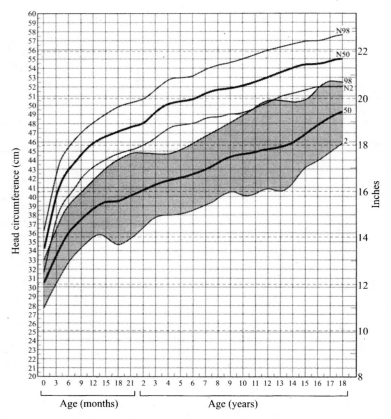

**Figure 17.18** Cornelia de Lange syndrome, head circumference, females, birth to 18 years, compared with normal females (N). Adapted from Kline et al. (1993).

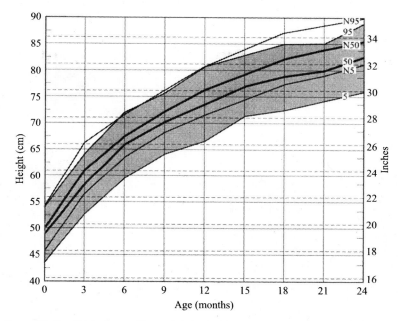

**Figure 17.19**   Cri du chat syndrome, height, males, birth to 2 years. Normal growth curves (N) are included. Adapted from Marinescu et al. (2000).

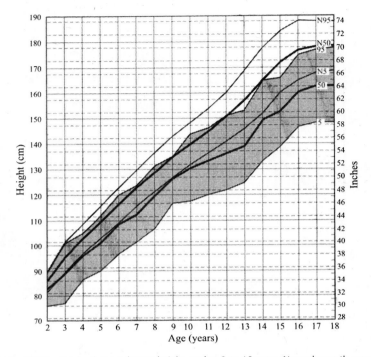

**Figure 17.20** Cri du chat syndrome, height, males, 2 to 18 years. Normal growth curves (N) are included. Adapted from Marinescu et al. (2000).

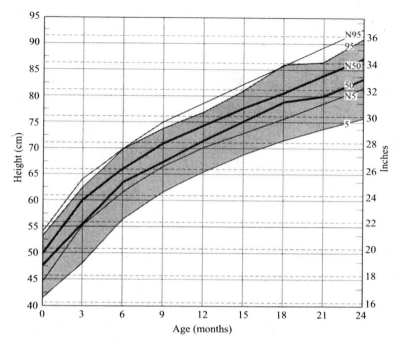

**Figure 17.21**   Cri du chat syndrome, height, females, birth to 2 years. Normal growth curves (N) are included. Adapted from Marinescu et al. (2000).

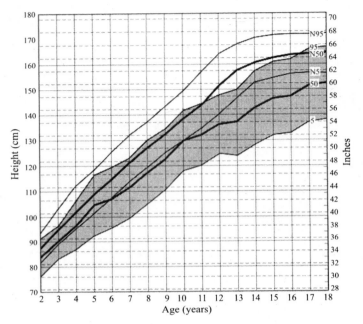

**Figure 17.22**  Cri du chat syndrome, height, females, 2 to 18 years. Normal growth curves (N) are included. Adapted from Marinescu et al. (2000).

**Figure 17.23**  Cri du chat syndrome, weight, males, birth to 2 years. Normal growth curves (N) are included. Adapted from Marinescu et al. (2000).

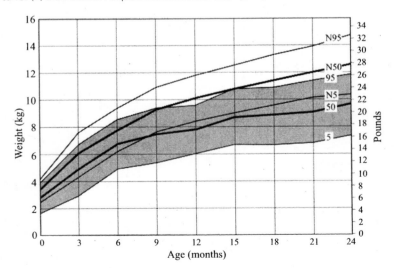

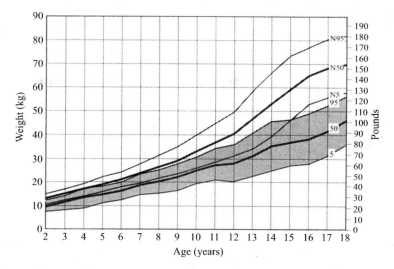

**Figure 17.24** Cri du chat syndrome, weight, males, 2 to 18 years. Normal growth curves (N) are included. Adapted from Marinescu et al. (2000).

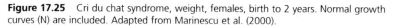

**Figure 17.25** Cri du chat syndrome, weight, females, birth to 2 years. Normal growth curves (N) are included. Adapted from Marinescu et al. (2000).

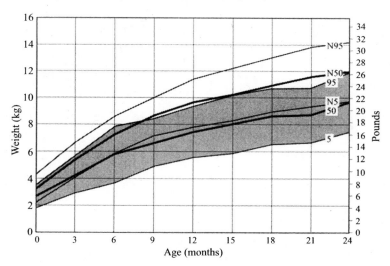

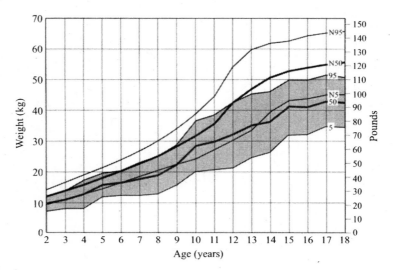

**Figure 17.26** Cri du chat syndrome, weight, females, 2 to 18 years. Normal growth curves (N) are included. Adapted from Marinescu et al. (2000).

**Figure 17.27** Cri du chat syndrome, head circumference, males, birth to 15 years. Normal growth curves (N) are included. Adapted from Marinescu et al. (2000).

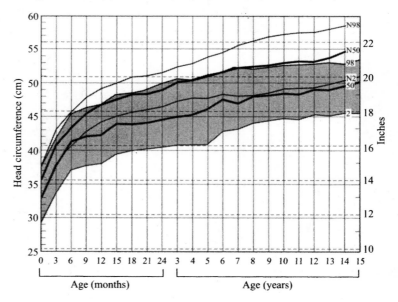
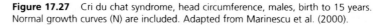

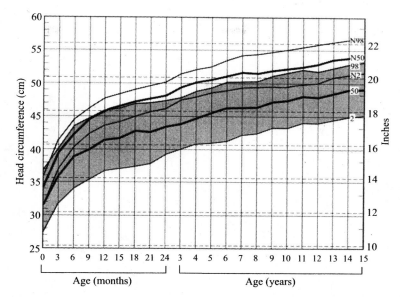

**Figure 17.28** Cri du chat syndrome, head circumference, females, birth to 15 years. Normal growth curves (N) are included. Adapted from Marinescu et al. (2000).

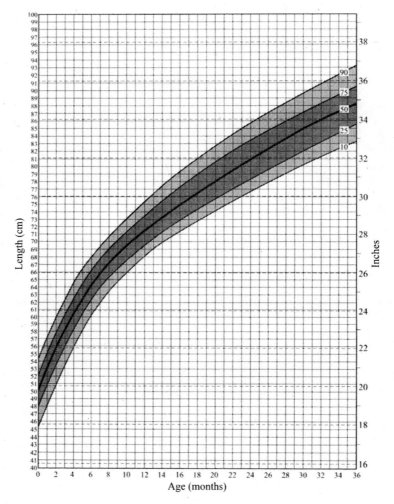

**Figure 17.29** Down syndrome, length, North American males, birth to 3 years. Adapted from Cronk et al. (1988) and http://www.growthcharts.com/.

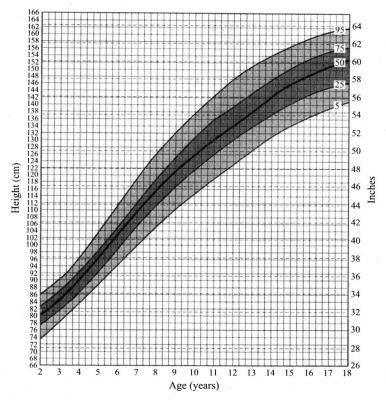

**Figure 17.30** Down syndrome, height, North American males, 2 to 18 years. Adapted from Cronk et al. (1988) and http://www.growthcharts.com/.

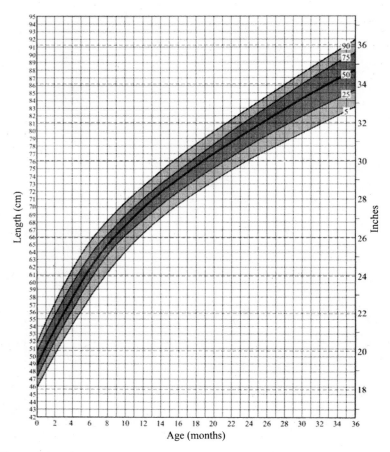

**Figure 17.31** Down syndrome, length, North American females, birth to two years. Adapted from Cronk et al. (1988) and http://www.growthcharts.com/.

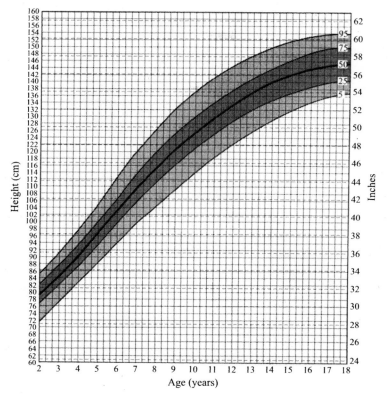

**Figure 17.32** Down syndrome, height, North American females, 2 to 18 years. Adapted from Cronk et al. (1988) and http://www.growthcharts.com/.

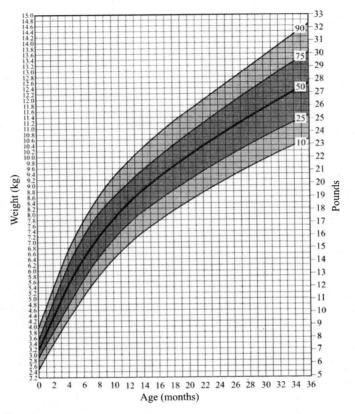

**Figure 17.33** Down syndrome, weight, North American males, birth to three years. Adapted from Cronk et al. (1988) and http://www.growthcharts.com/.

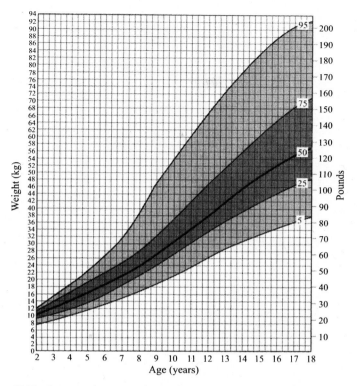

**Figure 17.34**   Down syndrome, weight, North American males, 2 to 18 years. Adapted from Cronk et al. (1988) and http://www.growthcharts.com/.

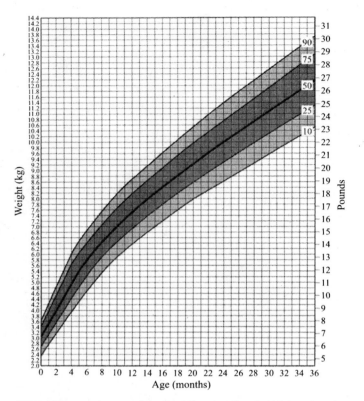

**Figure 17.35**   Down syndrome, weight, North American females, birth to three years. Adapted from Cronk et al. (1988) and http://www.growthcharts.com/.

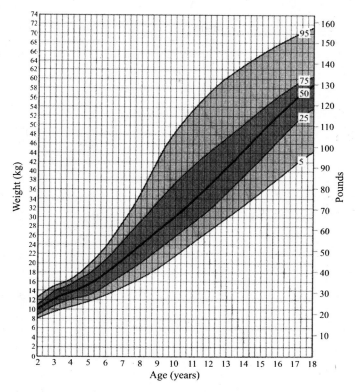

**Figure 17.36** Down syndrome, weight, North American females, 2 to 18 years. Adapted from Cronk et al. (1988) and http://www.growthcharts.com/.

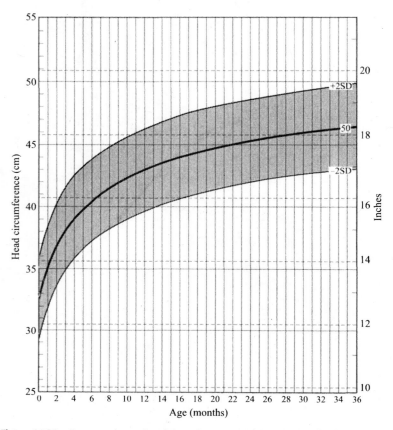

**Figure 17.37** Down syndrome, head circumference, North American males, birth to three years. Adapted from Palmer et al. (1992) and http://www.growthcharts.com/.

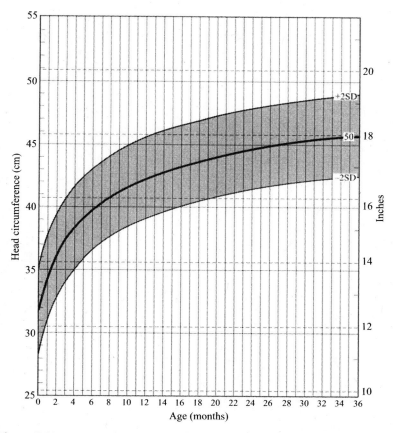

**Figure 17.38**  Down syndrome, head circumference, North American females, birth to three years. Adapted from Palmer et al. (1992) and http://www.growthcharts.com/.

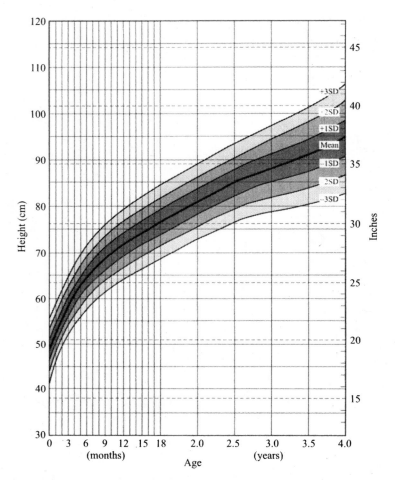

**Figure 17.39**  Down syndrome, height, North European males, birth to four years. Adapted from Myrelid et al. (2000).

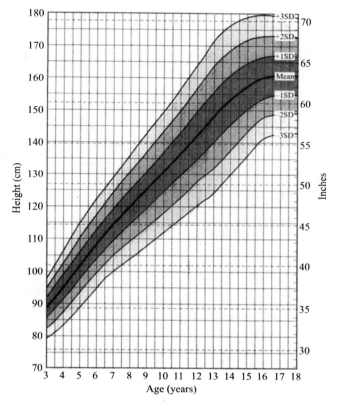

**Figure 17.40** Down syndrome, height, North European males, 3 to 18 years. Adapted from Myrelid et al. (2002).

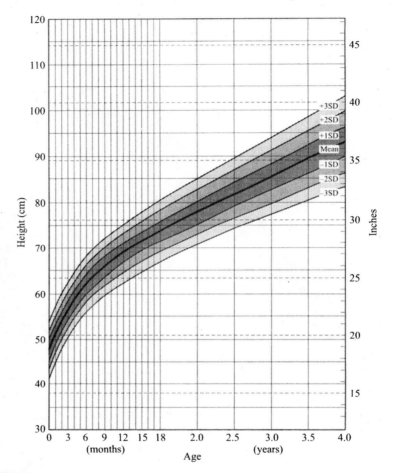

**Figure 17.41** Down syndrome, height, North European females, birth to four years. Adapted from Myrelid et al. (2002).

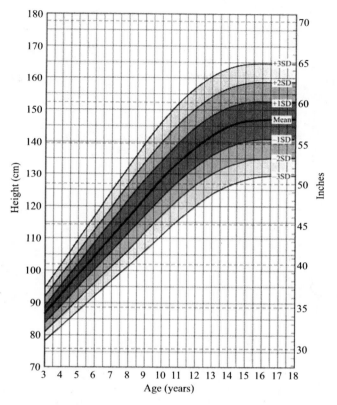

**Figure 17.42** Down syndrome, height, North European females, 3 to 18 years. Adapted from Myrelid et al. (2002).

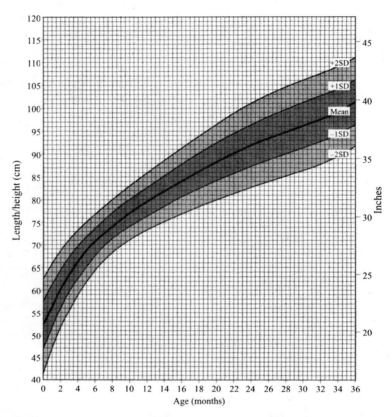

**Figure 17.43** Marfan syndrome, length/height, males, birth to three years. Adapted from Erkula et al. (2002).

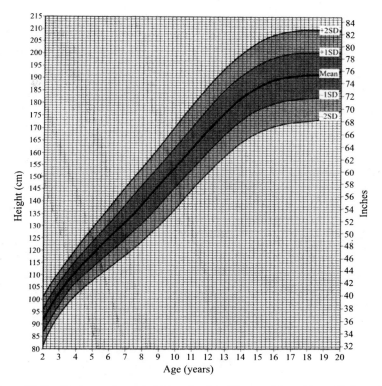

**Figure 17.44** Marfan syndrome, height, males, 2 to 20 years. Adapted from Erkula et al. (2002).

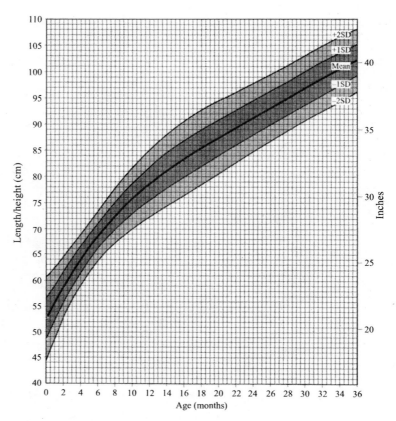

**Figure 17.45**  Marfan syndrome, length/height, females, birth to three years. Adapted from Erkula et al. (2002).

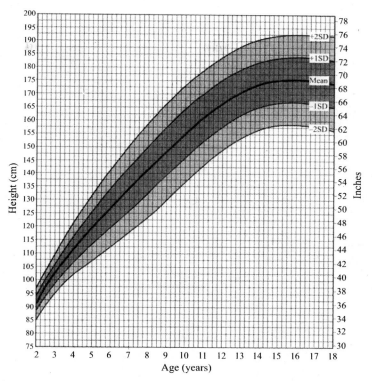

**Figure 17.46** Marfan syndrome, height, females, 2 to 20 years. Adapted from Erkula et al. (2002).

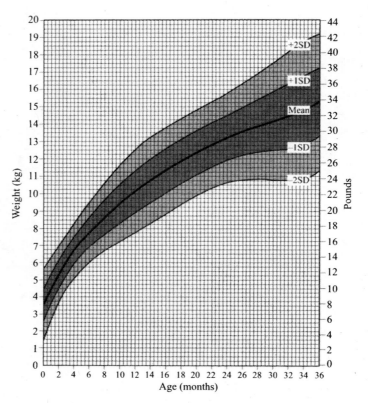

**Figure 17.47** Marfan syndrome, weight, males, birth to 3 years. Adapted from Erkula et al. (2002).

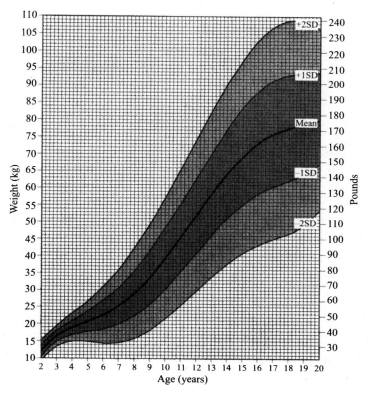

**Figure 17.48** Marfan syndrome, weight, males, 2 to 20 years. Adapted from Erkula et al. (2002).

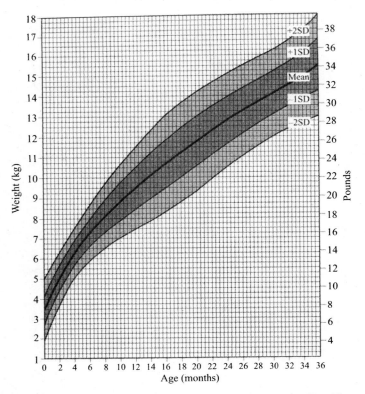

**Figure 17.49**   Marfan syndrome, weight, females, birth to three years. Adapted from Erkula et al. (2002).

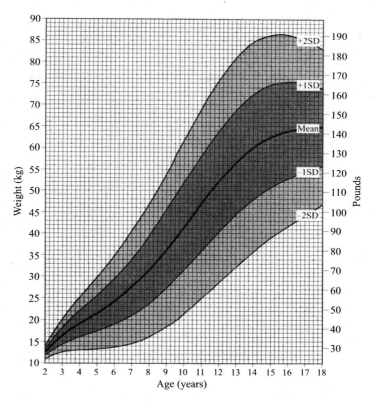

**Figure 17.50**    Marfan syndrome, weight, females, 2 to 20 years. Adapted from Erkula et al. (2002).

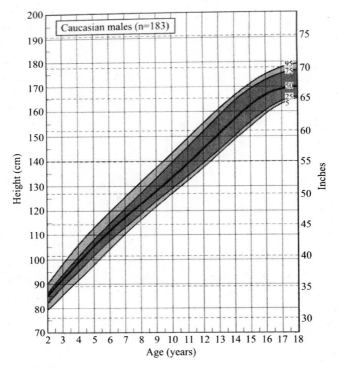

**Figure 17.51** Neurofibromatosis, type I, height, males, 2 to 18 years. Adapted from Szudek et al. (2000).

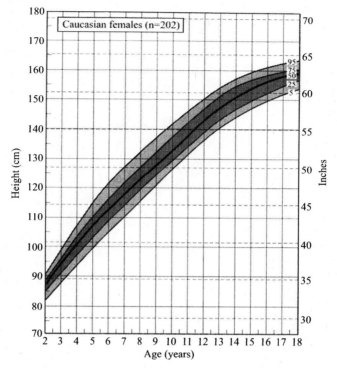

**Figure 17.52**  Neurofibromatosis, type I, height, females, 2 to 18 years. Adapted from Szudek et al. (2000).

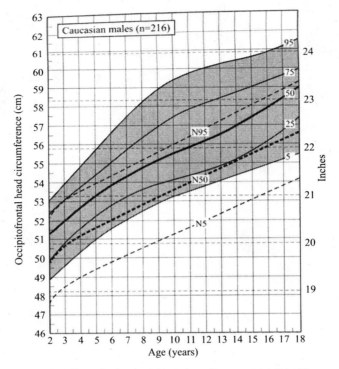

**Figure 17.53**   Neurofibromatosis, type I, head circumference, males, 2 to 18 years. Adapted from Szudek et al. (2000).

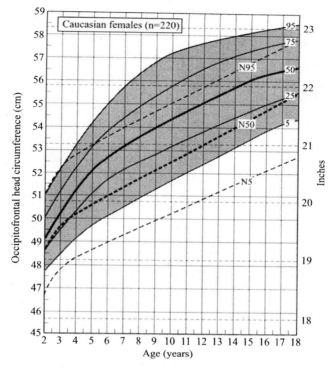

**Figure 17.54** Neurofibromatosis, type I, head circumference, females, 2 to 18 years. Adapted from Szudek et al. (2000).

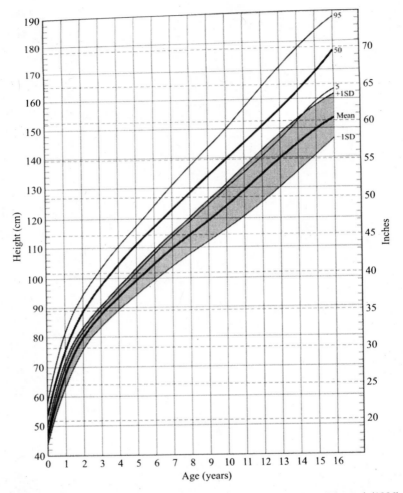

**Figure 17.55** Noonan syndrome, height, males, birth to 16 years. From Witt et al. (1986) and Ranke et al. (1988), by permission.

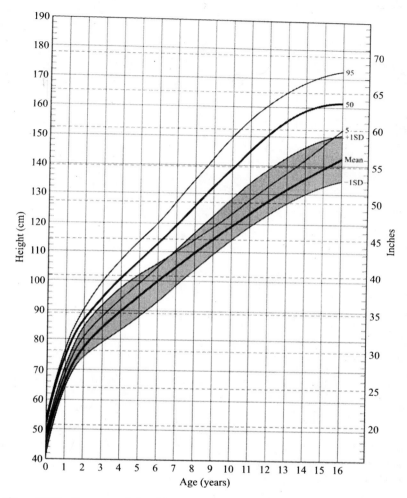

**Figure 17.56** Noonan syndrome, height, females, birth to 16 years. From Witt et al. (1986) and Ranke et al. (1988), by permission.

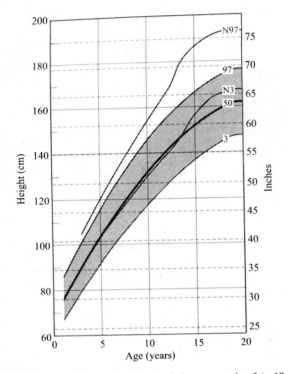

**Figure 17.57** Prader-Willi syndrome, height, North European males, 2 to 18 years. Adapted from Wollmann et al. (1998).

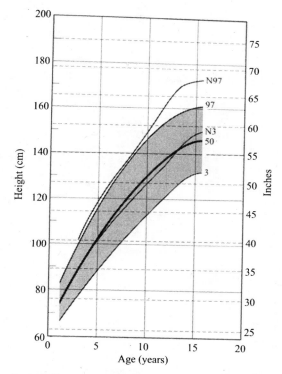

**Figure 17.58** Prader-Willi syndrome, height, North European females, 2 to 18 years. Adapted from Wollmann et al. (1998).

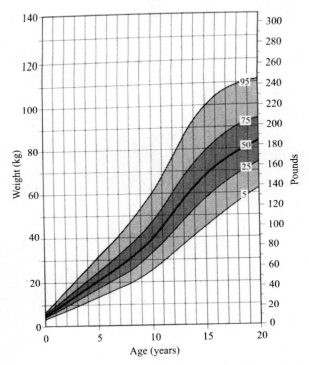

**Figure 17.59** Prader-Willi syndrome, weight, North European males, birth to 20 years. Adapted from Hauffa et al. (2000).

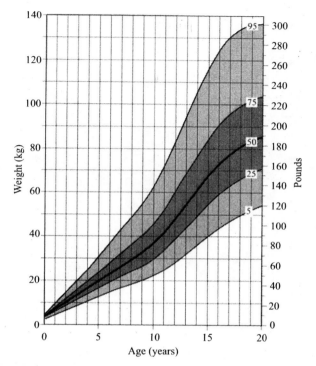

**Figure 17.60**    Prader-Willi syndrome, weight, North European females, birth to 20 years. Adapted from Hauffa et al. (2000).

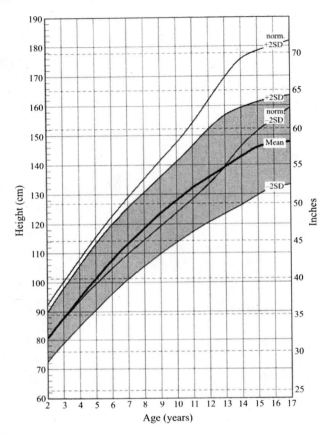

**Figure 17.61**   Prader-Willi syndrome, height, Asian males, 2 to 17 years. Adapted from Nagai et al. (2000).

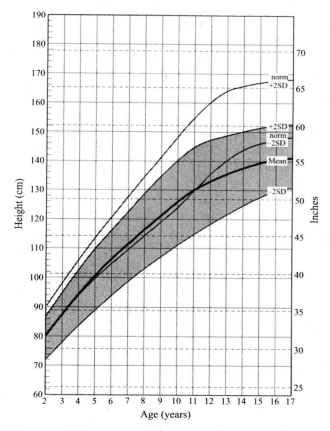

**Figure 17.62**　Prader-Willi syndrome, height, Asian females, 2 to 17 years. Adapted from Nagai et al. (2000).

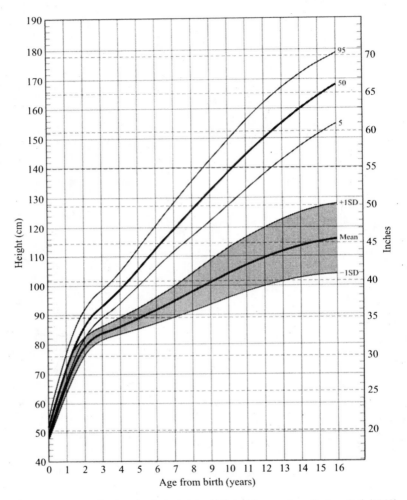

**Figure 17.63**  Pseudoachondroplasia, height, birth to 16 years. From Horton et al. (1982), by permission.

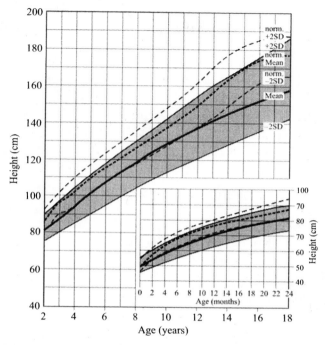

**Figure 17.64**   Rubinstein-Taybi syndrome, height, males, birth to 18 years. From Stevens et al. (1990).

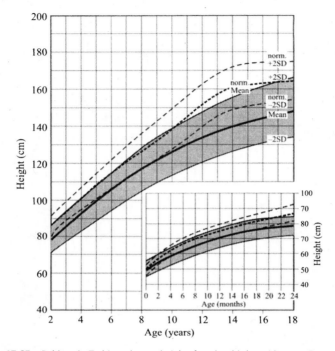

**Figure 17.65**   Rubinstein-Taybi syndrome, height, females, birth to 18 years. From Stevens et al. (1990).

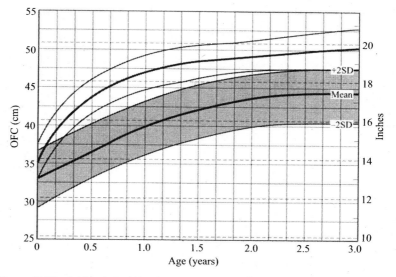

**Figure 17.66** Rubinstein-Taybi syndrome, head circumference, males, birth to three years. From Stevens et al. (1990).

**Figure 17.67** Rubinstein-Taybi syndrome, head circumference, females, birth to three years. From Stevens et al. (1990).

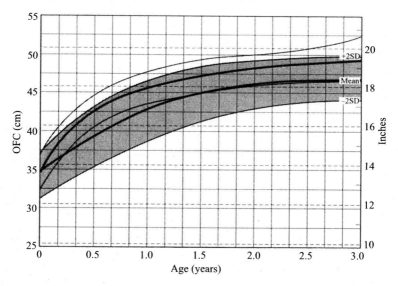

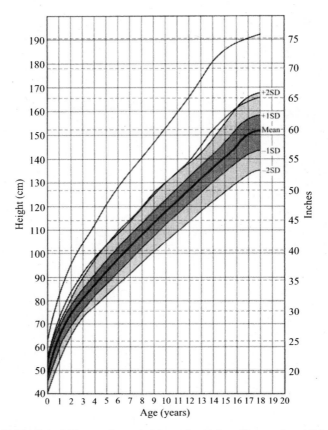

**Figure 17.68** Russell-Silver syndrome, height, males, birth to 20 years. From Wollmann et al. (1995).

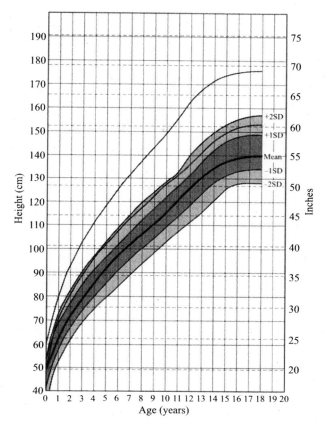

**Figure 17.69** Russell-Silver syndrome, height, females, birth to 20 years. From Wollmann et al. (1995).

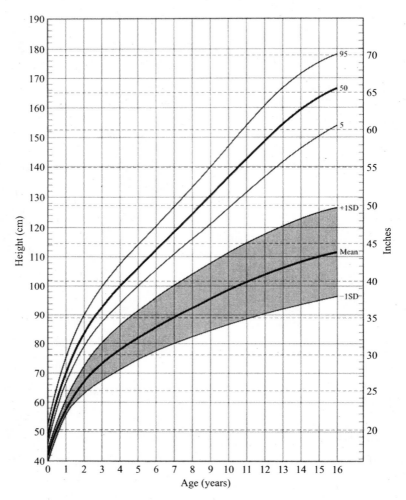

**Figure 17.70** Spondyloepiphysial dysplasia congenita, height, birth to 16 years. From Horton et al. (1982), by permission.

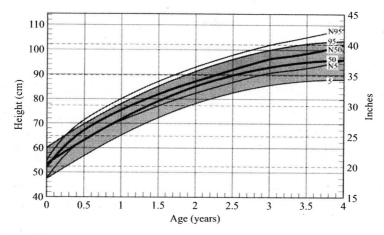

**Figure 17.71**   Height for males and females with trisomy 13, birth to seven years. Adapted from Baty et al. (1994).

**Figure 17.72**   Weight for males and females with trisomy 13, birth to seven years. Adapted from Baty et al. (1994).

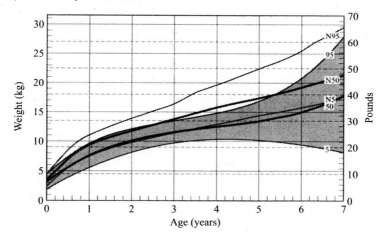

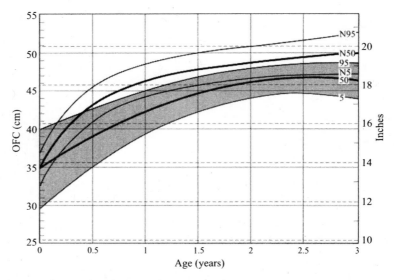

**Figure 17.73**   Head circumference for males and females with trisomy 13, birth to three years. Adapted from Baty et al. (1994).

**Figure 17.74**   Height for males and females with trisomy 18, birth to 18 years. Adapted from Baty et al. (1994).

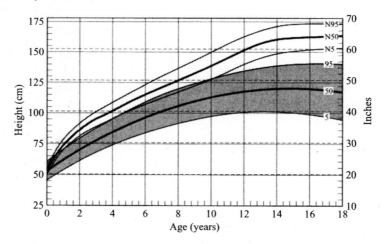

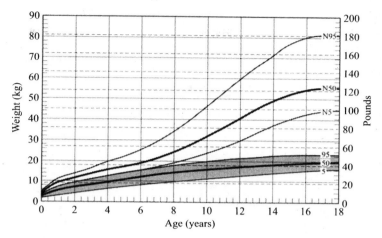

**Figure 17.75**  Weight for males and females with trisomy 18, birth to 18 years. Adapted from Baty et al. (1994).

**Figure 17.76**  Head circumference for males and females with trisomy 18, birth to three years. Adapted from Baty et al. (1994).

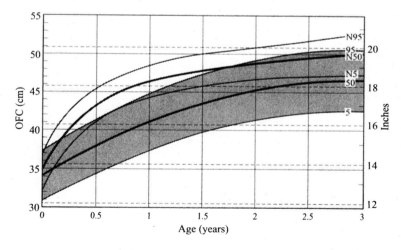

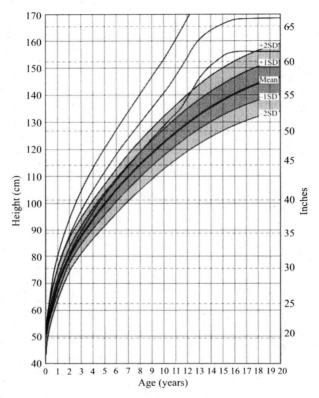

**Figure 17.77** Turner syndrome, height, North European females, birth to 20 years.
Adapted from Rougen–Weiterlaken et al. (1997).

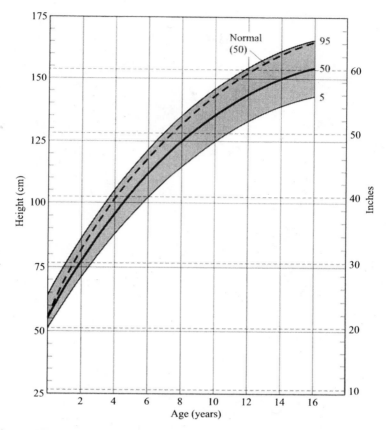

**Figure 17.78** Williams syndrome, height, males, birth to 16 years. From Morris et al. (1988), by permission.

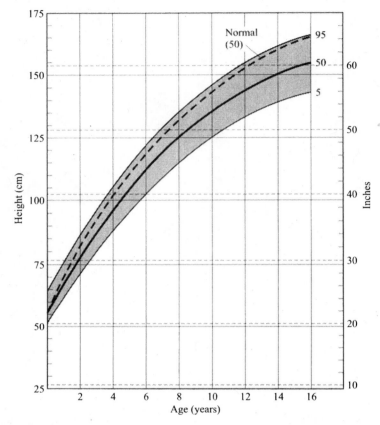

**Figure 17.79**  Williams syndrome, height, females, birth to 16 years. From Morris et al. (1988), by permission.

# Bibliography

Baty, B.J., Blackburn, B.L., and Carey, J.C. (1994). Natural history of trisomy 18 and trisomy 13: I. Growth, physical assessment, medical histories, survival, and recurrence risk. *American Journal of Medical Genetics*, **49**, 175–188.

Cronk, C., Crocker, A.C., Pueschel, S.M., Shea, A.M., Zackai, E., Pickens, G., and Reed, R.B. (1988). Growth charts for children with Down syndrome: 1 month to 18 years of age. (1988). *Pediatrics*, **81**, 102–110.

Erkula, G., Jones, K.B., Sponseller, P.D., Diele, H.C., and Pyeritz, R.E. (2002). Growth and maturation in Marfan syndrome. *American Journal of Medical Genetics*, **109**, 100–115.

Hall, J.G. (1985). A study of individuals with arthrogryposis. *Endocrine Genetics and Genetics of Growth*, pp. 155–162. Alan R. Liss, New York.

Hauffa, B.P., Schlippe, G., Roos, M., Gillessen-Kaesbach, G., and Gasser, T. (2000). Spontaneous growth in German children and adolescents with genetically confirmed Prader-Willi Syndrome. *Acta Paediatrica*, **89**, 1302–1311.

Holm, V.A. and Nugent, J.K. (1982). Growth in the Prader-Willi syndrome. *Birth Defects: Original Article Series*, **18(3B)**, 93–100.

Horton, W.A., Rotter, J.I., Rimoin, D.L., Scott, C.I., and Hall, J.G. (1978). Standard growth curves for achondroplasia. *Journal of Pediatrics*, **93**, 435–438.

Horton, W.A., Hall, J.G., Scott, C.I., Pyeritz, R.E., and Rimoin, D.L. (1982). Growth curves for height for diastrophic dysplasia, spondyloepiphyseal dysplasia congenita, and pseudoachondroplasia. *American Journal of Disease in Childhood*, **136**, 316–319.

Hunter, A.G.W., Hecht, J.T., and Scott, C.I. Jr. (1996a). Standard weight for height curves in achondroplasia. *American Journal of Medical Genetics*, **62**, 255–261.

Hunter, A.G.W., Reid, C.S., Pauli, R.M., and Scott, I. Jr. (1996b). Standard curves of chest circumference in achondroplasia and the relationship of chest circumference to respiratory problems. *American Journal of Medical Genetics*, **62**, 91–97.

Ikeda, Y., Higurashi, M., Egi, S., Ohzeki, N., and Hoshina, H. (1982). An anthropometric study of girls with the Ullrich–Turner syndrome. *American Journal of Medical Genetics*, **12**, 271–280.

Kline, A.D., Barr, M., and Jackson, L.G. (1993). Growth manifestations in the Brachmann–de Lange syndrome. *American Journal of Medical Genetics*, **47**, 1042–1049.

Marinescu, R.C., Mainardi, P.C., Collins, M.R., Kouahou, M., Coueourde, G., Pastore, G., Eaton-Evans, J., and Overhauser, J. (2000). Growth charts for Cri-du-chat syndrome: an international collaborative study. *American Journal of Medical Genetics*, **94**, 153–162.

Meaney, F.J., and Farrer, L.A. (1986). Clinical anthropometry and medical genetics: a compilation of body measurements in genetic and congenital disorders. *American Journal of Medical Genetics*, **25**, 343–359.

Morris, C.A., Derusey, S.A., Leonard, C.O., Dilts, C., and Blackburn, B.L. (1988). Natural history of Williams syndrome: physical characteristic. *Journal of Pediatrics*, **113**, 318–326.

Myrelid, A., Gustafsson, J., Ollars, B., and Anneren, G. (2002). Growth charts for Down's syndrome for birth to 18 years of age. Archives of Disease in childhood, **87**, 97–103.

Nagai, T., Matsuo, N., Kayanuma, Y., Tonoki, H., Fukushima, Y., Ohashi, H., Murai, T., Hasegawa, T., Kuroki, Y., and Niikawa, N. (2000). Standard growth curves for Japanese patients with Prader-Willi syndrome. *American Journal of Medical Genetics*, **95**, 130–134.

Palmer, C.G., Cronk, C., Pureschel, S.M., Wisniewski, K.E., Laxova, R., Crocker, A.C., and Pauli, R.M. (1992). Head circumference of children with Down syndrome (0–36 months). *American Journal of Medical Genetics*, **42**, 61–67.

Park, E., Bailey, J.D., and Cowell, C.A. (1983). Growth and maturation of patients with Turner's syndrome. *Pediatric Research*, **7**, 1–7.

Pelz, V.L., Sussmann, S., Timm, D., and Rostock, I. (1981). Ullrich-Turner syndrome. Kinderarztliche Praxis, **49**, 206–212.

Pyeritz, R.E. (1985). Growth and anthropometrics in the Marfan syndrome. Endocrine Genetics and Genetics of Growth, pp. 135–140. Alan R. Liss, New York.

Ranke, M.B., Heidemann, P., Knupfer, C., Enders, H., Schmaltz, A., and Bierich, J.R. (1988). Noonan syndrome: growth and clinical manifestations in 144 cases. *European Journal of Paediatrics*, **48**, 220–227.

Richards, G. Growth charts for children with Down syndrome. Available at: http://www.growthcharts.com/. Accessed March 30, 2006.

Stevens, C.A., Hennekan, R.C.M., and Blackburn, B.L. (1990). Growth in the Rubinstein-Taybi syndrome. *American Journal of Medical Genetics Supplement*, **6**, 51–55.

Szudek, J., Birch, P., Friedman, J.M., and the National Neurofibromatosis Foundation International Database Participants. (2000). Growth in North American white children with neurofibromatosis 1(NF1). *Journal of Medical Genetics*, **37**, 933–938.

Witt, D.R., Keena, B.A., Hall, J.G., and Allanson, J.E. (1986). Growth curves for height in Noonan syndrome. *Clinical Genetics*, **30**, 150–153.

Wollmann, H.A., Kirchner, T., Enders, H., Preece, M.A., and Ranke, M.B. (1995). Growth and symptoms in Silver-Russell syndrome: review on the basis of 386 patients. *European Journal of Pediatrics*, **154**, 958–968.

Wollmann, H.A., Schultz, U., Grauer, M.L., and Ranke, M.B. (1998). Reference values for height and weight in Prader-Willi syndrome based on 315 patients. *European Journal of Pediatrics*, **157**, 634–642.

# An Approach to the Child with Dysmorphic Features

18

The approach to the child with unusual physical features, multiple congenital anomalies, or a dysmorphic syndrome is a complex one. Careful physical measurements are not only important for determining the child's condition and present status, but are important as well for establishing baseline measurements in order to follow the affected individual over time and in order to define the natural history of the condition. If a child is seen repeatedly, careful serial measurements are invaluable for demonstrating the disproportionate growth of different parts of the body and the changing proportions that may occur with time.

As stated earlier in the book, a measurement really has meaning only in comparison with other measurements; therefore, all measurements need to be taken and recorded in a way that allows them to be compared with the norms for chronological age, the norms for height age, the bone-age–related norms, or the age-related measurement of some other part of the body. In each area of the body, there is a standard against which other measurements should be compared. For example, in the craniofacial area, the age-related head circumference (OFC) is used for the comparison with other measurements. Are the ears small or large for the age that corresponds to the head size? For example a six-year-old boy, who is 50th percentile for height with a head size that is 50th percentile for a two-year-old and an ear size that is 50th percentile for a four-year-old will appear to have large ears even though they are small for his age.

It is a general rule of thumb that any measurements that deviate more than two standard deviations from each other are considered to be outside the range of normal and need an explanation. Thus, if height is at the 10th percentile and weight is at the 90th percentile, although both measurements are normal, the child will be relatively overweight, and the physician should ask why. Similarly, if head circumference is at the 10th percentile and inner canthal distance is at the 90th percentile, the child will appear to have relative ocular hypertelorism, and the physician should ask why. Other measurements around and of the eye in such a child may allow the delineation of small palpebral fissures (as seen in the fetal alcohol spectrum disorder and blepharophimosis syndrome) or the delineation of laterally displaced inner canthus or telecanthus (as seen in Waardenburg syndrome).

As with any other medical evaluation a careful prenatal, medical, developmental, and family history; a thorough general physical examination, and appropriate laboratory evaluations should be obtained on any child with dysmorphic features or congenital anomalies. This book is aimed at providing data which allow the physician to describe and quantify physical anomalies as a meaningful and useful part of the evaluation. Most chapters deal with particular parts of the body. They outline the ways to describe and measure that area and provide graphs of normal values for frequently used measurements. Practically speaking, there are about 36 measurements that should be performed on all children being evaluated for dysmorphic features. These 36 measurements take less than 10 minutes to record. If a particular area seems to be disproportionate or abnormal, there are additional measurements or studies that can be performed. Photographs should be taken as well.

Figure 18.1 gives an example of an outline form for recording measurements. If the child is quiet, they can be done in a logical way. If the child is crying or agitated, it often pays to obtain distal measurements such as hands, feet and OFC first, before moving in toward the face and chest.

After the measurements are obtained, they should be compared with the normal age- and sex-related standards. Percentiles for the individual are generated. The measurements are then analysed. Any deviating percentile is evaluated. The next step is to compare the measurements with the norms for height age of that child. For example, if the chronological age of the child is four years but the child's height is that of the average (e.g., 50th percentile) two-year-old, the other body measurements need to be compared to the two-year-old standards. They may be completely normal for two years, suggesting that the child is growing like a two-year-old, or there may be marked disproportion. It may then be useful to compare particular parts of the body, such as comparing hand and foot measurements to the "age-related" or "height-related" hand and foot standards. These comparisons allow the physician to define better which body area, if any, is disproportionate. Finally, the child's measurements should be compared to bone-age–related norms. If the bone age was advanced in the four-year-old described above, the disparity between chronological age and height would be even greater.

In subsequent examinations, repeated measurements may be taken in the same way, allowing the construction of a longitudinal growth curve for various areas of the body. In many syndromes with disproportionate growth, the growth curves have not yet been defined. The definition of disproportionate growth in various body areas in these conditions should allow better understanding of the pathogenetic mechanisms leading to the disproportionate growth.

# Chapter 18 An Approach to the Child with Dysmorphic Features

Patient name _____ Date of birth _____ Hospital no. _____

Paternal ethnic origin _____ Height _____ Date of examination _____

Maternal ethnic origin _____ Height _____ Examiner _____

Patient age _____ Height age _____ Bone age _____

|  | Percentile | | | | | | Other anomalies |
|---|---|---|---|---|---|---|---|
|  | Right | Left | Chron-ologic age | Height age | Bone age | | |
| **Body** | | | | | | | |
| Length/height | | | | | | | |
| Weight | | | | | | | |
| Span | | | | | | | |
| Lower segment | | | | | | | |
| Upper segment (crown–rump or sitting height) | | | | | | | |
| U/L segment ratio | | | | | | | |
| Chest circumference | | | | | | | |
| Internipple distance | | | | | | | |
| Sternal length | | | | | | | |
| **Craniofacies** | | | | | | | |
| Head circumference (OFC) | | | | | | | |
| Anterior fontanelle | | | | | | | |
| Facial width | | | | | | | |
| Facial height | | | | | | | |
| Outer canthal distance | | | | | | | |
| Inner canthal distance | | | | | | | |
| Interpupillary distance | | | | | | | |
| Palpebral fissure length | | | | | | | |
| Nasal height | | | | | | | |
| Nasal protrusion | | | | | | | |
| Nasal width | | | | | | | |
| Ear length | | | | | | | |
| Ear width | | | | | | | |
| Ear position | | | | | | | |
| Ear rotation | | | | | | | |
| Philtrum length | | | | | | | |
| Mouth width | | | | | | | |
| **Limbs** | | | | | | | |
| Hand length | | | | | | | |
| Palm length | | | | | | | |
| Palm width | | | | | | | |
| Finger length | | | | | | | |
| Elbow angle | | | | | | | |
| Foot length | | | | | | | |
| Foot width | | | | | | | |
| **Genitalia** | | | | | | | |
| Labial size | | | | | | | |
| Testicle size | | | | | | | |
| Penile length | | | | | | | |

Development assessment _____

Summary of unusual/abnormal measurements _____

Any special techniques or instruments for measuring _____

Dermatoglyphics done  Yes/No     Photographs done  Yes/No     X-ray done  Yes/No     Bone age done  Yes/No

**Figure 18.1**  An example of an "easy to use" outline form for recording measurements.

476

# Glossary

**accessory nipple**  Additional nipple, unilateral or bilateral, on the trunk, lying on the "milk line" which runs caudally from the normal position of the nipples and cranially toward the axilla.

**acrocephaly**  Tall or high skull; the top of the head is pointed, peaked, or conical in shape; usually involving premature closure of the lambdoid and coronal sutures, with a vertical index above 77; also referred to as oxycephaly, turricephaly, and tower skull.

**acromelic**  Referring to the distal portion of the limb.

**ala nasi**  The most lateral part of the nose: the flaring cartilaginous area forming the outer side of each naris (nostril).

**albinism**  Deficiency or absence of pigment in the hair, skin, and/or eyes.

**alopecia**  Absence, loss, or deficiency of hair; may be patchy or total; transient or congenital, natural or abnormal.

**aniridia**  Absence of the iris.

**anisomastia**  Asymmetric or irregular size of the breasts.

**anisocoria**  Unequal pupil size.

**ankyloblepharon**  Adhesion of the ciliary edges of the eyelids to each other.

**anodontia**  Absence of teeth.

**anonychia**  Absence of nails.

**anophthalmia**  Congenital absence or hypoplasia of one or both eyes.

**anthropometrics**  The study of comparative measurements of the human body.

**aphakia**  Absence of the lens of the eye.

**arachnodactyly**  Long slender hands, feet, fingers, and toes; spider fingers, dolichostenomelia.

**areola**  Pigmented skin surrounding the nipple.

**arrhinencephaly**  Congenital absence of the rhinencephalon (hind brain).

**arrhinia**  Congenital absence of the nose.

**bathrocephaly**  A step-like posterior projection of the skull, caused by bulging of the squamous portion of the occipital bone.

**biacromial distance**  Maximum distance between the right and left acromion (shoulder width).

**bigonial distance** Distance between the lateral aspect of the angle of the jaw on the right and the same point on the left (mandible width).

**bi-iliac distance** Distance between the most prominent lateral points of the iliac crest.

**birth mark** Regionally limited alteration of skin color caused by vascular or pigment-distribution anomalies.

**bizygomatic distance** Maximal distance between the most lateral points on the zygomatic arches (zygion) (facial width).

**Blaschko line** Streak of pigmented skin reflecting embryonic migration of pigment-producing cells.

**blepharochalasis** Relaxation or redundancy of the skin of the upper eyelid, so that a fold of skin hangs down, often concealing the corner of the eye.

**blue nevus** Bluish macular area, mostly over the sacrum and back. More frequent in African, American, Hispanic, and Asian people.

**bone age** Radiological assessment of physiological age relating growth and skeletal maturation; stage of development of the skeleton as judged by X-rays and compared with chronological age.

**bony interorbital distance** The distance between the medial margins of the bony orbit, measured radiographically.

**brachycephaly** Shortening of the length of the skull; the cephalic index is 81.0 to 85.4

**brachydactyly** Short finger.

**brachyturricephaly** Combination of shortening of the skull (brachycephaly) along with towering of the skull (turricephaly, oxycephaly, or acrocephaly).

**Brushfield spot** Mottled, marbled, or speckled elevation of the iris due to increased density of the anterior border layer of the iris; white or light yellow iris nodule caused by deposition or aggregation of stromal fibrocytes; observed in 85 percent of patients with Down syndrome. Can be noted in the normal population (about 25 percent).

**buphthalmos** Congenital glaucoma; keratoglobus, or enlargement of the eye.

**café-au-lait macule** Macular area of increased pigment greater than 0.5 cm in diameter. More than five café-au-lait spots of 1.5 cm or greater can be a sign of neurofibromatosis.

**calipers** Instrument used for measuring distance or thickness.

**calvarium** Upper, dome-like portion of the skull.

**camptodactyly** Flexion contracture of a finger or toe; permanent flexion of one or both interphalangeal joints of one or more fingers; bent fingers.

**canthal distance, inner** Distance between the inner canthi (inner corners) of the two eyes.

**canthal distance, outer** Distance between the outer canthi (outer corners) of the two eyes.

**capillary hemangioma** Pink macular mark, localized over the forehead, face, or nape of the neck in the newborn (angel's kiss, salmon patch, stork bite, nevus simplex, erythema nuchae). Represents the fetal circulatory pattern in the skin and will resolve spontaneously.

**carpal angle** Angle made by the carpal bones at the wrist.

**carrying angle** Angle subtended by the forearm on the humerus; the deviation of the forearm relative to the humerus; the angle at the elbow joint.

**cavernous haemangioma** Elevated vascular nevus or strawberry nevus of solid red color.

**cebocephaly** Form of holoprosencephaly with ocular hypotelorism and a centrally placed nose with a single blind-ended nostril.

**cephalic index** The ratio of head width, expressed as a percentage of head length:

$$CI = \frac{\text{head width} \times 100}{\text{head length}}$$

**cephalometrics** The science of precise measurement of bones of the cranium and face, using fixed reproducible positions.

**cheilion** Most lateral point of the corner of the mouth.

**chest circumference** Circumference of the chest at the level of the nipples.

**chordee** Abnormal position of the penis caused by a band of tissue that holds the penis in a ventral or lateral curvature.

**clinodactyly** Permanent lateral or medial curve (deflection) of one or more fingers or toes.

**coloboma** Fissuring defect especially of the eye; may involve several layers (i.e., iris, retina, lid), usually congenital, but may be of traumatic origin.

**columella** Fleshy inferior border of the septum of the nose.

**concha** Structure resembling a shell in shape (e.g., hollow of the external ear, turbinate bone).

**cornea, transverse diameter** Distance between the medial and lateral border of the iris.

**craniorachischisis** Congenital failure of closure of the skull and spinal column.

**crown–rump length** Distance from the top of the head to the bottom of the buttock, with hips in flexion.

**cubitus valgus** Increased carrying angle at elbow.

**cuticle** Remnant of the eponychium at the base of a fingernail.

**cutis aplasia** Absence of skin in specific area; commonly of the scalp at the vertex.

**cryptophthalmos** Complete congenital adhesion of the eyelid; fused eyelid.

**cryptorchidism** Failure of the testis to descend into the scrotum.

**cystic hygroma** Sac, distended with lymphatic fluid, found usually in the neck.

**dental age** Physiological age of teeth as determined by the number and type of teeth that have erupted or been shed.

**Denver Developmental Screening Test** A screening test for gross motor, fine motor-adaptive, language, and personal–social skills.

**depigmentation** Area of absent or reduced pigment due to lack of functional melanocytes. Leaf-shaped area of depigmentation can be a sign of tuberous sclerosis.

**dermal ridge count** Number of dermal ridges in a particular dermal ridge pattern.

**dermatoglyphics** Pattern of ridges and grooves of the skin, best seen on the palms and soles.

**dermatome** Segmental area of skin defined by the distribution of sensory innervation.

**dermis** Underlying layer of the skin.

**developmental delay** Delay in acquisition of developmental milestones in comparison with age-related cohort.

**dimple** Indentation of the skin where the skin is deficient or attached to underlying structures, especially bone.

**dolichocephaly** Elongation of the skull; with narrowing from side to side. Cephalic index is 75.9 or less (*see also* scaphocephaly).

**dystopia canthorum** Lateral displacement of the inner canthi of the eye.

**ear length** Maximum distance from the superior aspect to the inferior aspect of the external ear (pinna).

**ear position** Location of the superior attachment of the pinna. Note that the size and rotation of the external ear are not relevant.

**ear protrusion** Protrusion of each ear, measured by the angle subtended from the posterior aspect of the pinna to the mastoid plane of the skull.

**ear rotation/angulation** Rotation of the longitudinal axis of the external ear (pinna).

**ear width** Width of the external ear (pinna), from just anterior to the tragus to the lateral margin of the helix.

**ectopia** Misplaced structure.

**ectopia lentis** Displacement of the crystalline lens of the eye.

**ectopia pupillaris** Abnormal eccentric location of the pupil.

**ectropion** Eversion or turning out of an edge (e.g., of an eyelid or of the lip).

**encephalocele** Herniation of the brain, manifested by protrusion through a congenital or traumatic opening of the skull; can be frontal or occipital.

**enophthalmus** Abnormal retraction of the eye into the orbit, producing a deeply set eye.

**entropion** Inversion of an edge (e.g., of the eyelid).

**epicanthal fold** Congenital fold of tissue medial to the eye consisting of a vertical fold of skin lateral to the nose, sometimes covering the inner canthus.

**epidermis** Superficial layer of the skin.

**epiphora** Abnormal overflow of tears down the cheek; mainly caused by stricture of the nasolacrimal duct.

**epispadias** Abnormal location of the urethra on the dorsal surface of the penis.

**eponychium** Epidermal layer which covers the developing fingernail prenatally.

**esotropia** Inward deviation of an eye when both eyes are open and uncovered; convergent strabismus.

**ethmocephaly** Form of holoprosencephaly in which there are two separate but hypoteloric eyes and a supraorbital proboscis.

**eurion** Most prominent lateral point on each side of the skull in the area of the parietal and temporal bones.

**exophthalmos** Abnormal protrusion of the eyeball.

**exotropia** Outward deviation of an eye when both eyes are opened and uncovered; divergent strabismus.

**facial height** Distance from the root of the nose (nasion) to the lowest median landmark on the lower border of the mandible (menton or gnathion); lower twothirds of the craniofacies.

**facial height, lower** Distance from the base of the nose (subnasion) to the lowest median landmark on the lower border of the mandible (menton or gnathion); length of the lower onethird of the craniofacies.

**facial height, upper** Distance from the root of the nose (nasion) to the base of the nose (subnasion); middle onethird of the craniofacies.

**facial index** Ratio of facial height (nasion to menton) to facial width (bizygomatic distance) used to assess a long, narrow face as compared with a short, wide face.

**facial width** *See* bizygomatic distance.

**finger clubbing** Enlargement of the distal part of the finger and nail, with abnormally curved nail and loss of the angle at the nail fold.

**flexion crease** Crease in skin overlying a joint; secondary to movement at that joint.

**fontanelle (fontanel)** Membrance-covered space remaining in the incompletely ossified skull of a fetus or infant.

**fontanelle size, anterior** Sum of the longitudinal and transverse diameters of the anterior fontanella along the sagittal and coronal sutures.

**fontanelle size, posterior** Length of the posterior fontanelle.

**forehead height** *See* skull height.

**Frankfort plane (FP)** Eye–ear plane that is a standard horizontal cephalometric reference. The Frankfort plane or Frankfort horizontal is established when the head is held erect, with the eyes forward, so that the lowest margin of the lower bony orbit (orbitale) and the upper margin of the external auditory meatus (porion) are in the same horizontal plane (the Frankfort plane).

**frenulum** Small fold of integument or of mucous membrane that may limit the movement of an organ or part, (e.g., beneath the tongue).

**frontal bossing** Prominence of the anterior portion of the frontal bone of the skull.

**gastroschisis** Congenital fissure of the abdominal wall not involving the site of insertion of the umbilical cord, and usually accompanied by protrusion of the small and part of the large intestine.

**genu recurvatum** Hyperextension of the knee.

**genu valgum** Outward bowing of knee; bow-leg.

**genu varum** Inward deviation of the knee; knock-knee.

**gibbus** Extreme kyphosis or hump; deformity of the spine in which there is a sharply angulated segment, the apex of the angle being posterior.

**glabella** The most prominent midline point between the eyebrows.

**glossoptosis** Downward displacement or retraction of the tongue; sometimes held by a frenulum.

**gnathion** The lowest median point on the inferior border of the mandible; *see* menton.

**gonion** The most lateral point of the posteroinferior angle of the mandible.

**head circumference** Distance around the head at its largest part.

**head length** Maximum dimension of the sagittal axis of the skull.

**head width** Maximal biparietal diameter.

**height** Distance from the top of the head to the sole of the foot in a standing position.

**heterochromia** Unequal color, usually used in reference to the iris.

**holoprosencephaly** Impaired midline cleavage of the embryonic forebrain, the most extreme form being cyclopia; a less severe form is arrhinencephaly.

**hydrocephaly** Abnormal increase in the amount of cerebrospinal fluid accompanied by dilatation of the cerebral ventricles.

**hyperextensibility** Excessive capability of the skin to stretch; excessive range of movement at a joint.

**hypertelorism** Abnormal distance between two organs or parts; commonly used to describe increased interpupillary distance (ocular hypertelorism).

**hypoacusis** Decreased perception of sound.

**hypodontia** Reduced number of teeth (*see* also oligodontia).

**hyponychia** Small dysplastic nails.

**hypospadias** Abnormal location of the urethra on the ventral surface of the penis; may be glandular (1°), penile (2°), scrotal (3°), or perineal (4°).

**hypotelorism** Abnormally decreased distance between two organs or parts, commonly used to describe decreased interpupillary distance (ocular hypotelorism).

**imperforate anus** Absence of the normal anal opening.

**intelligence quotient (IQ)** General intellectual functioning as assessed by special tests.

**interalar distance (nasal width)** Distance between the most lateral aspects of the alae nasi.

**intercommissural distance** Mouth width at rest; the distance between the two outer corners of the mouth (cheilion).

**internipple distance** Distance between the centers of both nipples.

**interpupillary distance** Distance between the centers of the pupils of the two eyes.

**inverted nipple** Inwardly directed tip of the nipple; nipple does not protrude from the areola.

**iridodonesis** Tremor of the iris on movement; usually due to dislocation of the lens.

**Kayser–Fleischer ring** Greenish-brownish pigment ring due to the deposition of copper at the outer edge of the cornea; as noted in Wilson disease.

**keratoconus** Conical protrusion of the cornea.

**koilonychia** Spoon-shaped nails.

**kyphoscoliosis** Abnormal curvature of the spinal column, both anteroposteriorly and laterally.

**kyphosis** Curvature of the spine in the anteroposterior plane. A normal kyphosis exists in the shoulder area.

**lagophthalmos** Condition in which the eyelid cannot be completely closed.

**lanugo** Embryonic or fetal hair; fine, soft, unmedullated.

**length** Distance between the top of the head and the sole of the foot when the individual is lying down (height).

**lentigo** Round or oval, flat, brown, pigmented skin spot caused by increased deposition of melanin, in association with an increased number of melanocytes at the epidermodermal junction.

**leukoma** Dense white opacity of the cornea.

**leukonychia** White spots or stripes on the nails.

**lingua plicata** Fissured tongue.

**Lisch nodule** Hamartomatous iris structure, usually visible only by slit lamp.

**lordosis** Curvature of the spinal column with a forward (ventral) convexity. A normal lordosis exists in the lumbar area.

**lower segment** Distance from the pubic bone to the sole of the foot.

**lymphangioma** Overgrowth of lymphatic vessels.

**macrocephaly** Abnormally large head.

**macrocranium** Abnormally large skull.

**macrodactyly** Abnormally large digit.

**macrocheilia** Abnormal or excessive size of the lip.

**macroglossia** Abnormally large or hypertrophic tongue.

**macromastia** Abnormally large breast.

**macronychia** Abnormally large nail.

**macrophthalmia** Abnormally large eye.

**macrostomia** Abnormally large mouth.

**mandible width** *See* bigonial distance.

**mandibular length, effective** Effective length and prominence of the mandible (cephalometric).

**manubrium** Cranial portion of the sternum which articulates with the clavicles and the first two pairs of ribs.

**maxillomandibular differential** Measurement determined by subtracting the effective midfacial length from the effective mandibular length (cephalometric).

**megalocephaly** Abnormally large head.

**melanocyte** Pigment cell in the skin.

**menton** The lowest medial landmark on the lower border of the mandible, identified by palpation, and identical to the bony gnathion.

**mesomelic** Referring to the middle segment of the limb.

**microcephaly** Abnormally small head.

**microcranium** Abnormally small skull.

**microgenia** Abnormally small chin; an alternative term for micrognathia.

**microglossia** Abnormally small tongue.

**micrognathia** Abnormally small jaw, especially with lower jaw recession (small chin).

**micronychia** Abnormally small nail.

**microphthalmia** Abnormally small eye.

**microstomia** Abnormally small opening of the mouth.

**microphallus** Abnormally small penis; micropenis.

**midfacial length, effective** Size and prominence of the maxilla (cephalometric).

**mid-parental height** Sum of parents' heights divided by two.

**miosis** Small, contracted pupil.

**mole** Circumscribed area of dark pigment which is often raised.

**monilethrix** Hair exhibiting marked multiple constrictions, with a beading effect and increased brittleness.

**mouth width** *See* intercommissural distance.

**mydriasis** Large, dilated pupil.


**nasal height** the distance from the nasal root (nasion) to base (subnasion).

**nasal width** *See* interalar distance.

**nasion** Midline point at the nasal root over the nasofrontal suture.

**nevus sebaceous** Raised waxy patch, with a mostly linear distribution.

**nipple** Papilla of the breast.

**Nystagmus** Involuntary rapid movement of the eyeball which may be horizontal, vertical, rotatory, or mixed.


**obliquity (slant) of the palpebral fissure** Slant of the palpebral fissure from the horizontal.

**occipitofrontal circumference (OFC)** Distance around the head, the largest obtainable measurement (head circumference).

**oligodontia** Less than the normal number of teeth (*see* hypodontia).

**omphalocele** Protrusion, at birth, of part of the intestine through a defect in the abdominal wall at the umbilicus. Protruding bowel is covered only by a thin transparent membrane composed of amnion and peritoneum.

**ONO angle** Angle subtended from the base of the nose in the midline to the outer canthi of the eyes.

**opisthocranion** Most posterior portion of the occipital bone in the midline.

**ophthalmoplegia** Paralysis of the eye muscles.

**orbital protrusion**  Degree of protrusion of the eye (exophthalmos).

**orbitale**  The lowest point of the inferior bony margin of the orbit, identified by palpation.

**orchidometer**  Measuring device for quantifying testicular size.

**oxycephaly**  *see* acrocephaly.


**pachyonychia**  long thickened nails.

**palpebral fissure length**  Distance between the inner and outer canthus of one eye.

**pattern profile**  Analysis of hand bone length, used to recognize particular syndromes.

**pectus carinatum**  Undue prominence of the sternum, often referred to as pigeon chest.

**pectus excavatum**  Undue depression of the sternum, often referred to as funnel chest.

**pes calcaneovalgus**  Dorsiflexion of the foot due to a contracture of foot (rocker bottom foot).

**pes cavus**  High arched foot with metatarsal heads pushed down (claw foot).

**pes equinovarus**  Planter flexion with internal rotation of ankle joint (club foot).

**pes valgus**  External rotation at ankle joint.

**philtrum**  Ventrical groove in the midline of the upper lip, extending from beneath the nose to the vermilion border of the upper lip.

**pili annulati**  Defect of keratin synthesis resulting in a irregular distribution of air-filled cavities along the hairshaft, which reflects the light differently and appears as alternating bands of white.

**pili torti**  Hair twisted by 180-degree angle.

**plagiocephaly**  Asymmetric head shape.

**Poland anomaly**  Absent or hypoplastic nipple and/or breast tissue in association with aberrant or hypoplastic pectoral development and limb deficiency.

**polydactyly**  Extra digit.

**polysyndactyly**  Extra digit with fused digits.

**polythelia**  Occurrence of more than one nipple on a breast.

**porion**  Highest point on the upper margin of the cutaneous external auditory meatus.

**postaxial**  Posterior or lateral to the axis (as in postaxial polydactyly where the extra finger is lateral to the fifth finger).

**portwine naevus**  Dark angioma, which can be purple in color and raised.

**preaxial**  Anterior or medial to the axis (as in preaxial polydactyly where the extra digit is medial to the thumb).

**prognathism** Protrusion of the jaw.

**prolabium** Prominent central part of the upper lip, in its full thickness, which overlies the premaxilla.

**pronasale** Most protruded point of the tip of the nose.

**pterygium** Wing-shaped web; with regard to the eye, a patch of thickened conjunctiva extending over a part of the cornea. The membrane is usually fan-shaped, with the apex toward the pupil and the base toward the inner canthus. With regard to the limbs, a skin web across a joint.

**pterygium colli** Thick fold or web of skin on the lateral aspect of the neck, extending from the mastoid region to the acromion.

**ptosis** Falling or sinking down of any organ (e.g., a drooping of the upper eyelid or breast).

**range of movement** Range of place or position through which a particular joint can move.

**retrognathia** Retrusion of the jaw back from the frontal plane of the forehead.

**rhizomelic** Referring to the proximal portion of the limb.

**saddle nose** Nose with a sunken bridge.

**scaphocephaly** Abnormally long and narrow skull as a result of premature closure of the sagittal suture (*see also* dolichocephaly).

**scoliosis** Appreciable lateral deviation from the normally straight vertical line of the spine.

**shawl scrotum** Congenital ventral insertion of the scrotum.

**single palmar crease** Single crease extending across palm.

**sitting height** Distance from the top of the head to the buttocks when in sitting position.

**skinfold thickness** Thickness of skin in designated areas (triceps, subscapular, suprailiac), used to assess subcutaneous fat and nutrition.

**skull height (forehead height)** Distance from the root of the nose (nasion) to the highest point of the head (vertex).

**span** Distance between the tips of the middle fingers of each hand when the arms are stretched out horizontally from the body.

**Sprengel deformity** Congenital upward displacement of the scapula.

**stadiometer** Upright measuring device.

**sternal length** Length of the sternum from the top of the manubrium to the inferior border of the xiphisternum.

**stellate iris** Iris pattern (star-like) with prominent iris stroma radiating out from the pupil.

**strabismus** Deviation of the eye; the visual axes assume a position relative to each other different from that required by physiological conditions. The various forms of strabismus are spoken of as tropias, their direction being indicated by the appropriate prefix, as in esotropia, exotropia, and so on.

**subalare** Point at the inferior border of each alar base, where the alar base disappears into the skin of the upper lip.

**submental** Situated below the chin.

**subnasale** Midpoint of the columella base at the apex of the angle where the lower border of the nasal septum and the surface of the upper lip meet.

**symblepharon** Adhesion of the eyelid to the eyeball.

**symphalangy** Extension contracture of a finger or toe with fusion of the joint.

**syndactyly** Webbing or fusion of fingers or toes.

**synechia** Adhesion of parts; especially, adhesion of the iris to the cornea or to the lens.

**syngnathia** Intraoral bands, possibly remnants of the buccopharyngeal membrane, extending between the jaws.

**synophrys** Confluent eyebrow growth across the glabella.

**talipes/clubfoot** Fixed abnormal position of foot due to contracture at ankle; equinovarus, calcaneovalgus.

**Tanner stages** Grading system to establish visual standards for the stages of puberty.

**telangiectasis** Prominence of blood vessels on the surface of the skin.

**telecanthus** Increased distance between the inner canthi of the eyes.

**testicular volume** Volume of the testis established by an orchidometer, or calculated from measurement or ultrasound.

**thoracic index** Ratio of the anteroposterior diameter of the chest to the chest width.

**torso length** Distance from the top of the sternum to the symphysis pubis.

**torticollis** Contracted state of the cervical muscles, producing twisting of the neck, resulting in an unnatural position of the head. The most common causes for this condition are trauma, inflammation, or congenital malformation involving the cervical vertebrae and/or the sternocleidomastoid muscle on one side.

**tragion** Superior margin of the tragus of the ear.

**trichoglyphics** Pattern of hair follicles.

**trichorrhexis** Nodular swelling of the hair. The hair is light colored and breaks easily.

**trigonocephaly** Triangular-shaped head and skull resulting from premature synostosis of the portions of the frontal bone with prominence of the metopic suture.

**triphalangeal thumb** Thumb with three phalanges.

**triradius** Dermatoglyphic pattern where three sets of ridges converge.

**turricephaly** *see* acrocephaly.

**umbilical cord length** Length of the umbilical cord from the insertion at the placenta to the abdominal wall of the neonate.

**upper segment** Distance from the top of the head to the pubic bone.

**vermillion border** Red colored edge of the lip where it meets the normal skin of the face.

**vertex** Highest point of the head in the midsagittal plane, when the head is held erect.

**weight** Heaviness of an object or individual.

**widow's peak** Pointed frontal hairline in the midline which may be seen with ocular hypertelorism.

**wormian bone** Small, irregular bone in the suture between the bones of the skull.

**xiphoid process** Most caudal bone of the sternum which articulates with the manubrium and the lowermost ribs.

**zygion** Most lateral point of each zygomatic arch.

# Index

Handbook asurement